D1505541

Therapeutic Touch

Therapeutic Touch

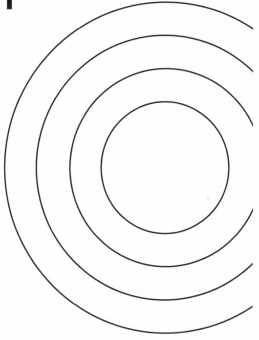

edited by
Béla Scheiber and Carla Selby

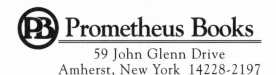 Prometheus Books

59 John Glenn Drive
Amherst, New York 14228-2197

Published 2000 by Prometheus Books

Inquiries should be addressed to
Prometheus Books
59 John Glenn Drive
Amherst, New York 14228–2197
VOICE: 716–691–0133, ext. 207
FAX: 716–564–2711
WWW.PROMETHEUSBOOKS.COM

04 03 02 01 00   5 4 3 2 1

Library of Congress Cataloging-in-Publication Data

Therapeutic Touch / edited by Béla Scheiber and Carla Selby.
        p.   cm.
Includes bibliographical references.
ISBN 1–57392–804–6 (alk. paper)
    1. Touch—Therapeutic use. 2. Imposition of hands—Therapeutic use.
3. Vital force—Therapeutic use. I. Scheiber, Béla. II. Selby, Carla.

RZ999.T48 2000
615.8'52—dc21   00–028604
                                                                      CIP

Printed in the United States of America on acid-free paper

This volume is dedicated to all the skeptics in the world who are committed to the quest for truth, wherever it may lead them. Members of Rocky Mountain Skeptics are most warmly thanked for their support and invaluable input throughout our decade-long investigation into Therapeutic Touch.

Béla Scheiber and Carla Selby

Béla Scheiber also dedicates this book to his parents who taught him the real life consequences when a society is ruled by ignorance and where individuals could have made a difference by their action but failed to act.

Contents

SECTION TWO: THE PHYSICAL SCIENCE OF THERAPEUTIC TOUCH

SECTION THREE: APPENDICES

Foreword

Ray Hyman

When a skeptic or an uninvolved, rational person encounters the topic of Therapeutic Touch he or she asks a simple question: Does it work? In this context the term *work* has a specific meaning. It does not refer to what people *believe* or what they would *like to be true*. Therapeutic Touch works only if it produces successful outcomes that surpass in quantity and quality what would be achieved by a placebo control condition. The issue for the rational skeptic, then, is: What is the evidence? Evidence, in this sense, consists of the outcomes of double-blind, randomized trials that include controls for placebos and other possible artifacts. Therapeutic Touch, as well as any other proposed treatment, should be accepted as a legitimate medical tool only if it has been supported by such evidence which has been replicated independently in more than one laboratory. In a rational and sane world this would be the central issue.

The practitioners of Therapeutic Touch and their supporters see things differently. For them the question of Therapeutic Touch's scientific validity is but a minor issue—if it is an issue at all. For many the central issue is one of empowerment. For nurse practitioners the practice is part of their turf battle with medical doctors. Many social and cultural themes condition the proponents. There is the "us-versus-them" mentality. There is the schizoid attitude toward science. On the one hand, the proponents want to gain the blessings of science, not through the rigors of scientific testing, but through the quasitheoretical associations of such terms as energy fields, quantum mechanics, and the like. At the same time, the movement appears to be motivated by a strong distrust and antipathy toward science and the scientific establishment. The proponents claim the high moral ground by appeals to openness, freedom of expression and choice, and concern

for humanity. Even gender issues and other appeals to political cor-
rectness are part of the mix. Given such a potent mix of ingredients, the
issue of scientific validity becomes almost irrelevant. Indeed, to raise
the issue of scientific validity in this highly charged atmosphere is to
risk being ostracized as a traitor to the cause.

Although I have devoted much of my career to observing and commenting upon various fringe and pseudoscientific movements, I have
not previously spent much time looking into Therapeutic Touch. Other
than reading an occasional article on the subject, I have not seriously
examined its claims. I am therefore grateful for the present collection
of articles. They are a welcome source of information about the various
issues, disputes, and evidential basis that underlie this controversial
subject. Here the reader will discover the historic roots of Therapeutic
Touch in theosophy and occult practices. Ethical, medical, scientific,
theological, theoretical, journalistic, and even political matters are
addressed.

As I read the various chapters, I was struck by how similar the
themes and issues are to those of many previous pseudoscientific and
fringe movements. Take phrenology as one example, one that superficially differs from Therapeutic Touch in many ways. Phrenology, which
was based on Gall's organology created in the late 1700s, had a widespread following throughout the 1800s.

It was highly controversial from its inception. The opponents were
mainly from the mainstream of the academic and scientific professions.
However, many supporters had either scientific or medical credentials.
Many prominent politicians, literary figures, and other celebrities were
strong adherents. Edgar Alan Poe, Walt Whitman, and Herman Melville
were among the many writers who used phrenological allusions in their
major works. A central issue was that of empowerment. Many of the
proponents felt that phrenology was not accepted because it was a
threat to those who controlled the status quo. Phrenologists became
allied with other outsiders and social movements, woman's suffrage,
penal reform, educational reform, mesmerism, the water cure, and
other movements and systems outside the establishment. According to
some historians, both the rise and eventual demise of phrenology had
nothing to do with its scientific validity. Like phrenology and some
other pseudoscientific movements, Therapeutic Touch encompasses
many of the same themes and forces. Certainly, the rise and widespread acceptance of Therapeutic Touch has had nothing to do with
whether it is scientifically valid or not. Whether its eventual fate will be
decided in the court of scientific methodology is yet to be known.

Who will read this book? What will be its impact on readers? In
what ways, if any, will the readers be changed? Will they come away

with altered beliefs? Will they behave in ways other than they would have if they had not read the book? The answers to such questions, we may surmise, will depend upon who the readers are. We might hope for certain effects if the reader is a practitioner or proponent of Therapeutic Touch. For example, we might hope that such readers will realize that the scientific case for the efficacy of the practice is weak or nonexistent. We might hope that such readers will urge the leaders in the field to make the collection of scientific evidence a top priority.

Realistically, we will probably not have such hopes fulfilled. Probably, very few proponents of Therapeutic Touch will read the book. If psychological research on attitude change is considered, those who do read the book can be expected to become even more attached to their belief in Therapeutic Touch. From the content of some of the chapters, we can anticipate the sorts of excuses and reasons they will use to dismiss the negative evidence of experiments. This is all part of what I have called self-sealing belief systems. No matter how many ways we find to puncture their beliefs, they have ways to automatically seal these punctures. This, of course, does not mean we should give up on our attempts to communicate with the believers.

What about readers who are already skeptical and critical of Therapeutic Touch? What impact, if any, might we hope the book will have upon them? The least impact would occur if the only effect is simply to reinforce the skepticism of such a reader. A more hopeful outcome, however, would produce some important changes in beliefs, attitudes, and behavior. At the very least, such a reader should come away with a better understanding and appreciation of the proponent's viewpoint. This, in turn, could produce alterations in behavior toward the proponents. Knowing something about the context of beliefs, issues, motivations, and politics underlying the practice of Therapeutic Touch might provide a basis for comprehending how otherwise sane and rational beings can become attached to an unsubstantiated system.

Of the many possible lessons for the critical reader, I will briefly discuss only one. With the exception of the five experiments done by Wirth, most of the adequately conducted tests of the claims of Therapeutic Touch were done by skeptics. I see many potential problems with this. The proponents can, and obviously do, dismiss such experiments on various grounds. Some of these grounds are that the test was unfair because it did not deal with Therapeutic Touch in its proper context; the test focused on only one, or on an irrelevant claim; a single negative outcome cannot discredit thousands of previously "successful" ones; the practitioners who were tested were inadequate in some way; the skeptic begins with a negative bias that could interfere with the successful application of the technique; and so on. In the ensuing debate, what gets lost is the very important point that the burden of proof should be on the claimant, not the critic.

The responsibility for demonstrating the efficacy of Therapeutic Touch rests squarely upon the shoulders of those who advocate the treatment. It is ethically irresponsible to advocate and use a treatment without first demonstrating, using the best scientific procedures, that the treatment, in fact, does work. Yet proponents have vigorously pushed this treatment on the public and governmental agencies for twenty-five years without first meeting this important obligation. Only belatedly have proponents attempted to carry out serious, double-blind experiments. As can be seen from the descriptions in this book, these experiments do not provide support for their claims.

Not only do attempts by skeptics to test Therapeutic Touch take attention away from the ethical obligations of the proponents, but they also have other negative consequences. Doing experiments, especially doing them correctly, requires precious resources and time. A single experiment rarely can settle whether a claimed treatment does or does not work. One reason is that the experiment cannot test or control for a variety of possibilities. A negative outcome by itself does not invalidate a treatment. For this, we would need a series of experiments done under a variety of conditions and involving a number of independent investigators.

For me, the important lesson to be drawn from the experiments by Emily Rosa and by the team of Long, Evans, and Bernhardt is not that they came out negative. Rather, the important point to be drawn is that these experiments should not have been necessary. If the proponents had been responsible citizens, they long ago should have conducted these and other experiments to evaluate their claims.

As I said, I think a careful reading of the chapters in this book can provide the skeptic and critic with other important lessons. Rather than trying to list some of these lessons, I want to comment on one additional point about these two sets of experiments that should give us pause. Emily Rosa's experiment, as everyone now knows, reported that all the participants did no better than chance in locating the position of Emily's hand. Rebecca Long and her colleagues found in their experiment that their participants could locate the correct position significantly better than chance. This was true even when the target hand was held even farther away from the participant's hand than was the case in Rosa's experiment. Investigating further, these latter researchers concluded that at least some of their participants were picking up clues, especially radiant heat from the experimenter's hand. They also showed that the participant's choices in this setup could be biased by other seemingly minor clues.

This, of course, raises the question of how come Rosa's participants did not also perform better than chance. At this time we do not know. However, given the outcome of the experiment by Long et al., it is reasonable to assume that Rosa's findings could easily have come out in favor of the participants. If this had been the case, we assume that Rosa and her associates would have been ethically bound to report that the outcome had come out in favor of the claims of Therapeutic Touch. Of course, if this had happened, we would expect that the skeptics would have immediately pointed to a variety of drawbacks in Rosa's experiment. Some almost surely would have suggested that she had not controlled for the possibility of other clues such as radiant heat.

I do not mean this to be a criticism of Emily Rosa's experiment. Given its original provenance, it was a commendable project. The problem, as I see it, is that skeptics and critics have to be careful not to claim more than is warranted. If we truly adhere to scientific rigor and standards, then we have to lean over backward to be scrupulously fair. If we are to succeed in our war against pseudoscience, we must not allow ourselves to fall into the trap of behaving like pseudoscientists just because some outcome fits our preconceptions.

I welcome this collection of papers on Therapeutic Touch. I hope that both proponents, critics, and other interested parties will read these papers and cogitate upon the various implications and lessons to be learned from them. Even if the readers are mainly skeptics, I hope that such readers will become more responsible and better skeptics as a result. As skeptics, we should always keep in mind that our goal is not to promote or discredit any particular system or claim. Rather, our goal is to promote rational and scientific inquiry, no matter what the outcome of that inquiry might reveal.

Introduction

In early October 1988, a call was received in the office of the Rocky Mountain Skeptics (RMS). Béla Scheiber took that fateful call. Dr. Bertram Rothschild, a longtime RMS member and psychologist at Colorado's Veterans' Administration Hospital, made a request for information: What did the Rocky Mountain Skeptics know about a nursing practice called "Therapeutic Touch" (TT)? Dr. Rothschild had been approached by a nurse seeking employment in the Pain Clinic at the VA hospital. Her credentials listed something that he had never encountered before: Therapeutic Touch. Béla agreed to investigate the practice and get back to him ASAP.

First, he searched through the literature. Had the accessibility to the internet come just a few years earlier, his search might have been simple—but all that was available were hard copies of books and journals. After hours of searching, he uncovered only one article printed in a Prometheus Books publication, *Examining Holistic Medicine* by P. E. and M. J. Clark. That's it. He found nothing else.

Next he called James Randi, a well-known student and investigator of the paranormal. The conversation was not very productive. Even James Randi had not heard of this nursing practice. Béla contacted other skeptics, only to be met with the same result.

Béla, who had founded RMS five years earlier, was baffled. What is Therapeutic Touch? Who teaches it? What are its origins? Most importantly, why had skeptics not heard of it? Skeptics were aware of acupuncture, iridology, homeopathy, magnetic therapy, phrenology, faith healing, psychic surgery, and more—but not Therapeutic Touch.

Three years passed. In October of 1991, Carol Galipeau, who fortuitously was both a nurse at one of the local hospitals and the wife of an RMS member, sent Béla a flyer that she had found at her place of work. She was aware of RMS's earlier interest in TT; her flyer alerted us that it was a practice freely taught in some hospitals. Indeed, the publication was clearly advertising a hospital-approved course in TT. What to do?

Béla contacted the only nurse in RMS, Linda Rojas. She was appalled at the infiltration into her chosen profession of what was to her an outrageous and scientifically baseless practice. It was soon clear that the two of them could not single-handedly tackle the situation but that others had to get involved. The rest is history laid out in detail in this book.

What did emerge from the hard work of the many people within RMS soon became widely known by the skeptic and the TT communities. Eleven years after Dr. Rothschild's inquiry, skeptics throughout the world have heard of TT, its claims and its personalities. They, too, began to conduct experiments and write papers and letters to the editor in newspapers from Boulder, Colorado to England, Canada, and Australia. No longer could TT practitioners fly under the radar of the skeptics. "Therapeutic Touch" could no longer simply be accepted in hospitals, taught in nursing schools, or be promoted by nursing boards. TT as a legitimate area of scrutiny by the skeptical community had arrived.

Many books have been written supporting the claims of Therapeutic Touch. This book is not one of those; it is unique in that aspect and in other ways. Not only is it the first one published by critics of TT, but it is also the first one that presents unedited papers describing the best case experiments conducted by TT advocates as well as articles describing the theoretical underpinnings of the discipline. In the best spirit of scientific inquiry, criticisms of the TT experiments are also included.

This book is written both for the skeptic and the nursing professional. We, the editors, believe that this volume will be a valuable addition to the library of anyone involved with or interested in TT. We are proud to bring to those interested in the state of our health care the best writings by those most knowledgeable about this subject.

After considerable evaluation of the evidence, the editors do not regard the "therapeutic" claim for TT to have been scientifically established. Furthermore, since touching is not required in TT, the term is misleading and vague. While it is customary to enclose such questionable phrases as Therapeutic Touch within quotes, this practice would be awkward in a book whose principal subject is Therapeutic Touch. Therefore, the editors have chosen to omit this punctuation in most cases when referring to TT throughout the book.

Béla Scheiber and Carla Selby
June 2000

Section I.

Social Science of Therapeutic Touch

I.

A Brief History of Therapeutic Touch

Jack Stahlman

THE ROOTS OF THERAPEUTIC TOUCH: EASTERN AND WESTERN TRADITIONS

In its contemporary form, Therapeutic Touch (TT) was developed in the late 1960s and early 1970s by cofounders Dolores Krieger, R.N., Ph.D., and Doris van Gelder Kunz. However, TT did not, of course, spring up out of whole cloth during this period. The roots of TT stretch back into the dim past of human history, drawing many of its tenets from Eastern thought and philosophy. Krieger (1975) reports that "energy-based healing" is recorded in ancient pictographs, cuneiform writings, and is found in Egyptian, Greek, Japanese, Chinese, and most importantly, Indian philosophy.

It is from Indian writings dating to at least 5000 B.C.E. that many of the basic concepts of TT are drawn, particularly from Hindu and Buddhist thought. The concept of infinite, universal *life-energy fields* are found both in Hinduism and Buddhism. The concepts of *chakras* ("energy centers"), *prana* ("life energy"), human consciousness as a transformer of matter, paranormal ideas such as clairvoyance and intuitive states of consciousness, action-at-a-distance via the notion of *akasha* (multidimensional space), and even some psychosomatic explanations of human health and disease, are all borrowed directly from Eastern religion and philosophy (Weber, 1991). These connections with Eastern traditions form an integral part of the theory underlying TT, and are embraced and heavily promoted by TT practitioners and theorists. Indeed, the concepts are ubiquitous throughout their writings (Carpenito, 1997; Krieger, 1975, 1997; Kunz, 1991).

The tradition of "healing" in Western culture also enjoys a long and varied history. The laying-on of hands encountered in the Christian tradition is based upon biblical accounts of miraculous healings performed by Jesus Christ. The New Testament contains forty-one references to Christ's ability to heal (Starn, 1998). The Christian view that certain people can heal by this means is derived from the New Testament description of the "Gift of Healing," one of the nine "Gifts of the Spirit" that are spoken of in 1 Corinthians 12. This tradition of divine healing through the laying-on of hands is further reinforced in Matt. 10:8 where Christ directs His disciples to "heal the sick, raise the dead, cleanse the lepers, cast out devils" (cited in Randi, 1987).

Healing continued as a part of the mission of the Catholic clergy until the twelfth century, when a papal edict ordered the practice halted. In spite of this edict and the subsequent burning of healers, heretics, witches, and midwives, the practice continued in wide usage (Starn, 1998).

European royalty adopted the laying-on of hands early in the fourteenth century. Healing through the "Royal Touch," as it came to be known, was seen as an extension of the Divine Right of kings and was performed as early as 1307 by the French monarch Philip the Fair. Soon afterward, the practice was adopted by English kings to supposedly cure scrofula, a tubercular inflammation of the lymph nodes of the neck that was also known as "The King's Evil" (Randi, 1987).

Healing via laying-on hands has not been limited to Catholicism and has also been part of Protestant traditions. Martin Luther, among others, practiced it in the sixteenth century. Luther took credit for numerous spontaneous and miraculous cures. By the mid-1600s, a practitioner named Valentine Greatraks, also known as "The Stroker," had become a sensation in England, drawing large crowds of both Catholics and Protestants who believed that he carried the "power of heaven" within his hands. Greatraks believed that disease was a result of demonic possession and claimed to cure the afflicted by the casting-out of demons. By the 1870s, London had become a center for healing via the laying-on of hands and remains so to this day (Randi, 1987).

In more modern times, the laying-on of hands was resurrected by nineteenth-century American and European evangelists. The Reverend William Branham, a former game warden *cum* fire-and-brimstone evangelist, is often credited with establishing the modern version of faith healing in the 1940s. Upon his death in 1965 as the result of an automobile accident, his followers refused to allow his burial for over four months in the expectation that he would rise from the dead on Easter Sunday. When the expected resurrection failed to take place, Branham was quietly buried (Randi, 1987).

The practice of TT is also mirrored in Wiccan healing massage rituals known as *auric* or *pranic* healing. This type of healing is nearly indistinguishable from TT in both technique and in the underlying concepts of balancing and manipulating energy fields. In fact, the technique describes an identical flicking-off of excess energy by shaking the hands, much in the manner that a cat shakes its feet after stepping in something distasteful (*Magickal Healing*, 1999). O'Mathúna (1996) lists some early theosophical writings that describe these techniques: Yogi Ramacharaka's *The Science of Psychic Healing* (1909), A. E. Powell's *The Etheric Double: The Health Aura of Man* (1925), and later occult books such as Janet and Stewart Farrar's *A Witches' Bible Compleat* (1981) and *Buckland's Complete Book of Witchcraft* (1987).

Advocates of TT for the most part studiously avoid the term faith healing, due in part to its religious connotations and in part to the negative images resulting from numerous charlatans. Janet Quinn, a well-known TT advocate, admits (National League for Nursing, 1992) that the laying-on of hands is a predecessor of TT, but states adamantly that TT is *not* a form of psychic healing, faith healing, or the laying-on of hands. According to Quinn, faith healing requires special abilities granted by God whereas TT, in keeping with its Eastern origins, is considered a natural human potential that can be learned and utilized by anyone. Quinn adds that faith healing requires complete faith on the part of the recipient, whereas TT does not. The recipient of TT is said to benefit even when unaware that the treatment is being performed. Another obvious difference is that faith healing is a literal laying-on of the hands, while TT is said to involve only the manipulation of energy fields with the practitioner's hands held two to four inches from the recipient's body.

It is important to note that the practice of laying-on of hands shares many fundamental attributes with TT. For example, much is made in TT literature of the intention of the healer; both in the practice of TT and in the laying-on of hands most practitioners exhibit a sincere desire to help the afflicted. Although some faith healers do practice the laying-on of hands, most practitioners of this art (and of TT) seem to lack the crass financial motives found in faith healing.

Although Quinn has pointed out differences between TT and laying-on of hands, they are subtle at best. For example, it is not entirely accurate to say that the laying-on of hands requires complete faith on the part of the recipient since this type of healing is also practiced on infants and the comatose. Even the differences in technique are not clear-cut. Also, a review of a widely distributed instructional videotape (National League for Nursing, 1992) reveals that TT is not entirely a "hands-off" technique. Quinn, who acts as the instructor on this tape, is seen to physically touch the recipient numerous times. Furthermore, Quinn states that it is quite appropriate to mix the nontouch of TT with actual physical contact and explains that the mix of the two is a matter of personal style on the part of the practitioner. Often TT is used as an adjunct to massage.

It is not a universally accepted idea that the laying-on of hands is a gift from God granted only to special individuals (MacNutt, 1974). As in TT, many who practice the laying-on of hands feel that it is a practice that can be used by anyone and they encourage its use. Krieger (1990, p. 86) states that in 1972 she "learned laying-on of hands and practiced it with some success." The practice of TT clearly shares much with the tradition of the laying-on of hands, perhaps as a secularized version or perhaps with Eastern religious concepts substituted for those of Christianity; nonetheless, the similarities are undeniable. Thus TT must be viewed as a descendant, an outgrowth, or at the very least, as a stepchild of the laying-on of hands.

It was the Theosophical Society that mixed science with Eastern and Western notions into a more contemporary form. Founded in New York City in 1875 by Madame Helena Petrovona Blavatsky, Henry Steele Olcott, and W. Q. Judge, the Society has been called the "Great Homogenizer" of ideas, blending such disparate "isms" as mesmerism, spiritualism, transcendentalism, Hinduism, Buddhism, and Darwinism into a somewhat cohesive form. The influence of this amalgamation continues today and is the source of the intellectual and philosophical framework into which TT was born.

Mesmerism is named after the eighteenth-century Viennese physician Franz Anton Mesmer (Carroll, 1999c). Mesmer had a background steeped in astrology and received his doctorate for a plagiarized dissertation on how the planets affect health. In the early 1770s, Mesmer met Fr. Maximillian Hell, a Jesuit priest and healer who claimed to have effected cures using magnetized steel plates. Mesmer promptly plagiarized Hell's methods, positing that the magnets cured people by restoring the flow of a universal magnetism that had become blocked as a result of disease. Mesmer later claimed that he could achieve the same cures without the use of magnetized steel plates, theorizing that he was able to restore balance through what he termed "animal magnetism." This idea has been compared to the "balancing of universal energies" encountered in TT (Fish, 1999).

Mesmer's cures soon became a sensation in Europe. By 1778 he had moved to Paris where, under the auspices of Louis XVI and Marie Antoinette, he set up the Magnetic Institute where he continued with his healing. However, Mesmer's success in Paris was relatively short-lived; in 1788 he was discredited by a royal commission that included Benjamin Franklin and was declared a fraud (Carroll, 1999c).

Despite having been officially discredited, by the 1820s Mesmerism had arrived in the United States and within a decade had become highly popular. Mesmerists toured the countryside performing miracles by making "magnetic passes" over the bodies of patients, a technique that later evolved into hypnotism (Brenneman, 1990). By 1829, the word *mesmerize* had entered the English language and it remains today in common usage, meaning "to hypnotize," "to fascinate," or "to be held spellbound" (Mish, 1990).

Mesmer's magnetic healing set the stage for the public's fascination with spiritualism. If magnetic and planetary energy could be transmitted through a healer, why couldn't the same be done with spiritual energy? Or, carrying this idea further, why could the dead not pass this spiritual energy to the living (Brenneman, 1990)?

The spiritualist movement officially began in upstate New York in 1848, when sisters Katherine and Margaret Fox (twelve and thirteen years old, respectively) claimed to be able to communicate with the dead through mysterious rappings. From these "spirit rappings," the "science" of spiritualism soon evolved and was endorsed by, among others, Mary Todd Lincoln, Sir Arthur Conan Doyle, and Sir Oliver Lodge, one of the premier physicists of the day. The Fox sisters became celebrities, and were later hired by P. T. Barnum to give public demonstrations. Spiritualism became a national craze, with religious, social, moral, and political overtones (Washington, 1995). The notoriety of the girls also spawned a host of imitators. Thousands of mediums were soon producing more and more marvels: words materializing on sealed slates, disembodied spirits of the dead speaking from floating trumpets, the ghostly touch of unseen hands, and spectral manifestations of the dead. Although the Fox sisters admitted some thirty years later that the spirit rappings were created by simply snapping the joints in their toes, a Pandora's box had already been opened and spiritualism had entered into the American psyche (Brenneman, 1990; Carroll, 1999a).

It was in the transcendental movement of 1836–1866 that we first find the blending of Eastern mysticism and Western thought that still flourishes in contemporary American society. Prior to the nineteenth century, interest in India was largely commercial, focusing on trade in silks, spices, precious metals, fine jewelry, valuable Dacca muslin, and occasionally rare books in Sanskrit. In 1812, Captain Heard of the brig *Caravan* set sail for Calcutta, with instructions from his friend Henry Pickering to secure a "Sanskrit Bible." Heard's return was the catalyst that sparked American interest in things Indian, with Sanskrit writings soon being in great demand. These new ideas found fertile ground in the bohemian Boston intellectual community, and as Indian thought permeated American writings and philosophy, the transcendental movement was born (Narasingha and Rosen, 1999).

The Transcendental Club, also known as The Circle, was founded in Concord in 1836 and included, among others, such luminaries and influential American writers as Henry David Thoreau, Ralph Waldo Emerson, teacher and philosopher Amos Bronson Alcott (father of Lousia May Alcott), the liberal Unitarian minister James Freeman Clark, and Margaret Fuller (great-aunt of R. Buckminster Fuller). In the Transcendental Club, the American version of mysticism was born. The Transcendental movement was "Yankee mysticism . . . Hindu detachment wed to American Manifest Destiny—prosperity with the Oversoul" (Brenneman, 1990, p. 15). The effects of this fusion of East and West echo in contemporary American society and are manifested in the teachings of the Theosophical Society.

The Theosophical Society was the crucible in which these disparate elements were fused. What remained was to tie faith to science, reason to revelation. The nineteenth century witnessed the rise of Darwin's theory of evolution, and despite the physical and rational basis of Darwin's theories, Theosophists saw in physical evolution a parallel to the spiritual. Just as mankind had evolved from the simple to the complex, from lowly, brutish, ancestors to a more "perfect" form, so, too, could he evolve to higher metaphysical and spiritual forms (Brenneman, 1990). It was this blending of evolutionary theory with mysticism that was the Society's most far-reaching achievement.

The Theosophical (from the Greek *theosophia*, literally "divine wisdom") Society was officially founded by Madame Blavatsky in the year 1875. In the previous year, Blavatsky had met Henry Olcott while investigating the Eddy brothers, a spiritualist duo operating out of Vermont. Finding a kindred spirit in Olcott, the two met with other occult-minded individuals; the Society was born. Previous to meeting Olcott, Blavatsky had worked as a circus performer and séance assistant and claimed to have spent several years in Tibet and India, where she claimed to have came into contact with the "Masters"—ancient teachers who possess astral bodies. According to Blavatsky, the Masters are not divine spirits, but rather a spiritually evolved form of humanity who possess great psychic powers and are the sacred keepers of "Ancient Wisdom" (Carroll, 1999b).

Several years after the Society was formed, Blavatsky and Olcott moved to India to establish the Theosophical Society Headquarters at Adyar. By 1885, however, Blavatsky had left India, accused of faking materializations of written teachings from the Masters (Carroll, 1999b). In 1888, she published her most influential work, *The Secret Doctrine*. The *Doctrine* was Blavatsky's reconciliation of the Ancient Wisdom with science and human culture—utilizing history, religion, and cosmology (Ellwood, 1996). In *The Secret Doctrine* we find the final mix of science,

Eastern mysticism, and philosophy that has had a profound influence on American thought and spawned, among other ideas, the New Age movement.

Membership in the Society increased exponentially in subsequent decades. By 1907, it claimed thirteen thousand members, which by 1911 had increased to sixteen thousand. New applicants continued to flood into the Society; by 1920, membership had risen to thirty-six thousand, peaking in 1928 at forty-five thousand.

Currently, despite the proliferation of interest in the occult and the popularity of New Age ideas, the Theosophical Society continues in a slow decline. The Society still functions from its headquarters at Adyar, but suffers from an elderly membership and a certain domesticity and lassitude. Concerned primarily with the study of esoteric wisdom and focusing on more dignified humanitarian enterprises (Theosophical Society, 1999), the Society maintains a low profile and seldom advertises or attempts to recruit new members. Hamstrung by respectability and the lack of new blood, classes continue and the sacred dances are passed on, but the Society lacks the drive of the heady days of its youth. The mantle of the New Age has been passed to its more modern and diverse offspring (Washington, 1995).

Against the background of this amalgam of Eastern mysticism and Western healing practices imbued with Darwinism, the stage was set for the arrival of TT.

KUNZ, KRIEGER, AND THE EARLY DEVELOPMENT OF THERAPEUTIC TOUCH

Dora van Gelder Kunz, who, along with Dolores Krieger, is credited as being a codeveloper of TT, reports a childhood steeped in mysticism and clairvoyant experiences. Born in 1904 into a Dutch family who managed a large sugar plantation in Java, Kunz (1991) reports that she was born fully encased in a caul, a fetal birth membrane that traditionally heralds clairvoyant and psychic abilities. According to Kunz, both her mother and grandmother had psychic abilities. Her mother was a strong believer in meditation; beginning at about five years of age, Kunz had been expected to meditate upon increasingly complex and abstract ideas in a special room set aside for just that purpose. Kunz relates that she first became aware of her own alleged psychic abilities at the age of six or seven, and was encouraged by C. W. Leadbeater, a fellow "clairvoyant" and a prolific theosophical writer. After moving to Australia at the age of twelve, Kunz states that she was in daily contact with Leadbeater for a number of years, although he did not specifically train her in developing her clairvoyant talents. However, it is clear from Kunz's published works and statements by Krieger (1979) that Leadbeater stood as a major influence.

Charles Webster Leadbeater was a controversial figure, even by Theosophical Society standards. He was a colorful figure with a penchant for confabulating fantastic tales of his personal adventures à la *The Adventures of Baron Munchausen*. Leadbeater's fantastic stories aside, the truth of the matter is that he was born in Stockport, England in 1854, the son of a poor railway clerk. In 1878 he secured a curacy in Bramshott, England, and by 1883 he was inducted into the Theosophical Society.

It was Leadbeater who first introduced Kunz to the ideas of theosophy, which became a lifelong interest of hers. Kunz later became the president of the Society, serving from 1975–1987. She has also served as the Chairman of the Theosophical Publishing House and as editor-in-chief of *The American Theosophist*.

It is interesting that Leadbeater was willing to act as a mentor to Kunz. His fear of women (some would say hatred) was such that he was reluctant to even shake hands with a female; he refused to remain in a room alone with them. It has been stated, perhaps rather waggishly, that Leadbeater's major interests in life were ritualism, spiritualism, elitism, and adolescent boys. At one point in his career, Leadbeater was ousted from the Society under allegations of inappropriate sexual contact with young boys; he was later reinstated through the influence of Annie Besant, a powerful ally in the Society hierarchy (Washington, 1995).

Like Kunz, Leadbeater claimed to be clairvoyant and to have the ability to read auras. Leadbeater's mysticism is evident in his writings. He claims to have used his occult powers to visit the mythical continents of Atlantis and Lemuria. Later he investigated what he termed the "true" history of Christianity, and he concluded that Christ was actually an Egyptian initiate who was born in the year 105 C.E. In *The Astral Plane*, considered by some to be his most important and far-reaching work, Leadbeater began documenting his studies into past lives and reincarnation. He was also a pioneer in the study of *psychometry*, which is a purported means of obtaining information about people and events associated with an object merely by touching, handling, or being near to the object. It is a technique currently in vogue among "psychic sleuths." From the standpoint of TT, however, Leadbeater's most notable work is undoubtedly *The Chakras* (1927), a testimony of clairvoyant observation that influenced both Kunz and Krieger (Washington, 1995).

By the early 1930s, Kunz, then in her twenties, was living in New York City where she worked with Dr. Otelia Bengtsson, a specialist in allergies and immunology. Kunz (1991) states that Bengtsson thought her clairvoyance would be helpful with patients who were difficult to diagnose or for whom conventional treatment was unsuccessful. Regarding her own role in treating these patients, Kunz writes:

> I would tell her what I thought the physical problems were, but I also explained the role that the patients' emotions played in the disease process, and gave advice about the ways in which they could help themselves. (p. 1)

According to Kunz, her collaboration with Bengtsson enabled her to become a careful observer and gave her the opportunity to study in depth the relationship between emotional patterns (as read in the aura) and physical disease. Additionally, Kunz felt that this period gave her the opportunity to study the relationship between disease processes and their psychological correlates (again, in the context of aura reading). Kunz has continued over her lifetime to use her clairvoyant abilities to study the human aura; she has stated that during the time period between the 1930s and 1991, she personally read hundreds, perhaps thousands, of auras (Kunz, 1991).

Subsequent to her work with Bengtsson, Kunz's interest shifted more to the phenomena of healing, particularly through the laying-on of hands, to the point that this became the main focus of her work. Although Kunz is typically cited as a cofounder of TT, she has remained somewhat of an enigma and a background figure, functioning primarily as a mentor and teacher to Krieger. Biographical information on her is scant: the Theosophical Society (of which she was president for twelve years) was unable to provide information, and attempts by the author to contact her in person were unsuccessful (perhaps understandably so, as Kunz was ninety-five years old at the time of the efforts to contact her).

A literature review reveals only three publications over Kunz's long career: a volume on chakras and human energy fields coauthored with Dr. Shafica Karagulla, an anthology dealing with healing arts which she edited, and *The Personal Aura*, published in 1991 when she was eighty-seven years old. This 1991 work is the only volume that was exclusively penned by Kunz and is based upon a study of fourteen "human auras" that were undertaken over fifty-five years ago. Kunz has given two reasons for the long lapse between her study and its publication: First, she was reluctant to publish a book based upon a minimal number of case studies. More importantly, she believed that the intellectual climate before 1991 was not conducive to any serious consideration of her controversial work. The precise reasons why she considered the intellectual climate to have become sufficiently more receptive to her ideas by 1991 can only be speculated.

More than any other individual, it was Dolores Krieger, R.N., Ph.D., who was the driving force in the development and early promotion of TT. It was Krieger, who at the time was the head of the Nursing Department at the New York University School of Nursing, who took an amalgam of Eastern mysticism and the overtly religious practice of the laying-on of hands and added an overlay of scientific respectability. It was Krieger who did the early research in TT, laid down a theoretical basis, and promoted it within the nursing establishment.

Krieger reports a wide variety of interests, among them organic gardening, mountain climbing, wood carving, rock collecting, and reading ancient petroglyphs. She has a background in comparative religion and is an avowed Buddhist.

Krieger's involvement in healing began in earnest in the late 1960s when she joined with Dora Kunz and Dr. Otelia Bengtsson (with whom Kunz collaborated in the early 1930s). At the time, Kunz and Bengtsson had been working with Oskar Estabany, a theosophical healer who employed the laying-on of hands. Estabany, who had been a Colonel in the Hungarian cavalry, began his career by "healing" ill horses. As his reputation as healer of animals spread, people began to seek his help with human afflictions and he soon began treating people with a combination of prayer and the laying-on of hands. Estabany believed that his healing powers were derived from channeling the spirit of Jesus Christ. Reminiscent of Mesmer, Estabany believed that he was able to "magnetize" inert objects such as cotton balls with his healing energy, a practice later adopted by TT practitioners (Krieger, 1979).

Estabany, who had retired to Canada, visited the United States for several weeks each year to set up temporary healing clinics. Krieger's function during these sessions was peripheral: she took case histories, monitored vital signs, and stood by in case nursing care was necessary. But this gave her the opportunity to observe Estebany closely (Krieger, 1990). She was quite impressed with Estabany, stating that "a felt energetic intensity built up in the rooms in which he did his healing, so that it was quite perceptible upon entering the house" (Krieger, 1979, p. 6). Her interest piqued by Estabany's apparent success with his patients, Krieger conducted a literature review and that the entire published literature on the subject of healing via the laying-on of hands consisted of two studies by Bernard Grad published in the *International Journal of Parapsychology* in 1961 and 1963.

These two studies by Grad, a Canadian biochemist at McGill University, were double-blind experiments involving the effects of healing through the laying-on of hands on mice and on barley seeds. In both studies, Estabany was the healer. In the mice experiments (Grad, 1961), 300 mice were wounded and randomly assigned to three groups: a control group that was allowed to heal naturally, a second control group held by medical students with no known prowess as healers, and a group treated by Estabany by the laying-on of hands. According to Krieger (1975), after two weeks Estabany's treatment group was found to have had accelerated wound healing, with a probability of one in a thousand that the results could have occurred by chance.

In Grad's barley seed experiments (1963), the seeds were soaked in saline to simulate unhealthy conditions, then assigned to one of three groups: a group watered with normal tap water, a group watered with flasks held by disinterested persons, and the treatment group, which was watered from flasks that had been held by Estebany. Krieger (1975, p. 784) reports that the group of seeds watered from the flasks held by Estebany "sprouted more quickly, grew taller, and had more chlorophyll than the seeds in the control group" (1975, p. 784).

Krieger (1975) also discusses work done by Sr. Justa Smith as being influential on her thinking in the late 1960s; because Smith's work, "Paranormal Effects on Enzyme Activity," was not published until 1972, it must be surmised that Krieger was privy to the results of Smith's work before actual publication. In Sr. Smith's study, flasks containing the enzyme trypsin were divided into four groups: one group of flasks was exposed to high levels of ultraviolet light to simulate an unhealthy condition and was held by healer Oskar Estabany for seventy-five minutes, a second group was not treated with ultraviolet light and was also held by the healer, a third group was exposed to a high magnetic field, and the fourth group (the control) was untreated. Krieger reports that both the samples held by the healer and those treated with a magnetic field displayed increased enzyme activity—effects that Krieger concluded would indicate a contribution to the improvement or maintenance of health.

Krieger states that the results of the studies by Grad and Smith, coupled with her own observations of patient healings performed by Estabany, "challenged me as a practitioner, teacher, and nurse researcher" (Krieger, 1975, p. 785). Krieger returned to the literature, searching for an explanation for this healing process. Unable to find a suitable explanation in Western literature, and having a strong background in comparative religion, Krieger turned to Eastern literature for illumination. She began a study of ancient healing practices, analyzed their underlying concepts, and attempted to correlate them with her contemporary findings (Krieger, 1975, 1990). Like Dora Kunz, Dolores Krieger was also heavily influenced by the occult writings of Leadbeater (Bullough and Bullough, 1998; Krieger, 1979).

It was in the Eastern writings that Krieger found her answers, and the rest, as they say, is history. The Eastern explanation of the process that occurs during the laying-on of hands lies in the Sanskrit concept of *prana*, or "human life energies," which Krieger posits is "intrinsic in what we call the oxygen molecule" (Krieger, 1975, p. 786). Illness is seen as a deficit of prana, while a healthy person carries an overabundance that can be transferred, given the proper intent, to another person. This nascent view of the healing process as a transfer of energy was later modified to become the current concept of "repatterning" or "rebalancing" energies (Carpenito, 1997).

The groundwork for the early theoretical basis of TT now complete, Krieger (1975) turned her attention to conducting research studies. Based upon her background in hematology, Krieger began her first pilot study into healing via the laying-on of hands in 1971, again using Estabany as the healer. Postulating that the mean hemoglobin values for an experimental group treated by the laying-on of hands would exceed their before-treatment values, Krieger conducted a study using nineteen ill people in the treatment group and nine ill people in the control group. Krieger reports that her hypotheses were confirmed. In 1972, Krieger conducted her first full-scale study of the phenomena, using much the same methodology and firmer controls; again, she reports that her hypotheses were confirmed.

Early in 1973, Krieger introduced the nursing profession at large to the subject of healing through the laying-on of hands when she reported the findings from these early studies at the American Nurses Association's 9th Council of Nurse Researchers. Later in 1973, she replicated her previous studies using forty-six subjects in the experimental group and twenty-nine in the control group, again with tighter controls, and again with similar findings. Krieger states, based upon her research up to that point, that she became convinced healing by the laying-on of hands is a natural human potential with two critical elements: the healer must carry an "intent to heal" and must be in good health, which is indicative of an overflow or prana (Krieger, 1975, 1990).

Based upon her understanding of healing as a natural human potential and what had been learned from previous research and clinical experience, Krieger (1990) concluded in 1974 that it was time to teach her methods to others; subsequently, Krieger and Kunz proceeded to teach the practice to a group of professional nurses. This represents a pivotal moment in the history of TT because, for the first time, the practice of the laying-on of hands was taught to those who did not profess to have inherent healing powers. The affiliation of TT with nursing quickly led to the proliferation of the practice. In addition, it was at this point that the terminology changed to *Therapeutic Touch*, shedding the religious connotations associated with the term "laying-on of hands." In effect, the practice become more secularized. This transition can be considered the birth of TT in its current form.

Next, Krieger undertook another study in New York City, again involving hemoglobin values. This time, however, the professional healers were replaced with sixteen nurses trained in TT. As in her previous studies, mean hemoglobin values of subjects were expected to increase following treatment with TT; as in previous studies, she reported that her hypotheses were confirmed (Krieger, 1975).

Based upon the favorable reception to her TT classes for nurses and her apparently successful research, Krieger submitted a proposal for a course on TT to the Division of Nursing at New York University. This proposal was passed by the curriculum committee and later approved by the Dean's Advisory Committee. In the fall of 1975, the first class in TT was taught at New York University, and TT has continued to be taught there ever since.

From these beginnings, TT propagated and was soon being taught at other universities. As more and more nurses became practitioners and advocated its use, TT became increasingly intertwined with the nursing profession. There remained only to be added an updated, twentieth-century "scientific" slant to the combination of Eastern mysticism with Western nursing practices: Enter Martha E. Rogers and her *science of unitary human beings*.

MARTHA E. ROGERS AND THE SCIENCE OF UNITARY HUMAN BEINGS

By 1979, nurse theorist Martha E. Rogers's rather esoteric theory of the *science of unitary man* (later changed to *science of unitary human beings*) had been incorporated into TT literature (Boguslawski, 1979; Miller, 1979). Rogers purported to offer a more "scientific" theoretical framework and an explanatory model of the energy fields encountered in the practice of TT. In the writings of Rogers, the relationship between TT and the science of unitary man involves circular reasoning: On the one hand, TT is seen as clinical application of the science of unitary man (Fitzpatrick, 1994) and as a real world demonstration of Rogers' theories. On the other hand, the science of unitary man has been used as the theoretical framework that forms the scientific basis of TT (Carpenito, 1997). Simply put, TT and the science of unitary man are often used to give validity to each other.

Beginning with the publication of "Nursing's Conceptual Model" in 1970, Rogers developed the science of unitary man in a series of papers over the next two decades (Rogers, 1970, 1980, 1986, 1990, 1992). Rogers defines a unitary human being as "an irreducible, indivisible, pandimensional energy field . . ." where *pandimensional* is defined as a "nonlinear domain without temporal or spatial attributes" (1990, p. 9). The science of unitary man is embodied in its three major principles: *resonancy*, *helicity*, and *integrality*. Briefly stated, the principle of resonancy holds that there is a continuous change from lower to higher frequencies in the human and environmental energy fields; the principle of helicity holds that these same fields progress to greater and greater diversity; and the principle of integrality is concerned with the mutual interaction between human and environmental fields.

It is the concept of metaphysical *energy fields* that is most pertinent to TT, since imbalances in these fields are said to be manipulated. Rogers identifies these energy fields as infinite and irreducible. Earlier versions of the theory of unitary man postulated that these fields are electrical in nature, but Rogers backed away from this idea as she refined her theories. With the publication of "Nursing Science and the Space Age" in 1992, Rogers had concluded that these fields are *not* of biological, physical, social, or psychological origin. Rather than humans and the environment *having* energy fields, they were seen as *being* energy fields. Although many TT theorists have linked universal energy fields to quantum physics, Rogers herself had little to say on the subject, preferring to discuss energy fields in vague generalities.

In 1990, Rogers proposed that the science of unitary human beings provides an explanation of paranormal events, such as precognition, telepathy, clairvoyance, and TT. According to Rogers, an infinite and pandimensional human energy field is in continuous mutual interaction with a pandimensional environmental field (the principle of integrality). She states that within this context, TT and the paranormal become rational and "normal" (Rogers, 1990).

Rogers has been a highly influential nursing theorist, generating an avid following among nurses and nursing researchers who subscribe to her holistic worldview. In 1988, the Society of Rogerian Scholars was chartered in the state of New York. The Society's mission statement contains the following fundamental objectives: to advance nursing as a basic science; to explore the meaning of a philosophy of wholeness for nursing; to foster the understanding and the use of the Science of Unitary Human Beings as a basis for theory development, research, education, and practice; and to provide avenues for dissemination of information related to the Science of Unitary Human Beings (Barrett, 1994). One of the major avenues used by the society to promote Rogers's ideas is the journal *The Rogerian*.

What were the philosophical and social contexts that primarily influenced Martha Rogers? Where did the ideas come from that led to her science of unitary human beings? In 1988, when questioned regarding the conceptualization of her theory, Rogers replied:

I started when I was born—collecting more and more facts. New knowledge began to come out—there was the dawn of the space Age. As for the framework, which comes first, the chicken or the egg? . . . There are new and old world views, ancient history, and the Indian philosophies. Things fell into place and grew. Now we're moving into recognizing that there are other ways of thinking. There are no closed doors in science. (Hecktor, p. 18)

Rogers's reply hints at an evolution of her thoughts over time rather than a moment of epiphany. However, she identifies only history and Indian philosophy as directly influencing her ideas. She has denied any single educational experience as being more influential than any other, saying that "they all contributed to many things. None was more important than any other" (Hecktor, 1994, p.18). Further, in 1989 Rogers stated that "no one philosophy or philosophers could be singled out as having influenced my writing" (Reeder, 1994, p. 317). These statements are consistent with Rogers's worldview of humankind as nonlinear, pandimensional beings and a universe in which all things are interrelated and in which all things influence all other things. To a Rogerian theorist, freed from the constraints of time and space, it is impossible to sort out just who influences whom. Indeed, some Rogerian scholars (Moccia, 1994; Reeder, 1994) have suggested that rather than Rogers being influenced by historical figures, it is the reverse that is true: It was through interactions with Rogers throughout time that "famous women and men develop[ed] their perspective on the world around them" (Moccia, 1994, p. 309). These encounters stretch across vast periods of human history, beginning with Greek antiquity, through the matriarchal Chumash tribe in the 1500s, to an aural encounter with Einstein at the turn of the century, to a meeting with Ghandi in 1986 (Moccia, 1994).

Despite Rogers's claims to the contrary, it appears that some philosophies have influenced her thought. Rogers reports that as a child she was a voracious reader, devouring dictionaries at age five and sets of encyclopedias by age eleven. As a teenager, she is known to have been preoccupied with Eastern philosophy, an interest that continued into later life. Her early interests included anthropology, archaeology, cosmology, ethnography, astronomy, ethics, psychology, and aesthetics (Reeder, 1994).

As an adult, Rogers was influenced (Reeder, 1994) by a number of writers, notably Nietzsche, Decartes, Alfred North Whitehead, and perhaps most importantly, Lancelot Law Whyte, an English theorist and author of *The Next Development of Man* (1961). It was Whyte who coined the term *unitary man*, later borrowed by Rogers. Although Whyte uses the term in the context of *unitary* (as opposed to *dualistic*)

thinking rather than in the context of the concept of energy fields postulated by Rogers, there are clear similarities. Rogers echoes many of
Whyte's ideas: Whyte describes a universal interelatedness and inter-
dependence of man and the environment, an idea that closely res-
onates with the writings of Rogers; Whyte states that man is "not subject to any fundamental division" (p. 38), and Rogers postulates that
man is "irreducible"; Whyte states that there is a progressive differen-
tiation of human behavior, thought, and social organization, and Rogers
theorizes a greater and greater diversity to the human energy field (the
principle of *helicy*); Whyte sees an acceleration of human development,
and Rogers sees an acceleration of human evolution, leading to the
development of "Homo spatialis," an evolutionary jump that Rogers
expects to take place within the next fifty years. Clearly, Rogers was
heavily influenced by the ideas and writings of Whyte.

THE MIDDLE YEARS:
THE PROLIFERATION OF TT

Moving beyond the early years of TT, we find a trend away from its religious and psychic roots and, with the addition of Rogers' theoretical
framework, toward a more scientific-sounding tone. Krieger (1979)
affirms the marriage of Eastern thought and Western science, stating
that TT has recaptured the "simple but elegant ancient mode of healing
and mated it with the rigor and power of modern science" (p. 16).
Although TT has never attempted to shed its Eastern connections,
retaining among others the Eastern concepts of prana and chakras,
practitioners prefer to consider this more as a philosophical than a religious basis.

In the intervening decades following Krieger's early research, the
TT movement has been characterized by a proliferation of practitioners and by an increasing "body of research" into the subject. As TT
has matured it has turned to a more Westernized research basis, primarily conducted by nurses and published in nursing journals. Examining several review articles and meta-analyses of quantitative research
into TT will give a useful overview.

Most research into TT has centered on its ability to reduce anxiety
and alleviate pain. Spence and Olson (1997) examined these two variables by reviewing the published literature from 1985 to 1995. Eleven
quantitative studies were examined. The authors conclude that these
studies offer support that TT is effective for the reduction of pain or
anxiety: Nine of the eleven studies indicated statistically significant
findings on at least some measures, although not always the on the

variables of interest, while seven of these studies either confirm the hypotheses, or show a trend toward expected results. They point out that some hypotheses were not supported and those studies that did report significant findings are in need of replication. The authors conclude that quantitative studies during this decade are few, lack replication, and are inconsistent, but that the results can serve as a springboard for directing future research.

Meehan (1998) likewise investigated the parameters of anxiety and pain. Reviewing ten studies which explored the effects of TT on anxiety, Meehan states that the findings of five indicate that TT was more effective than controls in reducing anxiety. In a review of several studies probing the relationship between TT and pain reduction, the author concludes that TT may have the potential to relieve mild, tension-related headache pain. However, she notes that no clinical studies have reported TT to significantly reduce postoperative pain or to act as an agonist for narcotic analgesics. There is some evidence that it may slightly decrease the need of postoperative patients for analgesic medications. Meehan concludes that although TT may not be significantly more effective than a placebo, inasmuch as it may enhance the placebo effect it may have some potential as an appropriate nursing intervention.

In reviewing Krieger's body of research developed over the past quarter century, McKinney states that the results of studies have been mixed, and that the direction of practice and research not always been clear. However, she concludes that Krieger's work has demonstrated support for an "intervention that produced hopeful but inconsistent findings" (McKinney 1995, cited in Spence and Olson, 1997, p. 3). She also points out the need for further qualitative studies to supplement quantitative research.

In addition to research into anxiety and pain reduction, a lesser body of research has focused on TT's ability to enhance wound healing in humans. Wirth, Richardson, and Eidelman (1996) reviewed a series of five clinical experiments previously conducted by Wirth that examined the effects of TT and other healing modalities on the reepithelization of full-thickness human dermal wounds. This series of studies found statistically significant results for two of the studies and nonsignificance or reverse significance for the remaining three. The authors of the 1996 review concluded that the inconsistent overall results of these experiments were inconclusive in establishing the efficacy of TT and the other alternative treatment methods in accelerating wound healing.

The growth of TT has also been characterized by a growing acceptance by professional nursing organizations and has been augmented by an increasing amount of public expenditure supporting continued research. As early as 1983, Krieger received a grant from the Department of Health and Human Services to conduct a comparison of TT and the Lamaze method for pregnant couples, with the dependent variable under consideration being anxiety. No statistically significant differences were identified (Krieger, 1990).

In 1992, the Division of Nursing at the D'Youville Nursing Center of Buffalo, New York, received a $200,000 grant from the U.S. Department of Health and Human Services to treat patients and train students in the technique of TT (Fish, 1999), in concordance with Krieger's assertion that the Society has the *duty* to permit the dissemination of training in TT (Krippner, 1992). In 1994, another large grant ($355,000) was made to a team of nurse researchers from the University of Alabama at Birmingham by the Department of Defense to conduct a study of the effects of TT on burn patients. Although this study concluded that patients receiving TT showed a reduction in pain and anxiety based upon questionnaires and visual analogue scales, there was no statistically significant reduction in medication usage in the experimental group. In addition, nosocomial (hospital-incurred) infections were more common in the group receiving TT (Turner, Clark, Gauthier, and Williams, 1998).

In 1987, the Board of Directors of the Order of Nurses of Quebec voted to accept TT as a bona fide nursing skill for their membership of 50,000 nurses (Krieger, 1990); by 1990, TT had been incorporated into the College of Nurses of Ontario Implementation Standards of Practice. Seven years later TT gained similar professional status in the United States with recognition granted by the North American Nursing Diagnosis Association (NANDA).

THE IMPRIMATUR OF NANDA

The year 1994 was a watershed for proponents of TT. In that year NANDA added the diagnosis of *energy field disturbance* to its widely used list of accepted nursing diagnoses, in effect granting its imprimatur to the practice of TT. The self-stated purpose of NANDA is to "define . . . and promote a taxonomy of nursing diagnostic terminology of general use to professional nurses" (NANDA, 1982, cited in Kozier, Erb, and Oliveri, 1991, p. 200). As such, NANDA is recognized as providing the official classification system—the gold standard of nursing diagnosis. As opposed to medical diagnosis, which describes a specific pathologic process, nursing diagnosis is concerned with the patient's response to disease and with actual or potential health problems. Typical nursing diagnoses would be impaired tissue integrity, ineffective airway clearance, chronic pain, or impaired gas exchange.

Energy field disturbance is defined as the "state in which a disruption of the flow of energy surrounding a person's being results in a disharmony of the body, mind, and/or spirit" (Carpenito, 1997, p. 344). Carpenito explains the "key concept" that TT is deeply rooted in Eastern philosophy; to the Eastern mind it is not necessary to understand how a therapy works or to conduct research, as research is an artifact of Western culture. The author goes on to explain that this diagnosis is unique for two reasons: First, it embodies a specific theoretical framework—Rogers's postulated energy fields. Second, it requires specialized training and supervised practice.

Two other factors also make energy field disturbance a unique diagnosis: First, the sanctioning of Therapeutic Touch by NANDA represents a turning point for both TT and nursing taxonomy; for the first time an "alternative modality" has been formalized into standard nursing practice. Second, it is the first and only nursing diagnosis that carries its own preemptive defense:

> This diagnosis may be considered unconventional by some. Perhaps each nurse needs to be reminded that there are many theories, philosophies, and frameworks of nursing practice. . . . Nursing diagnosis should not represent only the practices of nurses in the mainstream practice setting. . . . Rather than criticize a diagnosis as having little applicability to one's own practice, perhaps we should celebrate the diversity among us. Fundamentally, nurses are all connected as each of us and all of us seek to improve the condition of clients, families, groups, and communities. (Carpenito, 1997, p. 345)

THE RISE OF THE SKEPTICAL BACKLASH

The exponential growth of TT has not gone unnoticed or unchallenged by critics. It is beyond the scope of this brief history to delve deeply into the controversy surrounding the practice of TT, or to give thorough coverage to the challenges posed by critics. Nevertheless, as the skeptical movement is part and parcel of the history of TT, a brief synopsis of the major criticisms to date is provided.

Most criticisms of TT are centered around the following arguments: that there is little or no scientific evidence for either universal human energy fields or universal healing energies; that TT is based upon pseudoscientific interpretations of quantum physics that have little relation to science; that quantitative studies supporting the efficacy of TT suffer from poor sampling methods, are poorly controlled, use inadequate numbers of test subjects, or are poorly constructed and methodologically flawed; that studies supporting TT lack replication; that proponents misstate, overstate, misquote, or make unwarranted conclusions from existing quantitative studies; that the use of qualitative studies to support the efficacy of TT without the underlying support of quantitative work does little to support the case for TT; that much of the evidence offered by proponents of TT is anecdotal; that the body of scientific evidence is not sufficient to warrant the wide promotion and teaching of TT or funding using taxpayer money; that it seriously compromises the credibility and professionalism of nursing; that it has been heralded by the nursing establishment more out of a desire for empowerment and independence than as an efficacious treatment; that it may actually cause harm to patients; that in an era of cost-cutting and accountability it is a waste of time, resources, and talent; that it is a religious practice that has no place in the healthcare setting; that it offers a stamp of respectability to New Age practices that may lead patients away from traditional medical treatment; or that it is anti-Christian.

Criticism of TT arose soon after Krieger introduced the results of her early research and began promoting the practice. The earliest published critique found in a review of the literature was by Schlotfeldt (1973) and was written in response to Krieger's presentation of her hemoglobin studies at the 9th Council of Nurse Researchers. Schlotfeldt's critique praised Krieger for her creativity and imagination and her willingness to "seek scientific explanations for human interactions that heretofore have seemed to transcend science" (p. 59). Nonetheless, she pointed out several serious flaws in Krieger's research. Schlotfeldt questioned several of Krieger's basic assumptions, in particular her assertions that hemoglobin levels are a reliable measure of the state of a person's well-being, that hemoglobin levels are directly correlated to oxygen uptake, and that the transfer of prana from healthy to ill people actually does occur. Schlotfeldt also pointed out methodological flaws Krieger's work, most notably selection bias, nonequivalent control and experimental groups, and differing lengths of treatment for subjects in the experimental group. Schlotfeldt also pointed out that Krieger failed to discuss alternative explanations for her results.

The first critical response to TT found in a more widely circulated format was a lengthy letter in the *American Journal of Nursing* (Walike, et al. 1975), written in response to Krieger's 1975 article, "Therapeutic Touch: The Imprimatur of Nursing." This letter raised many of the objections later echoed by a growing number of TT opponents: Krieger's hemoglobin studies suffered from selection bias, unsound reasoning, overstatement of the results of Grad's work with Estabany, insufficient statistical analysis, and a failure to discuss alternative explanations or the limitations of her results. The authors went on to take the *American Journal of Nursing* to task for the credulous publication of an article that lacked scientific accuracy, bordered on sensationalism, and "attempts to embellish a totally unscientific process with the aura of science" (p. 1282).

A 1980 article entitled "A Skeptic's Guide to Therapeutic Touch" (Sandroff, 1980) gave a somewhat superficial overview of the skeptical viewpoint. In spite of the title, the bulk of this article presented TT in a highly favorable light, albeit with the addition of a few qualifiers. The majority of this article was spent quoting the "more open view" of TT proponents, detailing the procedure itself, and presenting the results of TT research at face value with little further commentary. Contact information was provided for workshops, seminars, and meetings for those who would "like to give therapeutic touch a try" (p. 82).

A relatively early and oft-cited review of TT research was published in 1984, by Clark and Clark. This paper critiqued much of the early research in TT and examined in detail several of the seminal studies conducted by Grad, Smith, and Krieger.

As discussed previously, Krieger reported that the 1961 study by Grad involving wound healing in mice demonstrated that after two weeks "healing in Estabany's group had accelerated to a degree that could have happened by chance less than once in a thousand times" (Krieger, 1975, p. 784). Although technically true, this statement is most disingenuous on the part of Krieger since she failed to report that these results were quite transient and that by the end of the study there was no significant difference in healing between any of the groups (Clark and Clark, 1984).

Clark and Clark also noted that Krieger overstated the effects of Grad's 1963 study reporting the effects of Estabany's healing on the growth of barley seeds treated with a weak saline solution. Krieger reported, "the seeds which were watered from the flasks held by Estabany sprouted more quickly, grew taller, and had more chlorophyll than the seeds in the control group." However, the dependent variables under consideration in this study were the number of plants per pot, the average height of plants per pot, and plant yield per pot; neither germination time nor chlorophyll content of the plants was studied. According to Grad's results, only on a single day did the experimental group contain a significantly greater number of plants. Although Grad reported statistically significant increases in height and yield in the experimental group in this study, he was unable to replicate these results in a series of four more experiments. None of the results of these replication studies were stable over time, a fact that Krieger failed to report (Clark and Clark, 1984).

Regarding Sr. Justa Smith's research in the early 1970s investigating the effects of Estabany and three other healers on the enzyme trypsin, Krieger stated that the results "all seem to contribute to improving or maintaining health" (Krieger, 1975, p. 785). Again, this appears to be an unwarranted conclusion, as Smith was unable to demonstrate increased enzyme activity in two of the three replication studies. In addition, her studies suffer from a lack of detail and insufficient statistical analysis (Clark and Clark, 1984).

Clark and Clark's analysis of Krieger's 1976 hemoglobin study identified several problems, including an inappropriate rationale for using hemoglobin as a measure of oxygen uptake, methodological problems, and the use of inappropriate statistical tests. Hemoglobin is a measure of oxygen capacity rather than oxygen uptake: a more appropriate and sensitive measure of oxygen uptake would have been the measurement of blood oxygen saturation. The use of meditation by some subjects was identified as a possible confounding variable. In addition, from the scant information provided, it does not appear that Krieger used random assignment to the control and experimental groups. Finally, Krieger's use of t-tests rather than an analysis of covariance was criticized as an inappropriate choice, especially since hemoglobin values increased in both the experimental and control groups, calling into question Krieger's interpretation of the results (Clark and Clark, 1984).

In 1996, James Randi, an outspoken critic of paranormal and psychic practices, in conjunction with the Philadelphia Association for Critical Thinking, posted a $742,000 award for any practitioner who could prove that he or she could detect a human energy field. A single practitioner agreed to be tested. In twenty trials during which she was asked to differentiate between an injured, painful limb and a healthy limb, the practitioner scored eleven out of twenty, statistically no better than chance (Glickman and Graceley, 1998) [see chapter 16 in this volume]. Although this result is insufficient to draw broader conclusions, Randi has continued to post this offer which has since grown to $1.2 million. No other TT practitioners have attempted to collect this award to date.

A more recent and widely publicized study conducted by opponents of TT was published in the *Journal of the American Medical Association* (Rosa, Rosa, Sarner, and Barrett, 1998). This study, with similarities to Glickman's 1996 test, attempted to explore one of the basic premises of TT—the ability of practitioners to perceive energy fields. Twenty-one TT healers were asked, under blinded conditions, to determine whether the investigator's hidden hand was posed over the healer's right or left hand. The results of this trial were calculated to be the correct hand only 44 percent of the time, results that are less than the 50 percent correct that could be expected by chance alone. The authors concluded that the failure of practitioners to substantiate one of the most fundamental claims of TT "suggest that TT claims are groundless and that further use of TT by health professinoals is unjustified" (p. 1009).

However, this study has been criticized by both advocates and at least one serious opponent of TT. Carpenito, an advocate of TT, questioned several aspects of the study including sample selection: "The description of the sample was limited to the number of years of experience and occupations, e.g., nurse, massage therapist, layperson, medical assistant, phlebotomist, chiropractor. Level of education and type of preparation for therapeutic touch were not addressed" (Carpenito, 1998, p. 3). Carpenito also raises the possibility of experimenter bias: "The adult authors were cited as associated with organizations such as Questionable Nurse Practitioners Task Force, National Council Against Health Fraud Inc., National Therapeutic Touch Study Group, and Quackwatch Inc." (Carpenito, 1998, p. 4; described in Rosa et al., 1998, p. 1005). She also raised the question of authorship not meeting *JAMA*'s published criteria: "From an editorial perspective, did Emily Rosa meet the criteria for authorship?" (Carpenito, 1998, p. 3).

Selby, a well-known opponent of the practice of TT, wrote that *JAMA*'s editor, George D. Lundberg made an unwarranted conclusion from a single study: "This simple, statistically valid study tests the theoretical basis for 'Therapeutic Touch': the 'human energy field.' This study found that such a field does not exist" (Lundberg, 1998, p. 1040). Selby noted that "the only conclusion that can be drawn from this report is that twenty-one people who accepted the challenge to be tested by the authors failed to produce outcomes necessary to convince us that HEF exists. They [Rosa et al.] do not prove that the HEF does not exist" (Selby, 1998, page 9). Selby further notes that the study suffers from experimenters' bias as was pointed out by Carpenito above (Selby, 1998, p. 9, 10). Nor was it double-blind: "Based on the description in the *JAMA* article, there was never any consideration given to an attempt to double-blind the experiment in any way" (Selby, 1998, p. 10). Additionally Selby objected to the lack of adequate controls: "The description of attempts to control for testable variables is very limited" (Selby, 1998, p. 11).*

---

*Editors' Note: Carpenito's (1998) position that the authorship of the *JAMA* article did not meet its own published criteria is supported by the AMA's published document, *JAMA Author Instructions*, updated January 5, 2000, which can be found on the internet at http:jama.ama-assn.org/info/auinst.html (retrieved February 8, 2000).

The section "Authorship Information" (page 3) states: "**1. Authorship Criteria and Responsibility**. All persons listed as authors must meet all the following criteria for authorship: I certify that (1) I have made substantial contributions to the conception and design or analysis and interpretation of data; (2) I have made substantial contributions to drafting the article or revising it critically for important intellectual content; and (3) I have given final approval of the version of the article to be published."

The group that originally focused critical attention on the practice of TT is the Rocky Mountain Skeptics (RMS). The group was founded in

The listed authors of the *JAMA* article are Linda Rosa, B.S.N., R.N.; Emily Rosa; Larry Sarner; and Stephen Barrett, M.D. On page 1005, the following roles are attributed to each: "Ms. E. Rosa designed and conducted the tests and tabulated her findings. Mr. Sarner did the statistical analysis. He and Ms. L. Rosa recruited the test subjects, performed the literature analysis, and drafted this report. Dr. Barrett added background material and edited the report for publication." There is no mention of nine-year-old Emily Rosa having "made substantial contributions to drafting the article or revising it critically for important intellectual content."

Carpenito's (1998) assertion that sample selection was not adequately addressed is supported by the *JAMA* article (page 1007, Methods section) where the authors state:

> In 1996 and 1997, by searching for advertisements and other leads, two of us (L.R. and L.S.) located twenty-five TT practitioners in northeastern Colorado, twenty-one of whom readily agreed to be tested. Of those who did not, one stated she was not qualified, two gave no reason, and one agreed but cancelled on the day of the test.
>
> The reported practice experience of those tested ranged from one to twenty-seven years. There were nine nurses, seven certified massage therapists, two laypersons, one chiropractor, one medical assistant, and one phlebotomist. All but two were women, which reflects the sex ratio of the practitioner population. One nurse had published an article on TT in a journal for nurse practitioners.

There is no mention of any effort to objectively verify any of the above qualifications. In fact Krieger introduced the concept of laying-on of hands to the nursing profession in 1973 and began teaching it as TT in 1974 (Krieger, 1975, 1990). In 1997 when the second test was conducted by E. Rosa, TT was no older than twenty-four years. Clearly the claim that the "reported practice experience of these tested ranged from one to twenty-seven years" is in conflict with the history of TT. What other self reported claims are in error? Nobody knows. Furthermore, there is no attempt at substantiating the claim that two out of twenty-one practitioners in the general population are in fact women.

Selby's criticism of experimenters' bias extends Carpenitio's concerns to actual statements made prior to the *JAMA* experiment. A few of these follow: "Therapeutic Touch is quintessential New-Age quackery" (Rosa, 1994, p. 41); "With no evidence whatsoever of a human energy field and no evidence of health benefits beyond placebo hocus-pocus, how do practices, such as TT, pass muster as continuing education?" (Rojas [Rosa], 1992); Linda Rosa, Corresponding Secretary of the National Therapeutic Touch Study Group, in 1995 received The Skeptics Society's annual Randi Award. The award ceremony was described in the April/May 1995 issue of the *Rational Skeptic*: "Earlier in the

Boulder, Colorado in 1983 by Béla Scheiber, with a policy of focusing on pseudoscience while remaining neutral on ideological and religious issues which are not testable by scientific procedures (Ingalls, 1998). In October of 1988, RMS became aware of the practice of TT when a psychologist from a pain clinic at the local Veterans Administration Hospital contacted the group regarding a nurse who, while applying for a job, expressed her desire to practice TT on patients. After consulting RMS, the psychologist wrote back to the organization: "Considering the shabby state-of-the-art of Therapeutic Touch I certainly won't permit it to occur in the Pain Clinic here" (Rothschild, 1998).

Although RMS has addressed numerous other issues in ensuing years, among them psychic surgery and alternative healthcare prac-

day, she [Rosa] gave an hour-long award speech to 150–200 people at the Californial Institute of Technology [Cal Tech] detailing FRS's [another group cofounded by Linda Rosa] multiyear struggle to expose TT as a pseudoscientific danger to nursing and public health. . . . Brandishing a manila envelope from the State Board of Nursing, Linda breathlessly opened it to reveal the eagerly awaited 'evidence' for TT's efficacy. It contained a large knife. . . . Laughter also ensued when Rosa characterized TT proponent's belief in human energy field as a symptom of 'physics envy.' "

Selby's criticism of inadequate controls can be supported best by what is missing from the Rosa et al. *JAMA* article: From the Methods section, the authors state that "the experimenter flipped a coin to determine which of the subject's hands would be the target. The experimenter then hovered her right hand, palm down, 8 to 10 cm above the target and said 'Okay.' The subject then stated which of his or her hands was nearer the experimenter's hand. Each subject was permitted to take as much or as little time as necessary to make each determination. The time spent ranged from seven to nineteen minutes per set of trial." There is *no* mention anywhere in the section about who documented the coin toss and the response following "Okay" or even how the subjects' response was recorded. If the documenter was the same person who flipped the coin, then clearly this would qualify as inadequate control. Further, there is no discussion about possible influence of "verbal cuing" by the experimenter (e.g. "Okay").

In the subsequent paragraph: "To examine where air movement or body heat might be detectable by the experimental subjects, preliminary tests were performed on seven other subjects who had no training or belief in TT. Four were children who were unaware of the purpose of the test. Those results indicated that the apparatus prevented tactile cues from reaching the subject." What is missing from the report are the data about the "control group" and any statistical treatment of those data. The description of the control sample testing lacks sufficient information regarding the means under which that portion of the experiment was handled. It also begs the question: Was the control group portion conducted in an identical manner and setting as the testing of the experimental subjects?

tices in general, the group has maintained a special interest in TT. Notable examples are (1) their confrontations with the Colorado Board of Nursing in 1992–1993 regarding the practice of awarding continuing education credits for TT classes and (2) demanding that the University of Colorado investigate the promotion of TT within its Health Sciences Center by some influential TT proponents within the "Center for Human Caring." As a direct consequence of RMS, the University of Colorado impaneled the Committee on Therapeutic Touch with Dr. Henry N. Claman as its Chair. With four other members of the committee, Dr. Claman reviewed all the literature, met privately with members of RMS, and held a public hearing and issued its *Report of the Chancellor's Committee on Therapeutic Touch* [see appendix 3].

Currently, RMS continues its vigorous opposition to the wholesale promotion of TT as a nursing practice, monitoring the use of TT in local hospitals and organizations, acting as a repository of literature, a source of credible information on the subject, publishing skeptical articles, and confronting healthcare facilities where the practice is promoted. However, RMS does support the scientific scrutiny (investigation) of TT—demanding that it be subjected to the same standards that is required of any new medical claim.

Not all criticisms of TT spring from the purely scientific point of view. In what could be described as a situation of strange bedfellows, conservative Christians have also been highly critical of it. Most of the criticisms generated by Christian opponents are centered around the assertions that it is a spiritually illegitimate practice (Fish, 1996), that practitioners usurp what is considered a power that should legitimately spring from God (Fish, 1996; O'Mathúna, 1998), that it is more a matter of faith than science and as such is similar to the teachings of Christian Science (Bullough and Bullough, 1998), that it stems from non-Christian traditions as opposed to prayer, and that there are similarities between TT and occult and Wiccan healing practices. The Watchman Fellowship, an activist Christian watchdog organization, points out that "all forms of divination or occult assessment are strictly forbidden in the scriptures," and that "spiritual and emotional healing can only occur in the context of a personal relationship with the living God, not through 'rebalancing energy' " (Fish, 1999, p. 4).

Perhaps the position of Christian opponents of TT is best summed up in the following statement by Bullough and Bullough (1998):

> Those that say they can practice the technique of therapeutic touch and divorce themselves from its occult associations need to be reminded that apart from the occult, therapeutic touch would cease to exist. It is rooted and grounded in psychic soil, and it bears related fruit. (p. 256)

TT *has* attempted to distance itself from its religious roots, to secularize itself, perhaps because of objections such as these. But it is a tenuous separation at best. The TT literature is rife with references to Eastern religious and philosophical concepts. Nor has TT entirely separated itself from its Christian roots. For example, in 1988, Krieger stated that while TT is not a miracle cure, it does fulfill six of the seven criteria of miraculous healing as delineated by Pope Benedict XIV, lacking only the criterion of being a "perfect" cure.

The discomfort of Christians (and secular humanists, for that matter) is no doubt further aroused when the developer of TT makes highly dramatic claims, such as that TT has been used to resurrect the dead. Krieger describes her memories of failure-to-thrive newborns:

> [The infants were] born prematurely and without robust vital signs, who rapidly lost all sign of crucial clinical indicators in spite of the intervention of heroic medical measures. Therefore, they had been extubated and declared dead. In several cases in the United States, nurses who were present in the neonatal intensive care units quietly picked up the apparently dead baby and did Therapeutic Touch. In too many instances to discount simply, the babies recovered and lived. As vital signs were reestablished, the children were reintubated, intravenous and other lifelines were reinserted, and the babies eventually went home to happy families. (1997, p. 12)

THE CURRENT STATE OF AFFAIRS

In spite of the heated controversy and the increasing attention of skeptics and opponents, the practice of TT continues to proliferate. Krieger (1997) states that she has personally taught the practice to over 43,000 health professionals and to several thousand laypersons. She points out that TT is the first alternative healing modality to be taught in fully accredited universities, is currently part of the curriculum of more than one hundred colleges and universities in the United States, and is being taught in over seventy-five foreign countries. In addition, Krieger lists one hundred healthcare facilities where TT is practiced, including hospitals, nursing homes, hospice centers, and psychiatric units. In many of the facilities, TT has become integrated into policies and procedures manuals (standards of care that are specific to individual institutions); TT is also being taught at many of these facilities.

TT continues to be actively promoted by the National League for Nursing, the American Theosophical Society, the Society of Rogerian Scholars, the Center for Human Caring at the University of Colorado, the

American Nurses' Association, the Nurse Healers and Professional Associates Cooperative, the American Holistic Nursing Association, and by thousands of practitioners. A search of CINAHL (a nursing database) for the period from 1982 to the present reveals a total of 353 hits; similarly, a search of MEDLINE (a more generalized medical database) for the period from 1966 to the present resulted in 109 citations, although most of these are repeats of those found in the CINAHL search. An *Alta Vista* search using the keywords "Therapeutic Touch" resulted in a staggering 4,356 hits; many of these are the websites of independent practitioners, although a portion are pages posted by skeptics.

The controversy surrounding the practice of TT is likely to continue unabated. The recent attention by the numerous, independent skeptic community throughout the world has made an impression on those that in the past were far too comfortable in making outrageous claims that went unchallenged. Perhaps now proponents will seek out the advice of responsible critics and do the experiments necessary to resolve the issues.

REFERENCES

Barrett, E. A. 1994. "On the Threshold of Tomorrow." In *Martha E. Rogers: Her Life and Her Work*. Edited by V. M. Malinski and E. A. Barrett. Philadelphia: F. A. Davis Company, pp. 271–75.

Boguslawski, M. 1979. "The Use of Therapeutic Touch in Nursing." *Journal of Continuing Education in Nursing* 10 (4): 9–15.

Brenneman, R. 1990. *Deadly Blessings: Faith Healing on Trial*. Amherst, N.Y.: Prometheus Books.

Bullough, V. L., and B. Bullough. 1998. "Should Nurses Practice Therapeutic Touch? Should Nursing Schools Teach Therapeutic Touch?" *Journal of Professional Nursing* 14 (4): 254–57.

Carpenito, L. J. 1997. *Nursing Diagnosis: Application to Clinical Practice*. 7th ed. Philadelphia: Lippincott.

———. "In Search of the Truth or Jerry Springer." *Nursing Forum* 33, no. 2 (April–June 1998): 3–4.

Carroll, R. T. Accessed April 26, 1999a. "Mesmerism." *The Skeptic's Dictionary*, at: http://www.dcn.davis.ca.us/go/btcarroll/skeptic/mesmer.html.

———. Accessed April 21, 1999c. "Theosophy." *The Skeptic's Dictionary*, at: http://www.dcn.davis.ca.us/go/btcarroll/skeptic/theosoph.html.

———. Accessed April 19, 1999b. "Spiritualism." *The Skeptic's Dictionary*, at: http://www.dcn.davis.ca.us/go/btcarroll/skeptic/spiritual.html.

Clark, P. E., and M. J. Clark. 1984. "Therapeutic Touch: Is There a Scientific Basis for the Practice?" *Nursing Research* 33 (1): 37–41.

Fish, S. 1996. "Alternative Therapies: Healing Science or Metaphysical Fraud." *Journal of Christian Nursing* 13: 3–11.

———. Accessed April 20, 1999. "Therapeutic Touch." *Watchman Fellowship Profile*, at: http://www.religioustolerance.org/ther_tou.htm.

Fitzpatrick, J. 1994. "Rogers' Contributions to the Development of Nursing as a Science." In *Martha E. Rogers: Her Life and Her Work*. Edited by V. M. Malinski and E. A. Barrett. Philadelphia: F. A. Davis Company, pp. 322–29.

Glickman, R., and Graceley, E. J. 1998. "Therapeutic Touch: Investigation of a Practitioner." *The Scientific Review of Alternative Medicine* 2 (1): 43–47.

Grad, B. 1963. "A Telekinetic Effect on Plant Growth." *International Journal of Parapsychology* 5: 117–33.

Grad, B., R. Caroret, and G. Paul. 1961. "An Unorthodox Method of Treatment of Wound Healing in Mice." *International Journal of Parapsychology* 3: 5–24.

Hecktor, L. 1994. "Martha E. Rogers: A life history." In *Martha E. Rogers: Her Life and Her Work*. Edited by V. M. Malinski and E. A. Barrett. Philadelphia: F. A. Davis Company, pp. 10–27.

Ingalls, H. 1998. "Huntley Ingalls on RMS." *Rocky Mountain Skeptic* 16 (1, 2): 3.

Kozier, B., G. Erb, and R. Oliveri. 1991. *Fundamentals of Nursing: Concepts, Process, and Practice*. Redwood City, Calif.: Benjamin/Cummings Publishing Co., Inc.

Krieger, D. 1975. "Therapeutic Touch: The Imprimatur of Nursing." *American Journal of Nursing* 75: 784–87.

———. 1979. *The Therapeutic Touch: How to Use Your Hands to Help or to Heal*. Englewood Cliffs, New Jersey: Prentice-Hall, Inc.

———. 1990. "Therapeutic Touch: Two Decades of Research, Teaching, and Clinical Practice." *Imprint* 37 (3): 83, 86–88.

———. 1997. *Therapeutic Touch Inner Workbook: Ventures in Transpersonal Healing*. Santa Fe, N.Mex.: Bear & Company Publishing.

Krippner, S. 1992. *Spiritual Dimensions of Healing*. New York: Irvington Publishers, Inc.

Kunz, D. 1991. *The Personal Aura*. Wheaton, Ill.: The Theosophical Publishing House.

Leadbeater, C. W. 1927. *The Chakras*. Wheaton, Ill.: The Theosophical Publishing House.

Lundberg, G. D. 1998. "Editor's Note." *JAMA* 279 (13): 1040.

MacNutt, F. 1974. *Healing*. Notre Dame: Ave Maria Press.

Magickal Healing: Healing Massage. Accessed April 21, 1999. Website of the Desert Wind Coven, at: http://www.geocities.com/Athens/Delphi/9533/past_howto_healing_0698.html.

McKinney, J. B. 1995. "Therapeutic Touch in Nursing Practice: Building the Knowledge." *Online Journal of Knowledge Synthesis for Nursing*. Website at: http://www.ref.oclc.org 2000.

Meehan, T. 1998. "Therapeutic Touch as a Nursing Intervention." *Journal of Advanced Nursing* 28 (1): 117–25.

Miller, L. 1979. "An Explanation of Therapeutic Touch Using the Science of Unitary Man." *Nursing Forum* 18: 278–87.

Mish, F, ed. 1990. *Webster's Ninth New Collegiate Dictionary*. Springfield, Mass.: Merriam-Webster Inc.

Moccia, P. 1994. "The Social Context within which Martha E. Rogers Developed Her Ideas." In *Martha E. Rogers: Her Life and Her Work*. Edited by V. M. Malinski and E. A. Barrett. Philadelphia: F. A. Davis Company, pp. 309–16.

Narasingha, B. G., and S. Rosen. Accessed April 24, 1999. "East Meets West." Website at: http://www.gosai.com/chaitanya/saranagati/html/nmj_article/east_west/index.html.

National League for Nursing. 1992. *Therapeutic Touch: Healing Through Human Energy Fields,* (videotape series), publication no. 42-2485, 42-286, 42-2487. National League for Nursing, New York.

O'Mathúna, D. 1996. "Nursing's New Alternative: Therapeutic Touch." *Ohio Council Against Health Fraud* 7 (winter): 2–4.

———. 1998. "The Subtle Allure of Therapeutic Touch." *Nurses' Christian Fellowship* 15: 4–13.

Randi, J. 1987. *The Faith Healers.* Amherst, N.Y.: Prometheus Books.

Reeder, F. 1994. "The Philosophical Context within which Martha E. Rogers Developed Her Ideas." In *Martha E. Rogers: Her Life and Her Work.* Edited by V. M. Malinski and E. A. Barrett. Philadelphia: F. A. Davis Company, pp. 317–21.

Rogers, M. E. 1970. "Nursing's Conceptual Model." In M. E. Rogers, *An Introduction to the Theoretical Basis of Nursing.* Philadelphia: Davis, pp. 89–94.

———. 1980. "Nursing: A Science of Unitary Man." In *Conceptual Models for Nursing Practice.* Edited by J. P. Reihl and C. Roy. 2d ed. New York: Appleton-Century-Crofts, pp. 239–331.

———. 1986. "Science of Unitary Human Beings." In *Explorations on Martha Rogers' Science of Unitary Human Beings.* Edited by V. N. Malinski. Norwalk, Conn.: Appleton-Century-Crofts, pp. 3–8.

———. 1990. "Nursing: Science of Unitary, Irreducible Human Beings: Update, 1990." In *Visions of Rogers' Science-Based Nursing.* Edited by E. A. Barrett. New York: National League for Nursing, pp. 5–11.

———. 1992. "Nursing Science and the Space Age." *Nursing Science Quarterly* 5: 27–34.

Rosa, L. A. 1994. "Therapeutic Touch: Skeptics in Hand to Hand Combat Over the Latest New Age Health Fad." *Skeptic* 3 (1): 40–49.

———. 1992. "Touchy Subject." *Rocky Mountain Skeptic* 9 (6): 4, 5.

Rosa, L., E. Rosa, L. Sarner, and S. Barrett. 1998. "A Close Look at Therapeutic Touch." *JAMA* 279 (13): 1005–1010.

Sandroff, R. 1980. "A Skeptic's Guide to Therapeutic Touch." *RN* (January): 25–30, 82–83.

Schlotfeldt, R. M. 1973. Critique of "The Relationship of Touch, with the Intent to Help or Heal to Subjects' In-Vivo Hemoglobin Values: A Study in Personalized Interaction." *Nursing Research Conference* 9: 59–71.

Selby, C. 1998. "The JAMA TT Article Critiqued." *Rocky Mountain Skeptic* 15 (6): 1, 10–12. (Available from the Rocky Mountain Skeptic, PO Box 7277, Boulder, CO 80306). Website at http://bcn.boulder.co.us/community/rms.

Smith. J. 1972. "Paranormal Effects on Enzyme Activity." *Human Dimensions* 1: 15–19.

Spence, J. E., and M. A. Olson. 1997. "Quantitative Research on Therapeutic Touch: An Integrative Review of the Literature 1985–1995." *Scandinavian Journal of Caring Science* 11: 183–90.

Starn, J. R. 1998. "Energy Healing with Women and Children." *Journal of Obstetric, Gynecologic, and Neonatal Nursing* 27 (5): 576–84.

Theosophical Society. Accessed April 22, 1999. "The Theosophical Society." Website at: http://www.garlic.com/~rdon/TS.html.

Turner, J. G., A. J. Clark, D. K. Gauthier, and M. Williams. 1998. "The Effect of Therapeutic Touch on Pain and Anxiety in Burn Patients." *Journal of Advanced Nursing* 28 (1): 10–20.

Walike, B., P. Bruno, S. Donaldson, R. Erickson, et al. 1975. ". . . attempts to embellish a totally unscientific process with the aura of science . . ." in Letters, *American Journal of Nursing* 75 (August): 1275, 1278, 1282.

Washington, P. 1995. *Madame Blavatsky's Baboon: A History of the Mediums, Mystics, and Misfits Who Bought Spiritualism to America.* New York: Schocken Books.

Weber, R. 1991. Foreword to *The Personal Aura.* Wheaton, Ill.: The Theosophical Publishing House.

Wirth, D. P., J. T. Richardson, and W. S. Eiedelman. 1996. "Wound Healing and Complementary Therapies: A Review." *Journal of Alternative Complementary Medicine* 2 (4): 493–502.

Whyte, L. L. 1961. *The Next Development in Man.* 2d ed. New York: Mentor.

2.

Therapeutic Touch as a Nursing Intervention

Therese C. Meehan

Therapeutic Touch (TT) is being proposed as a nursing intervention. Its proponents claim that it is integral to the art of nursing practice and can facilitate comfort and healing in a wide range of patients. However, the practice of TT *is* also controversial, primarily because it does not usually involve physical contact and is based on energy field theoretical frameworks. The development of TT and its conceptualization as an energy field interaction are reviewed, and points of controversy discussed. The method of practice is described. Review of controlled efficacy studies indicates limited and inconclusive scientific support for its proposed effects. The intrinsic relationship between TT and the placebo phenomenon is discussed. The potential of TT to enhance the placebo effect requires further exploration but should not be discounted in seeking to relieve discomfort and distress and facilitate healing. For some patients, TT may serve as a beneficial adjuvant nursing intervention.

INTRODUCTION

The nurturance of human life, the therapeutic use of self, and the specialized use of the hands have long been recognized as central characteristics of nursing practice. Thus, it should not be surprising that over the past twenty years therapeutic touch (TT) has been developed as a nursing intervention (McCloskey, Bulechek, 1996). Nurses who use TT

Originally published in *Journal of Advanced Nursing* 28, no. 1 (1998): 117–25. Copyright © 1998 by Blackwel Science Ltd. Reprinted with permission. The author wishes to thank Barbara J. Patterson, R.N., Ph.D., and Carol Wells Federman, R.N. MEd, for their critical review of an earlier draft of this article.

claim that it facilitates patient comfort and healing (Mackey, 1995; Sayre-Adams and Wright, 1995; Biley 1996; National League for Nursing 1992). Some schools of nursing in the United States include TT in their curricula, and funding agencies, including the U.S. National Institutes of Health and the U.S. Department of Defense, have supported efficacy studies. However, TT is also the subject of controversy. A number of nurses argue that it has no coherent theoretical basis, that proposed therapeutic outcomes are not scientifically verified, and that it seriously impugns nursing's development as a professional discipline (Clark and Clark, 1984; Oberst, 1995; Bullough and Bullough, 1995; Stahlman, 1995). This debate has also been reflected in the general press (Jaroff, 1994; Glazer, 1995). Controversy surrounding TT is most frequently prompted by its definition and explanation within energy field theoretical frameworks, and the fact that it does not usually involve actual physical contact. In addition, there is a range of views amongst its proponents regarding the operational definition of TT and the degree to which its proposed effects have been scientifically verified. This paper is intended to provide a critical review of the development and status of TT as a nursing intervention and to assist nurses in deciding when it may have an appropriate role in the care of their patients.

HISTORY AND DEVELOPMENT

TT was originally developed by Kunz and Krieger in the early 1970s (Krieger, 1979). Kunz had worked closely with physicians for a number of years observing and caring for chronically ill patients. She became especially interested in the laying-on of hands and observed its use by a number of well-known practitioners over a four-year period. Kunz was impressed with practitioners' ability to help ill patients by attuning to an inner spiritual dimension of themselves and focusing their compassionate intent to help through their hands. Although she observed that the laying-on of hands was done within a religious framework, she believed that it would be possible to develop a similar method of treatment within a broader philosophical framework, using different language, and thereby make it acceptable to a diverse range of people and medical institutions. She proposed that the ability to facilitate healing in others, through practices such as the laying-on of hands, was an innate human characteristic and could be learned by those who were sincerely interested, healthy, compassionate, and dedicated to helping others. Krieger participated in the development of the principles and practice of the new treatment and named it Therapeutic Touch.

Kunz chose to teach the new treatment primarily to nurses

because she believed that as a group they had the dedication necessary to learn and use it most effectively, and spent the most time with ill people. Krieger observed that nurses who learned TT appeared to be quite effective in helping ill patients and introduced TT to the nursing profession at-large in 1975.

THEORETICAL FRAMEWORKS

Two similar theoretical frameworks have been drawn upon to provide a rationale for TT. Weber (1981, 1990) has proposed a general energy field framework, developed from an interweaving of ideas from Eastern and Western philosophical thought and illustrated through reference to the writings of Patanjali, Govinda, Pythagoras, Plato, and Spinoza, among others. The framework is further illustrated through reference to a model of the relationship between an underlying energy field process and the world of ordinary experience, proposed by the theoretical physicist Bohm (1980, 1986). In this framework the universe is viewed as a unitary flow of energy within which all matter, consciousness, and events are interconnected. The human body is understood to be an expression of the underlying energy system, and consciousness, at its various levels, is considered to be part of physical matter. Fundamental to the energetic ground of the universe is a healing energy, a pure spiritual energy, composed of intelligence, order, and compassion, which gives rise to and permeates all living systems.

Integral with consciousness are three key concepts: compassion, intention, and nonattachment. It is proposed that in an orderly universe, when conscious intent to help or to heal is guided by compassion, it can have a powerful healing influence. While the practitioner's compassionate intent is to facilitate healing, it at the same time does not involve personal attachment to a patient or to specific therapeutic outcomes. Further, it is claimed that when an individual is in a state of calm and peace of mind, it is possible to sense the human energy field as it extends beyond the body using the natural sensitivity of the hands. It is also possible—through a feeling of compassion and intention to facilitate healing—to become consciously aware of and attuned to the universal healing energy, and to serve as an instrument for its healing influence.

A nursing theoretical framework developed by Rogers (1970, 1990), the Science of Unitary Human Beings, is also used as a rationale for TT (Malinski, 1993; Meehan, 1993; Biley, 1996). Drawing upon quantum theory, Rogers proposed that energy fields are the fundamental units of human beings and their environments. Energy field characteristics of openness, mutual process, dynamic unity, and capacity to establish patterns are regarded as fundamental to understanding the human life process and human-environmental interaction. Human consciousness and experience of health or illness are unitary and multidimensional in nature and a function of the mutual interaction between human being and environment. Therefore, within this framework, the aim of nursing practice is to strengthen the coherence and integrity of the patient as a unitary energy field process in order to maximize patient healing and well-being. From this framework Rogers derived a theory of paranormal phenomena which posits that in a unitary, multidimensional universe there is no linear time and no separation of human and environmental fields, and that action-at-a-distance phenomena, such as TT, are normal rather than paranormal.

Both frameworks are speculative and controversial, and continued critical evaluation of them in relation to TT is imperative. Both are based on abstract concepts which are extrapolated to the world of ordinary experience from complex philosophical systems on the one hand and the microscopic world of quantum physics on the other. In neither framework is the concept "energy field" precisely defined. It appears to mean a dynamic, unified, essential constituent which is present everywhere in space and within which everything in the universe is interconnected. Debate about the existence and nature of such a concept began with the earliest philosophers and continues today amongst philosophers of science. As critics are quick to point out, the existence of a human energy field has never been demonstrated scientifically. It is possible that a psychological-humanistic framework could provide an alternative explanation for TT. Although Weber (1990) has argued against this possibility, it cannot be ruled out. However, despite the speculation and controversy surrounding the concept of a human energy field, the North American Nursing Diagnosis Association has classified "energy field disturbance" as a legitimate nursing diagnosis, defining it as "a disruption of the flow of energy surrounding a person's being which results in disharmony of the body, mind, and/or spirit" (1994, p. 37).

It is clear that a spiritual dimension of human life and a universal healing energy are fundamental in the framework proposed by Weber. However, these concepts do not appear at all in Rogers' framework, although they are apparently assumed by many nurses who use the framework. Some writers state that TT involves direction of the practitioner's own excess energies for use by the person who is being treated, seeming to imply that the healing energy is a human characteristic alone. However, according to Kunz and most other literature, the practitioner's role as an instrument for a universal healing energy is a fundamental and inviolable assumption.

A related issue concerns the relationship between religion and TT. It has been claimed consistently in the literature that TT is not done within a religious context and that this characteristic helps differentiate it from the laying-on of hands. However, in a personal communication with the present author on 24 August 1995, Kunz pointed out that TT may certainly be done within a religious context. The important point is that a particular religious context is not necessary for TT to be effective. She explained that the broad philosophical background outlined by Weber may serve as a foundation for any practitioner, but that this background can also be clearly linked to most religious systems of thought. Thus, particular religious backgrounds can be drawn upon, naturally, to help practitioners facilitate their ability to practice TT effectively. Careful attention and further clarification in relation to these issues is needed in the literature. Confusion about them has led some nurses to debate whether or not they should practice TT (Wuthnow and Miller, 1987). It also leaves TT vulnerable to being swept under the umbrella of the "new age" movement and subject to its often superficial and pretentious forms of thinking.

A working understanding of the frameworks requires a good general knowledge of the history of philosophy. It also requires the ability to evaluate critically the on-going debate among quantum physicists about theories of nonlocality, and the debate among humanitarians and health professionals about the possible implications these theories may have for understanding the nature of consciousness and for promoting health and healing. While theories and discussions about the relationship between the microscopic and macroscopic world, such as those presented by Bohm (1980), Cushing and McMullin (1989), Josephson and Pallikari-Viras (1991) and Stapp (1993) offer some support for the frameworks, there is an urgent need for continued scholarly analysis in relation to their meaning for TT and nursing practice.

Overall, despite the provisional status of the frameworks, nurses who use TT accept them as axiomatic. Based on their experience in practice, the human energy field is a perceptible reality. Nurses who wish to gain some insight into this experience could experiment with a hand exercise developed by Krieger (1979) and reproduced in a recent practice-related journal article (Mackey, 1995). In considering these frameworks, nurses should not think of them as being radically different from or opposed to the biomedical physical-sensory framework. Rather, they should be thought of as placing the biomedical framework within a broader context enabling physical-sensory and psychological processes and human behaviour to be viewed from a different perspective and possibly to take on a new meaning. This could lead to more creative and effective approaches to patient care especially in situations where solutions are sought to chronic or intractable problems.

INTERVENTION PROCESS

The nurse prepares herself (or himself, of course) to administer TT by "centering" and remains centered throughout the intervention. In centering, she shifts her awareness from a direct focus on her physical environment to an inner focus on what she perceives as the center of life within herself—a center of calm, quiet, and balance through which she perceives herself and the patient as unitary wholes. She attunes to the universal healing energy so she may become an instrument for its healing influence. Her attitude becomes one of clear, gentle, and compassionate attention to the patient and of focused intent to help facilitate the patient's own natural healing tendency. At the same time, she is detached from any personal feelings or emotions. She remains quite aware of her physical environment but this is not the primary focus of attention. For the experienced practitioner, centering takes about ten seconds.

The assessment is done in relation to two principles: openness and symmetry. In a state of health, the patient as an energy field is perceived as a gentle, symmetrical, open flow from head to feet. In a state of illness, the flow is perceived as congested, asymmetrical and impeded. The nurse moves her hands, with the palms facing toward the patient and at a distance of about one to two inches, over the clothed body of the patient from head to feet in a smooth, gentle movement. She attunes to the patient's condition by perceiving the pattern of the energy flow through differences in sensory cues in her hands. These cues are extremely subtle and are typically described as warmth, coolness, tightness, heaviness, tingling, or emptiness. The nurse notes the overall pattern of the energy flow and any area of imbalance or impeded flow. Areas of congestion or imbalance are often but not always directly related to areas of illness in the patient's body. The initial assessment is done fairly quickly, in about thirty seconds, but assessment also continues throughout the intervention.

During the treatment phase, the nurse focuses her intent on the specific repatterning of areas of imbalance and impeded flow, using her hands as focal points. Her intention is to dissipate areas of imbalance and facilitate a gentle, symmetrical, open flow. She begins by moving her hands in gentle sweeping movements from head to feet. She then focuses her attention on areas of imbalance or congestion. For example, if she feels an area of heat over the left side of the patient's abdomen, she will project an image of coolness as she moves one hand repeatedly through that area, moving the other hand at the same time over the right side of the abdomen and bringing the left and right side into balance. If she perceives areas of heaviness or tingling over the patient's chest, she will project an image of a flowing or smoothing movement as she moves her hands repeatedly through the area until she begins to feel the quality of the energy flow change. To complete the treatment, she places her hands over the area of the solar plexus (just below the sternum) and focuses specifically on facilitating the flow of universal healing energy in the patient.

Physical touch can be incorporated into the treatment according to the wishes of the patient and at the discretion of the nurse. For patients who are chronically ill or have undergone extensive surgery, physical touch can facilitate the effect of the treatment. For example, for a patient who is recovering from cardiovascular bypass surgery, gentle massage of the neck and upper chest, shoulders, back, and feet can be very effectively incorporated into the treatment.

The length of time or "dose" of the intervention depends on the age and needs of the patient. It will range from about one to two minutes for a premature or small infant to five to ten minutes for an adult. In most efficacy studies a five-minute treatment has been used and Kunz proposes that generally, no more than a five-to-seven-minute treatment is needed. Hospitalized patients usually receive the intervention once or twice a day, or they may receive it with each dose of p.r.n. (as required) analgesic or sedative medication.

This description is adapted from established practice guidelines (Meehan, 1992), follows those of Krieger (1979), and is an elaboration of the standard operational definition used in efficacy studies. The practice is clearly subjective and changes in energy flow cannot be directly observed. Findings of descriptive (Heidt, 1990) and psychome-´ tric (Winstead-Fry, 1983; Ferguson, 1986; Wright, 1991) studies designed to investigate TT, indirectly suggest some beginning, tentative verification of the process.

Despite the standardized definition of TT, variations are reported in the way individual nurses practice TT (Lionberger, 1986). Minor variations in practice are acceptable and the practice may be incorporated naturally into other nursing interventions such as a back rub. However, some nurses make significant changes in practice based on their own personal beliefs about what it should be. It is claimed that "healing touch," "touch for health," and "magnetic unruffling" are either synonymous with TT or are variations of TT, but this is not the case. Some researchers, for example Wirth et al. (1993), purport to study TT but their operational definitions make it clear that it is not TT that is being tested. Significant changes from the standard practice of TT can result in practices which may or may not involve the therapeutic use of touch, but they are not TT.

PRACTICE LITERATURE

Observations reported by Krieger et al. (1979) suggested that TT could facilitate a relaxation response. This led to a widespread assumption that TT had the potential to modify physiological and psychological responses associated with stress. Anecdotal reports in the nursing literature document its use in promoting relaxation, comfort, and well-being in women during and after childbirth (Wolfson, 1990; Lothian, 1993), patients with AIDS (Newsham, 1989), hospitalized infants (Leduc, 1987) and children (Macrae, 1979; Kramer, 1990; Thayer, 1990), clinic patients (Wytias, 1994), the elderly (Fanslow, 1990; Simington, 1993), people who are dying (Jackson, 1981); in patients undergoing surgery (Jonasen, 1994), psychotherapy (Hill and Oliver, 1993), physical rehabilitation (Payne, 1989) and drug rehabilitation (Macrae, 1989); in patients with insomnia (Braun et al, 1986; Heidt, 1991; Dall, 1993), and pain (Boguslawski, 1980; Wright, 1987; Meehan, 1990; Mackey, 1995; Biley, 1996), and in patient care generally (Fanslow, 1983; Hospital Satellite Network, 1986; Jurgens et al, 1987; Wyatt, 1989). Descriptive studies have suggested its effectiveness in reducing stress (Olson et al., 1992), facilitating health-related changes in the immune system (Quinn and Strelkauskas, 1989), and facilitating a sense of personal growth and well-being (Samarel, 1992). Effective outcomes attributed to TT are reported to be significant and in some cases seem quite dramatic. Altogether, approximately 160 reviews or anecdotal reports have appeared in the nursing literature since Krieger's introduction of TT in 1975.

This literature has played a major role in disseminating knowledge of TT to nurses and other health professionals. Nurses find their experiences with TT in practice convincing. Lothian reflects that "the wealth of experiential evidence that 'something' is happening in [TT] is compelling" (1993, p. 35). Feltham writes that TT is a special way of showing empathy and caring and that "some things, like inner well-being and peace, are not measurable" (1991, p. 28). This literature has provided the impetus for a number of controlled efficacy studies.

CONTROLLED EFFICACY STUDIES

In 1975 Krieger reported that TT increased haemoglobin values in hospitalised patients. However, in subsequent experimental studies TT has been found to have no significant effect on haemoglobin values in postoperative patients (Meehan et al., 1991) or transcutaneous oxygen blood gas pressure in hospitalized premature infants (Fedoruk, 1984).

The claim that TT could facilitate a relaxation response (Krieger et al., 1979) led to a series of single-blind studies designed to test hypotheses that TT would reduce stress and situationally induced anxiety. Randolph (1984) reported that healthy females who received a modified version of TT while being subject to artificially induced stress in a laboratory setting had no significant decrease in physiological indicators of stress, compared with a control group who received casual touch. Heidt (1981) reported a significant decrease in situationally induced anxiety in hospitalized cardiovascular patients who received TT compared with patients who received casual touch or verbal interaction. Quinn (1984) replicated the Heidt study using a similar sample and two groups. One group received TT which involved no physical contact and the control group received mimic TT. Patients who received TT had a significant decrease in anxiety immediately following treatment compared with patients who received mimic TT.

Quinn (1989) conducted a further replication study using preoperative open-heart surgery patients and adding a third no-treatment control group. In this study she also sought to determine whether subtle communication between nurse and patient through eye and facial expression, rather than an energy field, could explain any therapeutic effect. Thus the TT and mimic TT treatments were done with patients in a side-lying position facing away from the treatment nurse. No significant differences in anxiety, systolic blood pressure, or heart rate were found between the groups immediately or one hour following treatment. While Quinn acknowledged that these findings suggested that eye and facial contact could play a role in mediating any therapeutic effect of TT, she concluded that the findings were probably due to overriding effects of tranquillising medications.

As part of a large study designed to test the effects of TT on surgical patients' stress reactions, Meehan et al. (1991) found that preoperative patients who received TT demonstrated approximately the same post-treatment mean decrease in anxiety as was found in the Heidt (1981) and Quinn (1984) studies, but the decrease was not significantly different from the mimic TT group. In the same study, postoperative patients who received TT morning and evening over a three-day postoperative period had no significant decrease in anxiety or fatigue or increase in vigour over the intervention period, compared with mimic TT and no-treatment control groups.

Hale (1985) tested the effects of TT on anxiety, blood pressure, and pulse rate in a sample of forty-eight hospitalized adults and found no significant differences compared with mimic TT and routine care. Parkes (1989) tested the effects of TT on anxiety in sixty elderly hospitalized patients and found no significant differences compared with mimic TT and no treatment. Simington and Laing (1993) reported that post-treatment anxiety scores of elderly institutionalized patients who received TT incorporated into a backrub procedure were significantly lower than patients who received a back-rub without TT. Using a small sample of thirty-one hospitalized psychiatric patients as subjects, Gagne and Toye (1994) compared the effects of two fifteen-minute sessions of TT, relaxation therapy, and mimic TT given over a twenty-four-hour period on anxiety and movement. Subjects demonstrated high levels of pretreatment anxiety and both the TT and the relaxation subjects experienced significant decreases in anxiety (twice as great as in the Heidt and first Quinn studies) compared with the mimic TT group.

Using a crossover design, Fedoruk (1984) found that when hospitalized premature infants were treated with TT they scored significantly lower on a behavioral indicator of stress compared with responses to mimic TT or the presence of a nurse. Also using a crossover design, Mersmann (1993) tested the effect of TT on milk letdown in mothers of nonnursing preterm infants. Mothers experienced significantly more leaking of milk during TT treatment and expressed significantly more milk following TT compared with mimic TT and no treatment.

These studies were conducted under a wide range of conditions, and designs varied considerably in their control for threats to internal and external validity. In all studies concerning anxiety, the same state anxiety instrument was used, and except where noted, sample sizes allowed for at least thirty subjects per group. A number of specific limitations confound the findings; for example, Randolph used a modified form of TT, the first Quinn study did not include a standard control group, Parkes encountered difficulty with the measurement of anxiety in her elderly subjects, and Fedoruk reported variability in intervention times and that differences in posttreatment stress were due in part to increases in stress following the mimic treatment. In some studies the investigators provided all of the experimental and control treatments. Of the ten clinical studies using adults as subjects, the findings of five indicated that TT was significantly more effective than controls. However, given the strength of the placebo effect, these findings provide no real evidence that any effects of TT are significantly greater than a placebo.

Keller and Bzdek (1986) initiated investigation of the effect of TT on pain with a study of the effect of TT on tension headache pain in healthy adults. Those who received TT were found to experience a significant reduction in headache pain immediately following treatment and four hours later, compared with those who received mimic TT. All treatments were done by the first author.

Meehan (1993) reported that patients experiencing postoperative pain demonstrated no significant decrease in pain one hour following treatment compared with patients who received mimic TT. In addition, the 13 percent decrease in pain experienced by the TT patients compared very unfavourably with the 42 percent decrease experienced by patients in a standard control group who received a narcotic analgesic. Secondary analyses indicated that patients who received TT waited significantly longer than mimic TT patients before requesting further analgesic medication.

In an extension of this work, Meehan et al. (1990, 1991) found that postoperative patients who received TT in conjunction with a p.r.n. narcotic analgesic had no significant decrease in pain over the first three hours following treatment, compared with patients who received mimic TT with their narcotic, or narcotic alone. But again, patients in the TT group waited significantly longer before requesting further medication. On average, patients in the TT group waited ten hours, the mimic TT group seven hours, and the narcotic alone group six hours. However, standard deviation scores for the TT group were 60 percent more variable than the mimic TT group and twice as variable as the narcotic group.

These findings suggest that TT may have the potential to relieve relatively mild, tension-related headache pain. They indicate that TT does not have a significant direct effect on postoperative pain and does not potentiate the short-term effect of a narcotic analgesic. TT may, however, decrease postoperative patients' need for analgesic medication. This apparent indirect effect requires further exploration and should be interpreted with caution due to the large standard deviation noted for the TT group. Again, any claims beyond a placebo effect would not be warranted, and further research is needed. A controlled trial of the effect of TT on pain in patients recovering from burns, a situation in which treatment could be particularly pertinent, is currently under way (Bonnie, 1995).

THE PLACEBO EFFECT

Controlled efficacy studies point to the need to differentiate between the effects of TT and the placebo effect. However, in TT research, complete control for the placebo effect is not possible because TT and the placebo phenomenon appear to be intrinsically interwoven. Quinn (1984) designed a mimic TT procedure to control for placebo effect. Mimic TT consists of a nurse who has no knowledge of TT mimicking the movements of a nurse doing TT while counting backward in his or her head from specified numbers by seven seconds. Quinn held that mimic TT was the same in appearance as TT but did not include its therapeutic properties. It could therefore be viewed as a single-blind control, and study results indicate that it has some validity. However, Quinn specifically viewed the procedure as "a control for the intent of the practitioner, and the effects of the presence of a helping person" (Quinn, 1984, p. 45), placebo components associated with double-blind control. But, considering the definition of TT, it is unlikely that the intent of the practitioner can be differentially accounted for through comparison with mimic TT, and standard double-blind control requires that the treatment be separated from the knowledge of the person administering the treatment. In effect, double-blind control is not possible in TT research.

Roberts et al. (1993) have suggested that the placebo effect is much more powerful than is commonly supposed and that its full force is best estimated from uncontrolled trials where both the person administering the treatment and the subject believe it will be effective. Under such circumstances, they have estimated that the placebo effect could account on average for 70 percent of positive outcomes: 40 percent excellent and 30 percent good. Possibly, TT effects reported in the practice literature should be considered against this standard. Roberts (1995) proposes that natural history and spontaneous recovery together constitute a powerful component of the placebo effect. If this is the case, and if the intent of the TT practitioner is to facilitate the natural healing potential present within the patient, then TT can be viewed as an effort to enhance significantly the placebo effect. Roberts also cites regression to the mean as a significant placebo component since patients often seek treatment when symptoms are worse, and the more severe a symptom, the more dramatic is its relief. It is not unusual for a nurse to be asked to provide TT as a last resort when nothing else seems to help and when a patient's symptoms are at their worst, thus this placebo component could account for some of the dramatic effects reported in the practice literature. Also, this factor could be operating in some controlled studies, despite random assignment and covariance analysis.

Roberts (1995) cautions that even in double-blind studies, the placebo effect is almost always a confounding factor in effects attributed to a specific treatment. He cites as an example a review by Moerman (1983) which indicated that in thirty-one double-blind trials of cimetidine, a drug of "proven" effectiveness, the placebo was just as effective as the active drug 60 percent of the time. Assuming that the placebo effect would have an even greater influence in single-blind studies, there is little remaining leeway within which to demonstrate any specific TT effects beyond a placebo effect. Nonetheless, TT is still judged scientifically according to this criterion.

The view that TT is only a placebo and nothing more has served as a rallying cry for critics. Providing as much control as possible for the placebo effect has posed a major challenge in TT research. However, ironically and in the long run, this problem has the potential to shed new light on the nature of TT, and possibly the placebo effect, and on what should be expected in terms of its therapeutic outcomes.

CONSIDERATIONS FOR THE USE OF TT IN NURSING PRACTICE

The literature suggests that TT may have potential as a nursing intervention, particularly for patients who are experiencing stress-related reactions. The adjuvant role of TT is emphasized and great care is warranted in ensuring that patients are medicated adequately and appropriately, especially for pain. Although it cannot be claimed with any confidence that TT is significantly more effective than a placebo, the meaning of this fact should be weighed carefully against the needs and wishes of individual patients. The use of TT should be considered in the light of the potential healing power of the placebo phenomenon and the extent to which a patient could benefit from enhancing the placebo effect as much as possible. If patients ask for TT, it is usually because they believe it will help them and it is therefore naturally likely to facilitate their recovery. In addition, data from studies indicate that even when patients do not believe TT will help them, it still can have a beneficial effect. In the case of a patient who is dying, experience has shown that it helps provide comfort and a sense of peacefulness. In extrapolating from data on placebo effectiveness, it could even be suggested that for a patient in a stress-related situation where the physician, nurse, and patient believe in TT, it could have at least a positive effect 70 percent of the time and an excellent effect 40 percent of the time.

There appear to be no risks to patients associated with TT when it is used appropriately as a nursing intervention, but there are some patient groups where caution is suggested. Treatments should be brief and particularly gentle for infants, very debilitated patients, and the elderly. Although one study is reported on the use of TT to decrease anxiety in hospitalized psychiatric patients, particular care should be taken in using TT with patients who have a psychiatric condition and may be extremely sensitive to close human interaction and its meaning. Care should also be taken when using TT with patients taking medications, in case of any potentiating interaction effects. Overall, in terms of risk-benefit ratio, when relief from stress-related reactions often engendered by illness is balanced against the fact that there are no reports of adverse effects from TT, the potential benefit appears to outweigh any risk.

Although other health professionals and laypeople may learn and practice TT, it is suggested that TT be offered to patients as a nursing intervention, within the context of professional nursing practice. Ideally, nurses have the most nurturing relationship with patients and the practice of TT fits naturally into nursing care. Likewise, given that nurses are constantly observing and assessing patients they are in the best position to provide TT at the most appropriate time and to monitor its effects.

There are as yet no professional standards or certification programs set for nurses who practice TT. In order to ensure an appropriate balance and integration of TT with medical care it is recommended that nurses who provide TT for patients be first selected as being already skilled and responsible clinicians in their practice area, have a good knowledge of medical care, good judgment, and be able to work well with a traditional healthcare team. They should have learned TT within a university, medical center, hospital, or a home care nursing or continuing education program. They should have had at least thirty hours of instruction in the theory and practice of TT, thirty hours of supervised practice with relatively healthy individuals, and have successfully completed written and practice evaluations (Meehan, 1992). They should carefully follow the practice guidelines developed by Krieger (1979).

CONCLUSION

The practice of TT has emerged as a specialized example of the therapeutic use of touch in nursing practice. Despite controversy engendered by its association with energy-field theoretical frameworks and the limited and inconclusive scientific support for its proposed effects, it may have some potential as a nursing intervention. It seems clear that TT is intrinsically interrelated with the powerful placebo effect and offers nurses a natural opportunity to better understand and use this phenomenal function of human interaction to facilitate patient healing and well-being. Further theoretical development and on-going efficacy studies are needed. Further debate and a certain degree of philosophical and scientific circumspection can only serve to sharpen nurses' insight into the nature and role of TT as a nursing intervention. In the meantime, some nurses in practice will remain convinced of its adjuvant effectiveness in facilitating comfort, peacefulness, and healing in a wide range of patients.

REFERENCES

Biley, F. 1996. "Rogerian Science Phantoms, and Therapeutic Touch: Exploring Potentials." *Nursing Science Quarterly* 9: 165–69.

Boguslawski, M. 1980. "Therapeutic Touch: A Facilitator of Pain Relief." *Topics in Clinical Nursing* 2 (1): 27–37.

Bohm, D. 1980. *Wholeness and The Implicate Order.* Boston: Routledge & Kegan Paul.

———. 1986. "The Implicate Order and the Super-Implicate Order." *Dialogues with Scientists and Sages: The Search for Unity.* Edited by R. Weber. New York: Routledge & Kegan Paul, pp. 23–52.

Bonnie, F. 1995. "Therapeutic Touch: How Effective for Pain Relief?" *The UAB Nurse Scientist* 1: 2–3.

Braun, C., J. Layton, J. Braun. 1986. "Therapeutic Touch Improves Residents' Sleep." *American Health Care Association Journal* 12 (1): 48–49.

Bullough, B., and V. L. Bullough. 1995. "More on Therapeutic Touch (Letter)." *Research in Nursing and Health* 18: 377.

Clark, P. E., and M. J. Clark. 1984. "Therapeutic Touch: Is There a Scientific Basis for Practice?" *Nursing Research* 33: 37–41.

Cushing, J. T., and E. McMullin, eds. 1989. *Philosophical Consequences of Quantum Theory.* Notre Dame, Ind.: University of Notre Dame Press.

Dall, J. V. 1993. "Promoting Sleep with Therapeutic Touch." *Addiction Nursing Network* 5 (1): 23–24.

Fanslow, C. A. 1983. "Therapeutic Touch: A Healing Modality Throughout Life." *Topics in Clinical Nursing* 5 (2): 72–79.

———. 1990. "Touch and the Elderly." *Touch: The Foundation of Experience.* Edited by K. E. Barnard and T. B. Brazelton. Maddison: International Universities Press, pp. 541–49.

Fedoruk, R. B. 1984. "Transfer of the Relaxation Response: Therapeutic Touch as a Method for Reduction of Stress in Premature Neonates." Doctoral dissertation, University of Maryland, Baltimore, (UMI no. 8509162).

Feltham, E. 1991. "Therapeutic Touch and Massage." *Nursing Standard* 5 (4): 26–28.

Ferguson, C. 1986. "Subjective Experience of Therapeutic Touch Survey (SETTS): Psychometric Examination of an Instrument." Doctoral dissertation, University of Texas, Austin (UMI no. 8618464).

Gagne, D., and R. C. Toye. 1994. "The Effects of Therapeutic Touch and Relaxation Therapy in Reducing Anxiety." *Archives of Psychiatric Nursing* 7 (3): 184–89.

Glazer, S. 1995. "The Mystery of Therapeutic Touch." *Washington Post* 19, H16–H17.

Hale, E. H. 1985. "A Study of the Relationship between Therapeutic Touch and the Anxiety Levels of Hospitalized Adults." Doctoral dissertation, Texas Women's University, Houston (U Microfilm no.8618897).

Heidt, P. R. 1981. "Effect of Therapeutic Touch on Anxiety Level of Hospitalized Patients." *Nursing Research* 30: 33–37.

————. 1990. "Openness: A Qualitative Analysis of Nurses' and Patients' Experiences of Therapeutic Touch." *Image: Journal of Nursing Scholarship* 22: 180–86.

————. 1991. "Helping Patients Rest: Clinical Studies in Therapeutic Touch." *Holistic Nursing Practice* 5 (4): 57–66.

Hill, L., and N. Oliver. 1993 "Therapeutic Touch and Theory-Based Mental Health Nursing." *Journal of Psychosocial Nursing* 31 (2): 19–27.

Hospital Satellite Network. 1986. "Therapeutic Touch: A New Skill from an Ancient Practice." (Videocassette no. 7538). New York: American Journal of Nursing Company.

Jackson, M. E. 1981. "The Use of Therapeutic Touch in the Nursing Care of the Terminally Ill Person." In *Therapeutic Touch: A Book of Readings*. Edited by M. A. Borelli and P. Heidt. New York: Springer, pp. 72–79.

Jaroff, L. 1994 "A No-Touch Therapy." *Time* 21: 88–89.

Jonasen, A. M. 1994. "Therapeutic Touch: A Holistic Approach to Perioperative Nursing." *Todays OR Nurse* 16 (1): 7–12.

Josephson, B. D., and F. Pallikari-Viras. 1991. "Biological Utilization of Quantum Nonlocality." *Foundations of Physics* 21: 197–207.

Jurgens, A., T. C. Meehan, and H. L. Wilson. 1987. "Therapeutic Touch as a Nursing Intervention." *Holistic Nursing Practice* 2 (1): 1–13.

Keller, E., and V. M. Bzdek. 1986. "Effects of Therapeutic Touch on Tension Headache Pain." *Nursing Research* 35: 101–106.

Kramer, N. A. 1990. "Comparison of Therapeutic Touch and Casual touch in Stress Reduction in Hospitalized Children." *Pediatric Nursing* 16: 483–85.

Krieger, D. 1975. "Therapeutic Touch: The Imprimatur of Nursing." *American Journal of Nursing* 75: 784–87.

————. 1979. *Therapeutic Touch: How to Use Your Hands to Help or Heal.* Englewood Cliffs, N.J.: Prentice Hall.

Krieger, D., E. Peper, and S. Ancoli. 1979. "Therapeutic Touch: Searching for Evidence of Physiological Change." *American Journal of Nursing* 79: 660–62.

Leduc, E. 1987. "Therapeutic Touch (Letter)." *Neonatal Network* 5 (6): 46–47.

Lionberger, H. 1986. "Therapeutic Touch: A Healing Modality or a Caring Strategy." *Methodological Issues in Nursing.* Edited by P. L. Chin. Gaithersberg, Md.: Aspen.

Lothian, J. A. 1993. "Therapeutic Touch." *Childbirth Instructor* 3 (2): 32–36.

Mackey, R. B. 1995. "Discover the Healing Power of Therapeutic Touch." *American Journal of Nursing* 95 (4): 27–32.

Macrae, J. 1979. "Therapeutic Touch in Practice." *American Journal of Nursing* 79 (4): 664–65.

————. 1989. "Principles of Therapeutic Touch Applied to the Treatment of Addiction." *Addiction Nursing Network* 1 (2): 4–5.

Malinski, V. 1993. "Therapeutic Touch: The View from Rogerian Nursing Science." *Visions* 1: 45–54.

McCloskey, J. C., G. M. Bulechek, eds. 1996. "Iowa Intervention Project." *Nursing Interventions* Classification 2d ed. St. Louis: Mosby, p. 564.

Meehan, T. C. 1990. "The Science of Unitary Human Beings and Theory-Based Practice: Therapeutic Touch." *Visions of Rogers' Science-Based Nursing.* Edited by E. A. M. Barrett. New York: National League for Nursing, pp. 67–81.

———. 1992. *Therapeutic Touch.* In *Nursing Interventions: Essential Nursing Treatments.* Edited by G. M. Bulechek and J. C. McCloskey. 2d ed. Philadelphia: W. B. Saunders, pp. 201–12.

———. 1993. "Therapeutic Touch and Postoperative Pain: A Rogerian Research Study." *Nursing Science Quarterly* 6 (2): 62–78.

Meehan, T. C., C. A. Mersmann, M. Wiseman, B. B. Wolff, and R. Magady. 1990. "The Effects of Therapeutic Touch on Postoperative Pain" (abstract). *Pain Supplement* 5: 149.

———. 1991. *Therapeutic Touch and Surgical Patients' Stress Reactions.* Final project report to the National Center for Nursing Research, National Institutes of Health, Washington, D.C.

Mersmann, C. A. 1993. "Therapeutic Touch and Milk Letdown in Mothers of Non-Nursing Preterm Infants." Doctoral dissertation, New York University, New York (U Microfilm no. 9333919).

Moerman, D. E. 1983. "General Medical Effectiveness and Human Biology: Placebo Effects in the Treatment of Ulcer Disease." *Medical Anthropology Quarterly* 4 (14): 313—16.

National League for Nursing. 1992. *Therapeutic Touch: Healing through Human Energy Fields* (videotape series), publication no. 42-2485, 42-2486, 42-2487. New York: National League for Nursing.

Newsham, G. 1989. "Therapeutic Touch for Symptom Control in Persons with AIDS." *Holistic Nursing Practice* 3 (4): 45–51.

North American Nursing Diagnosis Association. 1994. *NANDA Nursing Diagnosis: Definitions and Classifications 1995–1996.* Philadelphia: North American Nursing Diagnosis Association.

Oberst, M. 1995. "Our Naked Emperor" (editorial). *Research in Nursing and Health* 18: 1–2.

Olson, M, N. Sneed, R. Bonadonna, J. Ratliff, and J. Dias. 1992. "Therapeutic Touch and Post-Hurricane Hugo Stress." *Journal of Holistic Nursing* 10: 120–36.

Parkes, B. S. 1989. "Therapeutic Touch as an Intervention to Decrease Anxiety in Elderly Hospitalized Patients." Doctoral dissertation, University of Texas, Austin (U Microfilms no. 8609563).

Payne, M. B. 1989. "The Use of Therapeutic Touch with Rehabilitation Clients." *Rehabilitation Nursing* 15 (2): 69–72.

Quinn, J. F. 1984. "Therapeutic Touch as Energy Exchange: Testing the Theory." *Advances in Nursing Science* 6 (2): 42–49.

———. (1989) "Therapeutic touch as energy exchange: replication and extension." *Nursing Science Quarterly* 2 (2): 79-87.

Quinn, J. F., and A. J. Strelkauskas. 1989. "Psychoimmunologic Effects of Therapeutic Touch on Practitioners and Recently Bereaved Recipients: A Pilot Study." *Advances in Nursing Science* 15 (4): 13–26.

Randolph, G. L. 1984. "Therapeutic and Physical Touch: Physiological Response to Stressful Stimuli." *Nursing Research* 33: 33–36.

Roberts, A. H. 1995. "The Powerful Placebo Revisited: The Magnitude of Nonspecific Effects." *Mind/Body Medicine* 1: 1–7.

Roberts, A. H., D. G. Kewman, L. Mercier, and M. Hovell. 1993. "The Power of

Nonspecific Effects in Healing: Implications for Psychosocial and Biological Treatments." *Clinical Psychology Review* 12: 375–91.

Rogers, M. E. 1970. *An Introduction to the Theoretical Basis of Nursing.* Philadelphia: F. A. Davis.

———. 1990. "Nursing: Science of Unitary, Irreducible Human Beings: Update 1990." In *Visions of Rogers' Science-based Nursing.* Edited by E. A. M. Barrett. New York: National League for Nursing, pp. 5–11.

Samarel, N. 1992. "The Experience of Receiving Therapeutic Touch." *Journal of Advanced Nursing* 17: 651–57.

Sayre-Adams, J., and S. Wright. 1995. *The Theory and Practice of Therapeutic Touch.* London: Churchill Livingstone.

Simington JA. (1993) "The Elderly Require a 'Special Touch.' " *Nursing Homes* 4: 30–32.

Simington, J. A., and G. P. Laing. 1993. "Effects of Therapeutic Touch on Anxiety in the Institutionalized Elderly." *Clinical Nursing Research* 2: 438–50.

Stahlman, J. 1995. "Therapeutic Touch: Fuzzy Metaphysics" (letter). *American Journal of Nursing* 95 (7): 17.

Stapp, H. P. 1993. *Mind, Matter, and Quantum Mechanics.* Berlin: Springer-Verlag.

Thayer, M. B. 1990. "Touching with Intent: Using Therapeutic Touch." *Pediatric Nursing* 16: 70–72.

Weber, R. 1981. "Philosophical Foundations and Frameworks for Healing." In *Therapeutic Touch: A Book of Readings.* Edited by M. A. Borelli and P. Heidt. New York: Springer, pp. 13–39.

———. 1990. "A Philosophical Perspective on Touch." In *Touch: The Foundation of Experience.* Edited by K. E. Barnard and T. B. Brazelton. Madison, Wisc.: International Universities Press, pp. 11–43.

Winstead-Fry, P. 1983. "A Report to the Profession: Nursing Research Emphasis Grant: Families and Parenting." *Division of Nursing.* New York: New York University.

Wirth, D. P., Y. J. Richardson, W. S. Eidelman, and A. C. O'Malley. 1993. "Full Thickness Dermal Wounds Treated with Non-Contact Therapeutic Touch: A Replication and Extension." *Complementary Therapies in Medicine* 1: 127–32.

Wolfson, I. S. 1990. "Therapeutic Touch and Midwifery." In *Touch: The Foundation of Experience.* Edited by K. E. Barnard and T. B. Brazelton. Madison: International Universities Press, pp. 383–402.

Wright, S. M. 1987. "The Use of Therapeutic Touch in the Management of Pain." *Nursing Clinics of North America* 22: 704–15.

———. 1991. "Validity of the Human Energy Field Assessment Form." *Western Journal of Nursing Research* V13: 635–47.

Wuthnow, S. W., and A. Miller. 1987. "Should Christian Nurses Practice Therapeutic Touch?" *Journal of Christian Nursing* 4 (4): 15–19, 29–30.

Wyatt, G. 1989. "Keeping the Caring Touch in the High-Tech Maze." *Michigan Hospitals* 26 (5): 6–9.

Wytias, C. A. 1994. "Therapeutic Touch in Primary Care." *Nurse Practitioner Forum* 5 (2): 91–96.

3.

Should Nurses Practice Therapeutic Touch? Should Nursing Schools Teach Therapeutic Touch?

Vern L. Bullough and Bonnie Bullough

This article argues that in the current setting of nursing practice, Therapeutic Touch should be treated as a religious practice. The article examines the religious sources of the ideas and documents the connection with the teachings of particular religious groups. Recognizing Therapeutic Touch as a religious issue requires new kinds of approaches in the practice and teaching of Therapeutic Touch in nursing.

Should nurses practice Therapeutic Touch? Should nursing schools teach Therapeutic Touch? The answers to these two questions is not the same. Put simply, in the authors' opinion, (1) nurses who believe in Therapeutic Touch should be allowed to use it in their treatment modalities if the patient or client wishes them to do so and it does not otherwise take time away from their regular nursing duties, and (2) most schools of nursing should not teach Therapeutic Touch as part of their regular curriculum.

The contradictory answers come because of the nature and role of religion in the curriculum of secular nursing as well as in the personal belief systems of the individual nurse. The authors believe and advocate that Therapeutic Touch be regarded as a religious practice similar to prayer or to other healing techniques advocated by adherents of Christian Science. By labeling Therapeutic Touch a religious practice, a matter of faith rather than science, it changes the nature of the discussion, and this is what the authors hope to do in this article. The implications of this classification and their recommendations are summarized at the end.

Originally published in *Journal of Professional Nursing* 14, no. 4 (July–August 1998): 254–57. Copyright © 1998 by W.B. Saunders Company. Reprinted with permission.

RELIGION AND THE NIGHTINGALE VIEW OF NURSING

The place of religious practices in nursing is part of an old debate, dating at least from the time of Florence Nightingale and the founding of secular nursing. A deeply religious person herself, Nightingale believed that nurses' primary responsibility was to care for the physical needs, not the spiritual ones, of the sick and wounded. She worried that if nurses were charged with both, they might be too busy praying over their patients to observe their physical or even emotional needs (Bullough and Bullough, 1978; Bullough, Bullough, and Stanton, 1990).

This did not mean that she rejected religion. Nursing itself was conceived by her and others as an elevated "calling" or "vocation" (Bryant and Coling, 1990), and this demanded a kind of commitment that she believed only a religious person would have. This belief carried over to the United States and clearly appears in the final report of the committee to establish a hospital training school for nurses at Bellevue, one of the first three to be established in the United States.

> We wish our candidates to be religious women but do not require that they should belong to any given sect. To Catholic and Protestant our doors are equally open; we impose no vows: we say to all, in the words of the founder of the Sisters of Charity: "your convent must be the houses of the sick, your cell the chamber of suffering, your chapel the nearest church; your cloister the streets of a city or the wards of a hospital: your grate [motivation], the fear of God, and your womanly modesty your only veil. (Nutting and Dock, 1907–1912, vol. 2, p. 387)

Nurses could certainly silently pray over their patients if they wanted to, and nurses in Catholic hospitals, whatever their religion, learned to baptize and even if necessary hear final confessions and perform last rites. Most such exercises were for emergencies, and publicly praying over or with patients was normally done by those who had completed their shift work and with the consent of the patient. In general, however, spiritual issues increasingly came to be delegated to official or unofficial chaplains or to representatives of specific religious groups.

THERAPEUTIC TOUCH AND RELIGION

Therapeutic Touch, however, is not being pushed as a religious practice but as an alternate therapy; however, sometimes the lines between the two are confused because many religious practices such as prayer or laying-on of hands are alternative therapy but clearly recognized as religious practices. Therapeutic Touch also is clearly based on religious practices and beliefs, with roots in many religions. It came into nursing through the efforts of Doris Krieger (1975) who publicized her views in the *American Journal of Nursing*. As Krieger (1979) later amplified on her views, she explained that she had become interested in it through the influence of Dora Kunz (1991), then one of the leaders of the theosophical movement in America, and through the writings and teachings of two other theosophists: Charles W. Leadbetter, one of the more famous theosophist seers, and Oskar Estebany, a former Hungarian cavalry officer who retired to Canada and worked in theosophical healing with Kunz. Krieger, however, neglected to identify the theosophical connections of her own beliefs and practices.

Theosophy (literally "wisdom of god") developed in the nineteenth century as a syncrestic American religion, just as did Seventh Day Adventists, Mormonism, and Christian Science. It was founded in 1875 in the United States by Helena Petrovina Blavatsky, a Russian-born psychic, and a colleague, Col. Henry Steele Olcott, also a psychic. Madame Blavatsky, as she was known, claimed she had been sent to the United States by the Russian lodge of the Universal Mystical Brotherhood to share truth and unveil error. Many of her early followers came from Spiritualism, another American religious grouping, which had started in the Rochester, New York, area in 1848 with the mystical rappings of the Fox sisters and their alleged ability to communicate with the dead (Bullough, 1984). Blavatsky regarded her movement as a more sophisticated form of spiritualism and was highly critical of what she regarded as the primitive spiritualism of the Americans with its emphasis on contacting the dead. Instead, she conceived the job of the medium as one of contacting the superhuman adepts or "masters" eager to impart esoteric information to select human beings. These spiritual human beings had evolved in the next world to the point where they had merged into the universal environment, unseen but ever present, anxious to communicate with the earthly adepts who were chosen or set apart to carry out such contacts. Theosophists believed that because God was universal, truth could be arrived at either through intuition or through revelations given to mediums or adepts through contact with the seers and masters.

On the death of Madame Blavatsky in 1891, Annie Besant, an English woman, assumed a dominant role and moved the headquarters to India where Blavatsky earlier had established a society (Campbell, 1980). The American movement, however, remained separate from that of Besant, and there were several rival but more or less cooperating groups, in one of which, the Theosophical Society of America headquartered in Wheaton, Ill., Dora Kunz (1991) served as president. Key to Kunz's belief system was an understanding of divine wisdom, which included wholeness of the spirit and the body. Kunz personally emphasized the healing aspects of theosophy, and it was under her influence that many theosophists were encouraged to enter into various healthcare professions. Her disciples were influential in advocating and popularizing holistic medicine, although other groups were also active. Therapeutic touch was and is part and parcel of the religious teachings of the Theosophists (Campbell, 1980), although Kunz and Krieger, had slightly different versions.

In Krieger's (1979) view of Therapeutic Touch, it was not something that every nurse could do. She believed that before individuals could practice it, they needed to become aware of their interior experiences, that is, achieve the theosophical medium state necessary for communication with the masters, although she also sometimes expressed this in Jungian terms as entering into the archetypal journey (Jung, 1963, 1969). It was from her spiritual mentor, Dora Kunz (1991), that Krieger received the ideas of auras, the energy fields that surround individuals, which Therapeutic Touch was believed to direct. This was part of what might be called theosophical physics.

Helping to give political sanction in nursing to Therapeutic Touch was Martha Rogers (1970), chair of the department of nursing at New York University (NYU). Rogers, a nursing theorist, visualized a human being as an evolving four-dimensional energy field, a theory which in its essentials, was very similar to the physics being promoted by theosophy and which was later explained in some detail by Margaret A. Newman (1994). Rogers encouraged a whole generation of students and colleagues to study such favorite subjects of theosophists as clairvoyance, precognition, mysticism, out-of-body experiences, Kirlian photography, Therapeutic Touch, and so forth (Rogers, 1970). Her influence extended deep into nursing because many of the staff members of nursing organizations headquartered in New York and the staff of nursing journals published there studied under her at NYU or came into contact with her and proved receptive to ideas such as those advocated by Krieger (1979).

This perhaps led to a deemphasis on the religious nature of Therapeutic Touch, although it clearly remains part and parcel of theosophist and spiritualist ideas. One of the major centers for the study and practice is Lily Dale, a spiritualist center located near Chautauqua, New York, and run by the various spiritualist and theosophical groups. Lily Dale also serves as a training ground for mediums, a perhaps natural alliance because today's health-oriented mediums, following Blavatsky, are particularly interested in establishing contact with higher-order spirit guides who can instruct them in the finer points of healing through energy manipulation (Rogo, 1992). Lily Dale has some ties with the Pumpkin Hollow Center in Craryville, New York, which Krieger uses as her training ground for Therapeutic Touch. A nurse medium who attended both camps was asked if there were any differences between Therapeutic Touch and mediumship. She replied: "You can label it whatever you want, but they are basically the same" (Rogo, 1992, pp. 15–16).

There are, however, many different sources. Mary Jo Trapp Bullbrook, a nurse healing touch practitioner, who presented a workshop to nurses in Rochester, New York, stated that her techniques were "channeled to her" by such individuals as Alice Bailey, the deceased founder and former director of the Healing Light Center in Glendale, California (Fish, 1996).

Some have also associated Therapeutic Touch with the modern witchcraft religious movement known as Wicca. The Wiccan healing ritual views diagnosis as a mainly clairvoyant art, and treatment involves a laying-on of hands characterized by "electromagnetic passes" over the body almost identical to those taught by Krieger (Farrar, 1983). In fact, it is not much of an overstatement to say that Therapeutic Touch is found in many of the new religious groupings that have sprung up in the last part of the twentieth century.

Implications:

Accepting Therapeutic Touch as a basic religious belief has several implications that should help solve some of the controversies associated with it.

1. Like prayer, Therapeutic Touch is difficult to test, and this helps explain *why* different researchers get quite different results (Clark and Clark, 1984; Wilson, 1995) and why so many view the results in different ways. It becomes a matter of faith more than of science, and the authors believe that like in the case of other religious beliefs, nurses can agree with each other to allow individual nurses to follow their own conscience on such matters. Therapeutic Touch healers might well be classed as being similar to Christian Science healers, and those who want treatment under such a system should be allowed to seek it out.
2. It also means that we must be very conscious of the religious or philosophical beliefs of others and leave the teaching and practice of Therapeutic Touch to those *who* do believe. One of those

who wrote strongly about this was Sharon Fish, who held that Therapeutic Touch was helping bring to birth in nursing a host of spiritually illegitimate and dangerous practices, including mediumship and more. Those who say they can practice the technique of Therapeutic Touch and divorce themselves from its occult associations need to be reminded that apart from the occult, Therapeutic Touch would not exist. It is rooted and grounded in psychic soil, and it bears related fruit.

Therapeutic Touch is not a practice Christians can engage in without seriously compromising their faith and potentially endangering their relationship with God. He alone can reach the true meaning of the laying-on of hands to comfort, care, and cure (Fish, 1996).

The authors would argue that care and caution must be exercised by nurses who practice Therapeutic Touch and that they should only offer their treatment to those who believe or want it after it is explained to them. It is not only the nonbeliever humanists who refuse, but so will many dedicated religious people. Quite clearly many Christians regard it as the work of devil.

3. The authors believe that teaching therapeutic Touch in the curriculum of any tax-supported nursing school or in schools with federal or state grants given for other than research purposes violates the rights of students and raises serious constitutional issues. They believe that students should not be forced to sit through sectarian religious teachings, even those that claim to be syncretic. Students, however, should be told about the existence of such techniques, and if they want to learn it, to do so on their own but not in any credit-bearing class.

4. Although it is true that many of today's therapeutic techniques might be traced to religious assumptions of the past, generally these have been empirically verified and are no longer sectarian. Perhaps one day this will happen to Therapeutic Touch, and research on the topic should continue. Researchers, however, have to confront the religious background of Therapeutic Touch and take that into account in designing studies, something that has not been done very effectively.

5. Last, the authors urge all nurses, believers and nonbelievers in Therapeutic Touch, to realize that the United States is a nation of great religious and cultural diversity. Respect for the religious practices of others requires all of us to take care not to violate the belief systems of our patients. At this point in history, Therapeutic Touch has to be classified as one treatment modality

that does violate the belief system of others regardless of whether or not it helps.

REFERENCES

Bryant, J. L., and K. B. Coling. 1990. "Broken Wills and Tender Hearts: Religious Ideology and the Trained Nurse." In *Nightingale and Her Era*. Edited by V. L. Bullough, B. Bullough, and M. Stanton. New York: Garland, pp. 153–67.

Bullough, V. L. 1984. "Spiritualism Unmasked." *Skeptical Inquirer* 4: 60–68.

Bullough, V. L., and B. Bullough. 1978. *The Care of the Sick*. New York: Prodist, Science History.

Bullough, V. L., B. Bullough, and M. Stanton. 1990. *Florence Nightingale and Her Era*. New York: Garland.

Campbell, B. F. 1980. *Ancient Wisdom Revived: A History of the Theosophical Movement*. Berkeley, Calif.: University of California Press.

Clark, P. O., and Clark, M. J. 1984. "Therapeutic Touch: Is There a Scientific Basis for the Practice?" *Nursing Research* 33 (1): 37–41.

Farrar, S. 1983. *What Witches Do*. Custer, W.Va.: Phoenix.

Fish, S. 1996. "Alternative Therapies: Healing Science or Metaphysical Fraud?" *Journal of Christian Nursing* 13: 3–11.

Jung, C. J. 1963. *Memories, Dreams, Reflections*. Translated by R. and C. Winston. New York: Random House.

———. (1969) *Four Archetypes*. Translated by R. F. C. Hull. Princeton, N.J.: Princeton University Press.

Krieger, D. 1975. "Therapeutic Touch: The Imprimatur of Nursing." *American Journal of Nursing* 75: 784–87.

———. (1979) *The Therapeutic Touch*. New York: Prentice Hall.

Kunz, D. van G. 1991. *The Personal Aura*. Wheaton, Ill.: Theosophical.

Newman, M. A. 1994. *Health as Expanding Consciousness*. St Louis, Mo.: Mosby.

Nutting, M., and L. Dock. 1907–1912. *History of Nursing*. 4 vols. New York: Putnam.

Rogers, M. 1970. *An Introduction to the Theoretical Basis of Nursing*. Philadelphia: Davis.

Rogo, D. S. 1992. *Techniques of Inner Healing*. New York: Paragon.

Wilson, D. F. 1995. "Therapeutic Touch: Foundation and Current Knowledge." *Alternative Health Practitioner* 1 (1): 54–66.

4.

Ethical Issues Concerning Therapeutic Touch

Dónal P. O'Mathúna

Practicing any healthcare therapy, whether called "conventional," "alternative," or "complementary," raises important ethical issues. Discussions of healthcare ethics are made difficult by the variety of values and world views held in pluralistic societies. The on-going debate over abortion and the growing public discussion about physician-assisted suicide reflect very different views on the right thing to do in response to certain medical circumstances.

In spite of the perennial debate over some issues in healthcare ethics, there is overwhelming consensus on other issues. This chapter will illuminate the ways that some of these widely accepted bodies of ideas within healthcare ethics might have impact on the practice of Therapeutic Touch. Because TT was developed and popularized within the nursing profession, specific references will be made to the American Nurses Association Code of Ethics (ANA, 1985). However, the general principles delineated here are most likely to be accepted by all practitioners of TT.

One of the central ethical principles in healthcare today is that of *informed consent*. Although sometimes viewed as no more than getting patients to sign a consent form, it is a rich ethical concept since it reflects two precepts widely valued in healthcare today. One is the respect healthcare providers should have for the autonomy of others. The other is the important role that healthcare providers have as advocates for their patients. I shall discuss both of these ideas and show how they lead to informed consent as a decision-making process, rather than a form-signing event.

A definition of informed consent which reflects the views of many scholars writing about healthcare ethics is given by Norton: "Informed consent should be a voluntary, uncoerced decision based on adequate information and deliberation by a sufficiently competent person" (1995, p. 345). To examine how these ideas should influence the practice of TT, consider the following case (Young, 1998).

Marcelyn, a nurse in a busy hospital, went to check on Sally, one of the patients assigned to her, and found Helen, another nurse, standing over her bed. Helen held a crystal over Sally's body with one hand, and moved her other hand back and forth along Sally's body. Startled, Marcelyn asked Helen what she was doing.

"I'm performing Therapeutic Touch to relieve her pain," Helen replied, dropping her hands to her sides and shaking them as if she was flicking water from them. "This removes the negative energy so positive energy can flow through her chakras."

Sally was in severe pain related to multiple sclerosis for which she was receiving morphine through an infusion pump. The drug left her sedated, so Marcelyn asked if Sally had consented to TT treatments.

Helen replied that she hadn't wanted to wake Sally up but she knew the TT treatment would help her feel better because "it works."

"You shouldn't do this without her permission," Marcelyn replied. "Please leave her in my care and go back to your own patients."

Leaving the room, Helen muttered something about how "unenlightened" Marcelyn was for being close-minded about new therapies like TT.

PATIENT ADVOCACY

This case illustrates the tension which arises between a patient's autonomy and a provider's desire to be an advocate. This tension underlies the importance of informed consent, which seeks to balance both concepts. Helen, like almost all healthcare professionals, has good intentions. She wants to bring relief to patients, and sees TT as one way to do so. In doing so, she seeks to be an advocate for her patients.

In the *Code for Nurses with Interpretive Statements*, patient advocacy is viewed as one of the foremost roles of the professional nurse. Advocacy generally means to protect and advance the interests of others, and should therefore be important to all healthcare providers. As such, advocacy should go hand-in-hand with respect for autonomy. The ethical principle of autonomy is the belief that people should be free to make their own choices about their futures, within the limits of respecting others' autonomy. In other words, an advocate is one who helps promote another's autonomy. In the above case, Helen and Marcelyn are advocates for Sally because they desire to help her obtain relief from her pain (assuming that this is why she came to the hospital).

Conflict can arise, however, when it comes to determining a person's best interests. Alternative therapists who adhere to a "holistic" approach to health care generally promote themselves as patient advocates as opposed to paternalistic providers (Daniels, 1994). Paternalism lies beneath the old adage that "doctor knows best." Hence, paternalistic physicians would tell their patients they were going to have surgery with little involvement of the patients in the decision. People would assume that physicians had their patients' best interests in mind, as well as the experience and knowledge required to make those decisions.

The same problems and limitations in medical care that have led people to explore alternative therapies have also led to the rejection of paternalism. Patients have the right to refuse any medical treatment, regardless of whether or not healthcare providers believe this is in the patients' best interests. Advance directives help ensure that even if patients become unable to communicate, their healthcare decisions are made according to their wishes. Patient autonomy is valued so much that even if physicians believe refusing a treatment will lead to a patient's death, the patient may legally refuse that treatment.

When Marcelyn saw Helen practicing TT she may have been disturbed by the paternalism reflected in Helen's actions. Helen had decided that she knew what was best for Sally in this situation: TT. She had decided she did not need to get permission from Sally to proceed. Although impossible to quantify, there are growing reports of TT being practiced this way in hospitals. Apparently, some nurses believe it is ethical to give TT to patients who are sleeping, unconscious, or under the influence of anesthesia (Fish, 1995). Yet because of the value placed on informed consent, practicing TT without first obtaining permission is unethical.

Paternalism is at one end of a spectrum of ways to determine patients' best interests. In the paternalistic view, patient advocacy means getting patients to do what the healthcare providers believe they should do. At the other end of the spectrum is a view growing in popularity within nursing called *existential advocacy*. According to this approach, "the patient is the one who decides what is in her or his 'best interest' in any situation" (Gaylord, 1992, p. 13). Existential advocacy assumes that people's best interests are promoted by self-actualization or self-empowerment:

> Human advocacy does not just give the patient information and await his decision, it helps the patient to authentically exercise their [sic] freedom of self-determination. It helps them to become clear about what *they* want to do. Human advocacy insists that it is *the patient* who must ultimately decide what is in the patients [sic] best interests. (Darbyshire, 1989, p. 22; emphasis in original)

While appearing to promote patients' autonomy, existential advocacy is part of a broader worldview that actually undermines autonomy. It fits in with the belief held by many alternative therapists that people can, and should, 'create their own reality.' Thus, for example, Deepak Chopra, M.D., claims: "The mind makes reality. Outside our perceptions, thought, and experiences, reality has no validity. . . . We create our reality." By implication, when people decide that a therapy works for them, that decision becomes part of their reality. Others have no right to claim that this reality is not valid. Critiquing an alternative therapy then becomes much more than a discussion about evidence: it becomes a personal insult to someone's view of reality. An existential advocate, then, should not place barriers in the way of patients obtaining the alternative therapies they have decided they want. "The nurse is obliged to act in the patient's best interests on the basis that only the patient can define his or her best interests" (Ellis, 1995, p. 206).

There should be little surprise, then, that existential advocacy is used by some nurses to promote alternative therapies, including TT. Dolores Krieger claims that "the concept of multiple realities is valid. . . . TT has benefited from being perceived in this more liberal perspective" (1993, pp. 6–7). Other nurses claim that when choosing an alternative healer, "the patient should be encouraged to trust her or his own intuition and judgment about whether that individual healer is appropriate at that time. The encouragement to rely on her or his own ability to decide what is best is a type of personal growth and healing in itself" (Engebretson, 1993, p. 55).

Patients should be the ones making their own decisions about healthcare and the practitioners that they visit. This is what is meant by autonomy. But one major problem with existential advocacy and 'reality creation' is that it unhinges the decision-making process from the limits imposed on everyone by objective reality (which does exist). Chopra and Krieger may claim they create their own realities but if they step off a ten-story building, gravity will pull them and their view of reality down to earth.

We all have difficulty accepting the limitations and boundaries we face. As healthcare professionals, it is important to recognize our own limitations and to help patients come to terms with theirs. To accept, or even promote, a patient's false view of reality is unethical. In our case study, imagine that Sally woke up while Helen was administering TT. After Helen explained what she was doing, Sally gave her permission to continue, and asked her to return. Two days later, Sally's physician informs her that some of her pain is caused by a malignant tumor. He believes he has found it early enough that surgery could remove it completely and prevent further spreading. After thinking about it for a day, Sally declares that she believes TT and guided imagery can cure her cancer and she wants no medical treatment. According to existential advocacy, Marcelyn and Helen should support Sally's decision.

> There are times when what is in the patient's best interests, as perceived by the healthcare professionals, is in conflict with the view of the patient, but that does not mean that the professionals should impose their own views. Patients' best medical interests are not necessarily their best interests as people. . . . Overruling patient wishes in such situations is blatantly paternalistic. (Ellis, 1995, p. 207)

Ironically, though, existential advocacy is also paternalistic. Allowing patients to create their own healthcare reality is deciding for them that their interests are best-served by total self-determination, even when the patient lacks sufficient information for appropriate decision-making. The evidence that self-determination is automatically what is best or is even what patients want, does not exist. Many patients come to healthcare professionals because they don't know what is best and they want advice. They don't necessarily want to be told what to do but want help and guidance in making their decisions. Illness, by its nature, sets up a situation in which power is unequally distributed. Advocacy assumes that people with more power look out for the interests of those who are less powerful and therefore vulnerable. This places a burden on advocates to exercise their power within ethical boundaries. Informed consent is highly regarded because it provides a method of keeping the advice-giving process as ethical as possible. At its core is the belief that the advice given should be based primarily on objective evidence. Other subjective and value-laden advice may be given but in those cases, patients should be clearly informed of the nature of the evidence or the lack of any.

INFORMED CONSENT

The process of informed consent is designed to protect patients' autonomy from the two extremes given above. On the one hand, they are protected from paternalists who deny their autonomy by taking responsibility for decision-making away from them. On the other hand, they are protected from those who would leave them believing in false ideas and implausible therapies, guided only by intuition. The informed consent process respects and promotes people's autonomy by actively engaging them in discussions involving all the information needed to make a truly informed decision. People are shown respect by assuming that they can understand the basics of how to weigh evidence and balance the risks and benefits of a particular therapy.

There is broad consensus that the informed consent process involves five general aspects. Whether a therapy is conventional or alternative should make no difference in whether patients are given the opportunity to provide informed consent. The five aspects of achieving informed consent are:

1. Competence: the patient should be alert and oriented and able to understand all the relevant information being presented by the healthcare provider.
2. Information: the patient should be given a reasonable amount of information about the established benefits and risks of the treatment and ones of similar effectiveness and safety.
3. Understanding: the patient should be able to understand the information presented. This should take into account the patient's language skills, educational level, and experience with the healthcare system. Patients should be able to express in their own words the information they have been given, and should be given the opportunity to ask questions.
4. Lack of Coercion: the patient should not be overtly pressured into choosing one therapy or subtly manipulated or deceived into accepting one course of action.
5. Authorization: the patient should conclude the informed consent process by given written or verbal consent to treatment which is witnessed by an uninvolved party.

Ethicists disagree over certain aspects of the informed consent process. Debate occurs, for example, over how many different therapies patients should be informed about before consenting to one. Others disagree about how many of the risks a patient should be told about, especially if some are extremely rare. In spite of these differences, the overall process is not controversial and all five aspects are important to ensure that decisions to accept or reject therapies are arrived at ethically. In applying these criteria to TT, we will not refer further to the first and fifth. Issues of mental competence are beyond the scope of this chapter. Clearly, though, nurses who give TT to sleeping or unconscious patients, like Sally, without first obtaining informed consent, are acting unethically. If someone is no longer competent to give informed consent, ethical and legal guidelines exist for determining who can give consent for treatment.

PRESENTATION OF INFORMATION

Central to the process of informed consent is the disclosure and discussion of information. When advocates act ethically and professionally they provide "correct, objective information rather than unrealistic promises" (Fletcher, 1992, p. 1353). Patients often learn about alternative therapies through word-of-mouth, the Internet, and advertisements. Needless to say, this information spans the whole spectrum of quality, is often incomplete, and at times is distorted and even deceptive.

Promoters of alternative therapies should accept ethical responsibility to ensure the accuracy of their advertisements. The media should also accept their ethical obligation to ensure veracity in its reporting on alternative therapies. Nurses and other providers must take this responsibility very seriously. The *Code for Nurses* states: "The nurse participates in the profession's effort to protect the public from misinformation and misrepresentation and to maintain the integrity of nursing" (ANA, 1985). Nurses should critically examine all the information they pass on to patients and withstand the pressure to recommend alternative therapies based on media releases, hearsay, and testimonials. Informed consent requires information based on the most accurate and reliable evidence available. "Nurses have both a professional and moral obligation to base their clinical practice on recent and valid research findings" (Norton, 1995, p. 346).

An example of testimonial information is when Helen was confronted by Marcelyn. She replied confidently that TT "works." She did not elaborate on this but promoters of TT frequently claim it has dramatic effects in several areas.

Information provided for informed consent should include the benefits a patient can most *reliably* expect. According to Krieger, TT's most reliable clinical effect is causing a relaxation response in the patient within two to four minutes. The second most reliable clinical effect "is the amelioration or eradication of pain. . . . For TT's third most reliable clinical effect, I would choose the facilitation of the healing process per se" (1993, pp. 83–84). As an example of the latter, she claims (without citation) that several replicated studies found that bone fractures heal more than twice as quickly when treated with TT.

In general, Krieger states that more than twenty years of "basic, formal, and clinical research" supports the efficacy of TT (1993, p. 8), and Thorpe claims that TT "is among the most well-researched of the alternative touch healing techniques" (1993, p. 10).

Although much "research" has been conducted by proponents of TT, most of these have been limited and the results unsupportive of the claims made. None of their studies have examined the nature, properties, or even the existence of the alleged human energy field (HEF) that is so central to their practice. Prominent proponents admit that no one has managed to measure the interactions between HEF or demonstrate that energy is actually directed during TT (Krieger, 1979; Quinn, 1989). Two studies conducted by those skeptical of TT's effectiveness found that practitioners could not detect an HEF (Rosa et al., 1998; Glickman and Gracely, 1998). In the Rosa study, practitioners could not even correctly identify the location of the experimenter's unseen hand at levels predicted by chance. Glickman tested one practitioner, whose result was consistent with chance [see chapter 16 in this volume]. In a third skeptical study (Long et al., 1999), essentially using the same protocol as the Rosa study although with test subjects who were not TT practitioners, subjects reliably achieved scores significantly greater than chance. However, when body heat and other cues were eliminated the results fell to the chance level [see chapter 15 in this volume]. Throughout the history of TT's promotion, independent reviews of its research have found little or no objective evidence to support the effectiveness of the therapy (Schlotfeldt, 1973; Walike, 1975; Clark, 1984; Claman, 1994). Yet Meehan, a prominent researcher in the field, concluded her 1998 review by stating that TT "may have some potential as a nursing intervention" despite "the limited and inconclusive support for its proposed effects" (Meehan, 1998, p. 123).

The goal here is not to review TT research but to point to its relevance for the informed consent process. When experts in the field claim a therapy has "limited" and "inconclusive" research support, it is unethical to tell others that the therapy is research supported. Patients being offered the therapy and those being introduced to it in training sessions should be told clearly of its controversial and experimental nature. Institutional policies and procedures should point out the lack of high-quality, supportive research. Only when people are informed of these important factors can they truly be sufficiently informed to consent to receive or decline TT.

Going back to our case study, Helen may not have participated in any TT research herself. Like most busy healthcare professionals, she may not have had time to read the original research reports. She probably relied instead on nursing journals, which publish general reviews of developments affecting nursing. Many of these journals regularly print reviews about TT. However, these reviews are often written by TT practitioners and read like promotional advertisements rather than objective reviews. This itself raises ethical issues about conflict of interest in writing reviews, but of greater concern here is the way some of these articles interfere with the informed consent process.

Reviews of TT sometimes misrepresent the original research

studies they are discussing. The sweeping claims made about research on TT, in general, are not valid. More specific problems also occur. Quinn's 1984 study, which found that TT relieved anxiety, is often cited without mentioning that her 1989 study failed to replicate those findings. Reviewers often cite two studies by Wirth, which found that TT hastened wound healing, but rarely mention his three later ones which found no such hastening (Wirth, 1995) [see chapters 9 and 17 in this volume]. Meehan (1993) is cited to support a pain-relieving ability for TT when in fact the pain relief found in her study was not statistically significant. She herself stated in 1998 that any alleged pain relief from TT could be the result of random factors or the placebo effect. What is more problematic ethically is the way some reviewers actually distort the results of some research. For example, two review articles cited Parkes's dissertation in support of TT's ability to reduce anxiety (Jonasen, 1994; Hughes, 1996). That research actually found increased anxiety among those receiving TT (Parkes, 1985). Other examples are documented elsewhere (O'Mathúna, in press).

Inaccurate reviews of TT adversely affect nursing practice. Nurses incorporate TT into the profession based on misinformation. The public hears of its acceptability within nursing and becomes interested in trying the therapy. Well-meaning but poorly informed (or misinformed) practitioners give inaccurate information to those considering TT. These patients and trainees are then denied the opportunity to make informed decisions about the therapy. The overall effect is the very opposite of what the *Code for Nurses* calls for; misinformation and misrepresentation is fostered.

INFORMING ABOUT HARM

The informed consent process should also include a description of the adverse effects most likely to be experienced. Many proponents of TT make claims like, "Therapeutic touch has no reported adverse effects" (Benor, 1996, p. 204), yet others describe numerous potentially harmful effects. Indeed, even seemingly innocuous interventions such as the hand motions of TT have the potential for, at minimum, psychological harm.

No research exists on adverse incidences associated with TT, nor is there information on their frequency. Claims for and against the safety of TT are all presented anecdotally, this being the least reliable form of evidence. Anecdotal evidence of safety or effectiveness should lead only to further research, not firm statements that the therapy is safe or that it works. Anecdotal reports of harm should similarly be treated cautiously and lead to research.

Given the lack of actual research on the safety of TT, as well as the clear limitations of reports on potential adverse effects, it remains unethical to place people at risk without good reason. Since the benefits of TT are highly tentative, placing patients at any risk from the therapy is highly suspect. Until the potential harms can be more reliably ascertained and documented, and until they are understood, patients should be informed about the concerns of prominent TT practitioners.

HARM TO PATIENTS

As early as 1979 Krieger cautioned that "energy" should be sent carefully to the patient during treatment. "It is not enough to channel energy to an ill person; as a matter of experience, it seems that one can actually do more harm than good by simply flooding a weakened person with energy" (p. 60). She stressed the importance of practicing TT according to her guidelines to maintain its safety record (pp. 55, 89). By 1993, Krieger was much more specific: "Human energies are not well understood at this time, but we do know that indiscriminate and persistent interaction can overload the human system; a healee can overdose on human energies" (p. 169). She described some symptoms: "The progressive signs of overload to be aware of include increasing restlessness, irritability, and anxiety that may be expressed as hostility or felt as pain by the healee" (p. 75). She noted that two people doing Therapeutic Touch simultaneously on one patient must do so carefully. "Otherwise, the healee may experience ill effects such as nausea, dizziness, or irritability" (p. 128).

Other TT proponents have given similar general warnings (Mackey, 1995). Deborah Cowens was more specific: "By performing a long healing touch session on someone with a cold, you can trigger an even deeper discharge or elimination of waste products, and thus intensify the symptoms and cause more suffering. . . . In other words, you will increase the suffering of the patient significantly" (1996, pp. 56–57). She then warned that when patients have a fever or inflammation, "do not send life force into the body initially. This will serve to further inflame the condition" (p. 208). And again: "When treating people with cancer, *do not send energy to the area of the tumor*. This will only serve to strengthen the disease and make it more virulent" (p. 209; emphasis in original).

While no studies were given to support these cautions, they demonstrate the serious concerns some proponents have about TT's potential harm. When Wirth's later studies found statistical significance for slower wound healing rates after TT, he hypothesized: "Prior anecdotal research has indicated that if the healer is emotionally upset or physically ill, a transference of the state from practitioner to the patient might occur, thereby resulting in not only a nonsignificant treatment effect but, in extreme cases, a disturbance or inhibition of the patient's normal rate of healing" (1995, p. 51). Patients should be told of this risk.

Leading proponents also claim that certain groups of patients are more sensitive to TT than others. In 1979, Krieger reiterated a warning from Dora Kunz that TT ought to be done very gently and for no more than two to three minutes on children, very old people, very debilitated people, and in treating any person's head (p. 55). Macrae claimed, "However, children's systems are very sensitive, and as with medication, Therapeutic Touch must be given in smaller, more gentle doses. Too much or incorrect repatterning can cause discomfort, so it is extremely important to be sensitive to the patient's responses" (1979, p. 665). Concerns for these same groups of patients were reiterated more recently (Wytias, 1994). Again, no studies have been cited to support these concerns, although one study found increased anxiety among elderly hospitalized patients given TT compared to a control group, and cautioned against using TT with the elderly (Parkes, 1985).

All these cautions indicate that research into potential harmful effects of TT is needed. Until rigorous studies show that these concerns are not warranted, TT providers should inform trainees, patients, and research subjects about these harmful effects. Yet precisely the opposite occurs. For example, Krieger specifically cautioned those using TT with burn victims: "Burns are very sensitive to energy overload, so Therapeutic Touch must be done very gently at the site of burned tissue. Do the work for very short periods—two to three minutes at a time—and keep your hands moving so that your hand chakras do not focus energy too intensely at the burn site" (1993, p. 75). The U.S. Department of Defense funded a study on the use of TT with burn victims (Selby, 1996; Scheiber, 1997) [see chapters 19 and 20 in this volume]. No mention of these potentially harmful effects was made in the grant proposal although Krieger's book with the warnings was cited in the grant application. Treatment lengths from five to twenty minutes were proposed with no mention of Krieger's concerns. The informed consent given to research subjects stated: "There is no risk of injury from the administrations of TT" (Turner, 1994).

The same problem has been seen with the informed consent in other TT research. One form from a research project involving children stated: "In no case have there ever been any negative effects associated with TT. . . . There are no known risks" (France, 1991, p. 211). Another from a project with the elderly stated: "Therapeutic touch has no known negative side effects" (Parkes, 1985, pp. 95–96). These statements contradict TT's own literature and violate the ethical standards required of research.

HARM TO PRACTITIONERS

In addition to harmful effects on patients, statements have been made that practitioners may experience negative effects. These are explained on the basis of a two-way flow of energy. "It is also important for you to remain centered and aware of your own reactions to the healing process to not absorb any unbalanced energy from your patient" (Wytias, 1994, p. 94). Another proponent stated: "If you're not centered, you may actually absorb the patient's negative energy. That's why novices to this modality sometimes report posttreatment headaches" (Mackey, 1995, p. 28).

Further, proponents instruct trainees in "centering" as a form of meditation, thus centering could produce the side effects of meditation. One study found that 48 percent of Transcendental Meditation (TM) practitioners reported adverse effects from meditation (Otis, 1984). The most common negative effects in this study were anxiety, depression, confusion, frustration, mental and physical tension, and inexplicable outbursts of antisocial behavior. These were reported by TM trainers who persisted with the method, not by people who had stopped practicing. Other studies report similar findings with documented cases of adverse effects as serious as attempted suicide and psychiatric hospitalization (Shapiro, 1992). All these occurred from "simply" practicing meditation. *Qigong*, another Eastern therapy based on manipulating human life energy through meditation, breathing, and exercise, has also been found to precipitate psychological problems (Sampson, 1996; Ng, 1999).

Krieger wants TT to become a common event in every family. Before introducing people to TT and its form of meditation, the possible dangers and discomforts must be investigated further. Those responsible for offering courses in TT should be aware of these dangers, inform those in training about them, and know how to respond to any psychiatric problems. Informed consent requires that these harms be discussed before people consent to participate in TT.

AVOIDING COERCION

Overt coercion is unlikely to be a problem with TT but this aspect of informed consent can be violated more subtly. The informed consent process is designed to prevent people from being manipulated into making decisions that violate their beliefs or consciences. This can happen through unethical manipulation of the information presented.

For example, Helen's mutterings about Marcelyn being unenlightened and close-minded could pressure Marcelyn into accepting TT. She might even try TT herself but not as a result of an informed decision. An isolated incident will not put much pressure on Marcelyn but repeated incidents, especially if they involve several colleagues, could generate a coercive environment. Ethical resolution of such controversies and conflicts, possibly leading to appropriate policies regarding TT, should involve both sides presenting their cases. A process similar to informed consent should be used with the focus remaining on objective research evidence. Policies will then be based primarily on evidence for effectiveness and safety with the patients' best-interests remaining central.

Similar issues arise when discussing therapies with patients. Informed consent discussions should be clear and open, avoiding covert ways of influencing people. Subtle influences like body language and one's tone of voice could easily bias the presentation of information. Practitioners should describe TT to potential patients, emphasizing the way that it differs from physical touch or massage and stressing that it is based on human life energy, not physical phenomena. Other covert tactics occur in written presentations about TT, and are inappropriate. For example, TT is often compared to massage, biblical laying-on of hands, and everyday touch. Cowens opens her book with this description:

> Therapeutic touch is perhaps the first form of health care ever utilized. Every parent since Adam and Eve has used this practice instinctively when he or she has placed a loving hand on a child to reduce discomfort, help heal a wound, or alleviate a fever. Therapeutic touch is the most human of all forms of healing, using the hands to reach out in service to another person in a gesture of peace, balance, and love. (1996, p. 1)

Yet TT is completely different from comforting a child through physical touch, or holding her hand during a fever. These descriptions go beyond the use of metaphors or word-pictures employed in order to help people understand the nature of a treatment. Patients would rightly feel misled if a surgeon told them she would make "a little cut" when discussing something like open-heart surgery. The description and the actual procedure would be so fundamentally different that the patient would not have consented to the actual procedure involved. Instead, she or he would have been subtly coerced and manipulated into accepting a therapy without being fully informed of its nature.

Another area of coercion arises from the fact that TT originated in several religious practices. Proponents remain adamant, however, that TT is not religious as currently practiced. Most articles state that it does not require "a religious context" but the authors do not explain what this means. Roman Catholic priests bring Holy Communion to hospitalized parishioners, and Native American shamans conduct religious ceremonies in some hospitals. These remain religious practices even if done in hospitals for healing purposes. Prayer is a religious exercise no matter where it is conducted. Practices are religious because of the meaning given them, the powers called upon, and the purposes for which they are performed.

TT is one of a number of practices seeking to address spirituality in health care. Spirituality is often viewed as distinct from religion but in reality the two have much in common. One nursing article defined religion as beliefs and practices "that nurture a relationship with a superior being, force, or power" while spirituality inspires or harmonizes answers to questions about the "meaning and purpose of life and one's relation to the universe" (Emblen, 1992, p. 43). A more recent definition of spirituality as used in nursing literature reveals how much overlap occurs between these two concepts. "Spirituality is defined as experiences and expressions of one's spirit in a unique and dynamic process reflecting faith in God or a supreme being; it is connectedness with oneself, others, nature, or God; and an integration of the dimensions of mind, body, and spirit" (Meraviglia, 1999, p. 24). Until very recently, religion would have been defined in exactly these terms.

The point here is not to attempt to resolve the question of whether religion differs from spirituality. Rather, it is to point out that promotion of TT raises ethical issues concerning the promotion of religion in the guise of healthcare. Proponents claim that TT brings people into contact with their true selves and nature. "Thus, to center oneself means to approach the sacred or divine within" (Cowens, 1996, p. 131). At the same time TT purports to allow people to connect with the universal energy which pervades all things:

> In the end, healing touch is a challenge to the most fundamental beliefs of our society, to our modern world, and to each of us. Yet, it is the most liberating of practices and among the most powerful because it puts you in harmony with a greater reality, one that has sustained the world from the very beginning and will go on sustaining it forever. (Cowens, 1996, p. 219)

The purposes of those promoting TT overlap in many areas with those who promote religious views. One particular perspective on the deeper, spiritual aspects of life is presented and promoted. Having a religious base or being a religious practice does not necessarily mean that TT has no place in modern health care. Patients who want to participate in religious practices like prayer, communion, and other religious ceremonies ought to be able to do so to the extent that they are practical within the confines of the institution. However, when these practices are offered to patients it should be clear that they are religious.

In spite of claims to the contrary, TT remains identical in all essential aspects to the religious practices upon which it is based (Fish, 1995; O'Mathúna, 1998b). Krieger, a Buddhist, admits that TT is based on the same principles as Buddhism (Calvert, 1994). A practice identical to TT but called *auric* or *pranic* healing is found in Western occult and Wiccan religions (Farrar, 1981; Buckland, 1987). One nursing commentator views TT as integral to what she calls New Age nursing. "Is the practice of the New Age nurse deceptive? Do patients' weakened conditions simply make them targets of opportunity? If New Age nursing is care of the soul, is it also usurping the field of those perceived to be more prepared for that task, namely, religious priests, ministers, and rabbis? Or is the nurse a representative of a new religion?" (Barnum, 1996, p. 81).

Refusing to inform patients of this religious background is the equivalent of coercing them into a religious practice they may find offensive. Informed consent would insist that patients and trainees be told of these religious concerns ahead of time. The Equal Employment Opportunity Commission ruled in 1988 that employees cannot be required to learn or practice TT if they believe it conflicts with their religious beliefs. Other New Age practices integral to TT, such as meditation, guided visualization, and inducing altered states of consciousness, are also specified in this policy. "New Age training programs have the potential to create an intimidating work environment. According to judicial interpretation, the term 'religious' includes the New Age philosophy and New Age training programs. Although New Age consultants and employers argue that such training programs are not religious, the courts will likely hold otherwise. Most New Age training courses are derived from Eastern religions such as Buddhism and Hinduism" (Brierton, 1992, p. 419–20).

CONCLUSION

The process of informed consent is integral to the ethical, legal, and professional practice of health care. It ensures both the autonomy of the patient and the role of the healthcare provider as an advocate for the patient. Those offering TT to patients or training others in its practice should adhere to the five aspects involved in informed consent. Of central importance here is the information given to prospective recipients of TT. This information should accurately and clearly describe the practice and its theoretical basis. The research findings, both supportive and nonsupportive, should be described. The lack of evidence for its efficacy based on high quality clinical research should be stressed. The concerns expressed by some regarding the numerous potential adverse effects should be described, as well as the religious underpinnings of the practice. While making these presentations, care should be taken to avoid subtly influencing the prospective patient or biasing the information in order to coerce the patient into accepting the therapy. Only when patients and trainees have been clearly and accurately informed of all these aspects before participating in the therapy can practitioners be confident that they have acted ethically.

REFERENCES

American Nurses Association. 1985. *Code for Nurses With Interpretive Statements*. Kansas City: American Nurses Association.

Barnum, B. S. 1996. *Spirituality in Nursing: From Traditional to New Age*. New York: Springer Publishing Company.

Benor, R. 1996. "Therapeutic Touch." *British Journal of Community Health Nursing* 1 (4): 203–208.

Brierton, T. D. 1992. "Employers' New Age Training Programs Fail to Alter the Consciousness of the EEOC." *Labor Law Journal* (July): 411–20.

Buckland, R. 1987. *Buckland's Complete Book of Witchcraft*. St. Paul, Minn.: Llewellyn Publications.

Calvert, R. 1994. "Dolores Krieger, Ph.D. and Her Therapeutic Touch." *Massage* 47 (January–February): 56–60.

Chopra, D. 1995. *Creating Health*. Rev. ed. Random House Audio Publishing, audiocasette.

Claman, H. N. 1994. *Report of the Chancellor's Committee on Therapeutic Touch*. Denver: University of Colorado Health Sciences Center.

Clark, P. E., and M. J. Clark. 1984. "Therapeutic Touch: Is There a Scientific Basis for the Practice?" *Nursing Research* 33: 37–41.

Cowens, D. 1996. *A Gift for Healing: How You Can Use Therapeutic Touch*. New York: Crown Trade Paperbacks.

Daniels, G. J., and P. McCabe. 1994. "Nursing Diagnosis and Natural Therapies: A Symbiotic Relationship." *Journal of Holistic Nursing* 12 (June): 184–92.

Darbyshire, P. 1989. "Responsibility, Accountability, and Advocacy: Student Nurse Dilemmas, Part II." *Irish Nursing Forum and Health Services* 7 (May–June): 18–22.

Ellis, P. A. 1995. "The Role of the Nurse as the Patient's Advocate." *Professional Nurse* 11 (3): 206–207.

Emblen, J. D. 1992. "Religion and Spirituality Defined According to Current Use in Nursing Literature." *Journal of Professional Nursing* 8 (1): 41–47.

Engebretson, J., and D. Wardell. 1993. "A Contemporary View of Alternative Healing Modalities." *Nurse Practitioner* 18 (September): 51–55.

Equal Employment Opportunity Commission. 1988. *Notice* (September 2) N-915.022.

Farrar, J., and S. Farrar. 1981. *The Rituals.* Volume 2 of *A Witches' Bible Compleat.* New York: Magickal Childe.

Fish, S. 1995. "Therapeutic Touch: Healing Science or Psychic Midwife?" *Christian Research Journal* (summer): 28–38.

Fletcher, D. M. 1992. "Unconventional Cancer Treatments: Professional, Legal, and Ethical Issues." *Oncology Nursing Forum* 19 (9): 1351–54.

France, N. E. M. 1991. "A Phenomenological Inquiry on the Child's Lived Experience of Perceiving the Human Energy Field using Therapeutic Touch." Ph.D. diss., University of Colorado.

Gaylord, N., and P. Grace. 1995. "Nursing Advocacy: An Ethic of Practice." *Nursing Ethics* 2: 11–18.

Glickman, R., and E. J. Gracely. 1998. "Therapeutic Touch: Investigation of a Practitioner." *Scientific Review of Alternative Medicine* 2: 43–47.

Hughes, P. P., R. Meize-Grochowski, and C. N. D. Harris. 1996. "Therapeutic Touch with Adolescent Psychiatric Patients." *Journal of Holistic Nursing* 14 (1): 6–23.

Jonasen, A. M. 1994. "Therapeutic Touch: A Holistic Approach to Perioperative Nursing." *Today's O.R. Nurse* 16 (January–February): 7–12.

Krieger, D. 1993. *Accepting Your Power to Heal: The Personal Practice of Therapeutic Touch.* Santa Fe, N.Mex.: Bear & Company.

———. 1979. *The Therapeutic Touch: How to Use Your Hands to Help or to Heal.* Engelwood Cliffs, N.J.: Prentice-Hall.

———. 1997. *Therapeutic Touch Inner Workbook: Ventures in Transpersonal Healing.* Santa Fe, N.Mex.: Bear & Company.

Mackey, R. 1995. "Discover the Healing Power of Therapeutic Touch." *American Journal of Nursing* 95 (4): 27–32.

Macrae, J. 1979. "Therapeutic Touch in Practice." *American Journal of Nursing* (April): 664–65.

Meehan, T. C. 1998. "Therapeutic Touch as a Nursing Intervention." *Journal of Advanced Nursing* 28 (1): 117–25.

———. 1993. "Therapeutic Touch and Postoperative Pain: A Rogerian Research Study." *Nursing Science Quarterly* 6: 69–78.

Meraviglia, M. G. 1999. "Critical Analysis of Spirituality and Its Empirical Indicators." *Journal of Holistic Nursing* 17 (1): 18–33.

Ng, B. Y. 1999. "Qigong-Induced Mental Disorders: A Review." *Australian and New Zealand Journal of Psychiatry* 33 (2): 197–206.

Norton, L. 1995. "Complementary Therapies in Practice: The Ethical Issues." *Journal of Clinical Nursing* 4 (6): 343–48.

O'Mathúna, D. P. 1998a. "Therapeutic Touch: What Could Be the Harm?" *Scientific Review of Alternative Medicine* 2 (1): 56–62

———. 1998b. "The Subtle Allure of Therapeutic Touch." *Journal of Christian Nursing,* 15 (1): 4–13.

————. In press. "Misrepresentation of Therapeutic Touch Research in Reviews." *Image: Journal of Nursing Scholarship.*

Otis, L. S. 1984. "Adverse Effects of Transcendental Meditation." In *Meditation: Classic and Contemporary Perspectives.* Edited by Deane H. Shapiro Jr. and Roger N. Walsh. New York: Aldone, pp. 201–207.

Parkes, B. S. 1985. "Therapeutic Touch as an Intervention to Reduce Anxiety in Elderly Hospitalized Patients." Ph.D. diss., University of Texas at Austin.

Quinn, J. F. 1984. "Therapeutic Touch as Energy Exchange: Testing the Theory." *Advances in Nursing Science* 6 (1): 42–49.

————. 1989. "Therapeutic Touch as Energy Exchange: Replication and Extension." *Nursing Science Quarterly* 2 (2): 79–87.

Rosa, L., E. Rosa, L. Sarner, et al. 1998. "A Close Look at Therapeutic Touch." *Journal of the American Medical Association* 279: 1005–10.

Sampson, W., and B. L. Beyerstein. 1996. "Traditional Medicine and Pseudoscience in China: A Report of the Second CSICOP Delegation (Part 2)." *Skeptical Inquirer* 21 (1).

Scheiber, B., and C. Selby. 1997. "UAB Final Report of Therapeutic Touch—An Appraisal." *Skeptical Inquirer* 21 (3): 53–54.

Schlotfeldt, R. M. 1973. "Critique of the Relationship of Touch with Intent to Help or Heal to Subjects' in-vivo Hemoglobin Values: A Study in Personalized Interaction." In American Nurses' Association, *Proceedings of the Ninth ANA Nursing Research Conference.* New York: American Nurses' Association, pp. 59–65.

Selby, C., and B. Scheiber. 1996. "Science or Pseudoscience? Pentagon Grant Funds alternative Health Study." *Skeptical Inquirer* 20 (4): 15–17.

Shapiro, D. H., Jr. 1992. "Adverse Effects of Meditation: A Preliminary Investigation of Long-Term Meditators." *International Journal of Psychosomatics* 29: 62–66.

Thorpe, B. 1994. "Touch: A Modality Missing from Your Practice?" *Advance for Nurse Practitioners* 2 (February): 8–10.

Turner, J. G. 1994. *The Effect of Therapeutic Touch on Pain and Infection in Burn Patients.* Tri-Service Nursing Research Grant # MDA 905-94-Z-0080 and Application # N94-020.

Walike, B. C., et al. 1975. ". . . attempts to embellish a totally unscientific process with the aura of science . . ." in Letters, *American Journal of Nursing* 75 (August): 1275, 1278, 1282.

Wirth, D. P. 1995. "Complementary Healing Intervention and Dermal Wound Reepithelialization: An Overview." *International Journal of Psychosomatics* 42 (1–4): 48–53.

Wytias, C. A. 1994. "Therapeutic Touch in Primary Care." *Nurse Practitioner Forum* 5 (June): 91–97.

Young, M. A. 1998. "What Are You Doing to My Patient?" *Journal of Christian Nursing* 15 (1): 11.

5.

The Distortion of Martha Rogers's Theory by Therapeutic Touch Practitioners*

Michael Stanwick

Throughout the Therapeutic Touch literature (Benor, 1996; Daley, 1997; Meehan, 1985, 1998; Quinn, 1989; Sameral et al., 1998; Turner et al., 1998) it is often claimed that Martha Rogers's "Science Of Unitary Human Beings" (SUHB) (Rogers, 1970, 1986, 1990, 1992) provides a theoretical rationale for TT.

The essential question becomes: Does the "nursing theoretical framework developed by [Martha] Rogers (1970, 1990)," as Meehan (1998) describes it, truly provide the theoretical foundation for the central claim on which TT is based? In other words, are the "energy fields" that Rogers describes concordant in any way with the "energy" that TT practitioners claim to manipulate?

Central to this question is what Rogers intended her SUHB to be used for. Her conceptual system "provides a way of perceiving people and their world" (Rogers, 1986, 1992). Essentially, Rogers' SUHB is a framework of her beliefs which amounts to an attempt *to provide a way of viewing or conceptualizing the world as being organized in a certain way for the purpose of controlling certain processes within it.* It is clear from this context that "perceiving" has a precise meaning, that is, to apprehend with the mind, to comprehend or understand—to conceive. It does not apply to the act of apprehending through one of the senses, such as sight or touch. As Turner states, for example:

> Our present technology does not allow measurement of the human energy field, but to a trained sense, primarily touch, the human energy field can be perceived and assessed. (1994, p. 40)

---

*The author would like to make it known that the use of Rogers's theory in this chapter should not be taken in any way as either and endorsement or as an evaluation of the scientific validity of her theory.

It is difficult to comprehend how Rogers's abstract notion can be sensed by touch. This is an important distinction with respect to the use of energy fields in the practice of TT which will, we hope, become clear in the course of this discussion.

Returning to Rogers' notion of "energy field" a clear description may be found in her various publications describing the SUHB. For example:

> Unitary human beings are specified to be irreducible wholes. A whole cannot be understood when it is reduced to its particulars. . . . The unitary nature of environment is equally irreducible. The concept of *field* provides a means of perceiving people and their environments as irreducible wholes. (Rogers, 1986 p. 4)

Further:

> Energy fields are postulated to constitute the fundamental unit of the living and the nonliving. Field, then, is a unifying concept and energy signifies the dynamic nature of the field. Energy fields are infinite and pandimensional; they are in continuous motion. (Rogers, 1992, p. 30)

Here, Rogers uses the concept of "field" as a means of perceiving the conditions or "states of being" of an individual and his or her environment. This is achieved by considering that it has, among others, the qualities of "infiniteness," "openness," "pandimensionality," "irreducibility" and "indivisibility."

Thus, in Rogers's scheme, in order to be able to understand an individual, his or her environment, and the relationship between the two, she or he must first be perceived as infinite, open, pandimensional, irreducible, and indivisible wholes, that is, as fields.

In her scheme therefore, there are two "irreducible wholes" or fields—the human, as an individual or as a group (Rogers, 1990, 1992), and the environmental, and both of these irreducible wholes are considered to be openly and continuously involved in a mutual interplay, or what Rogers calls a mutual process (Rogers, 1990), so that they become integral with one another. For the purpose of this analysis it is not necessary to examine the nature of this "process," as Rogers would have it. All that is required is a recognition that Rogers' fields are meant to interact in some way or another. This continuous mutual activity or process is another facet of a field and is also a constituent of a key Rogerian concept—"energy."

Thus, fields are also perceived or considered to be dynamic or in continuous motion (Rogers, 1990, 1992). This additional quality of a field is denoted by the term energy. This quality indicates the "dynamic nature" of the field (Rogers, 1992) and is described by Rogers in her

"Principles of Homeodynamics" (Rogers, 1986, 1990, 1992). Here, the dynamism or continuous motion of a particular field involves continuous change, continuous, innovative, and unpredictable diversity, and continuous mutual interplay or interaction with other fields. Again, it is not necessary for the purpose of this analysis to examine the nature of this dynamism. All that is required is a recognition that, for Rogers, the term "energy" indicates that her fields are dynamic—in other words, her fields are "energetic."

All of these attributes of the dynamic nature of a field, summed up by the descriptive term "energy," affect another key abstract quality of a field, that of "pattern." In Rogers's scheme, each field is postulated to have its own unique pattern which is inferred from the manifestations or outcomes of interacting fields. According to Cowling in Samarel et al.,

> manifestations of field pattern are experienced or observed. These manifestations emerge out of the human and environmental field mutual process and take the form of individuals experiences, perceptions, and expressions. (1998, p. 1370)

In this study, these manifestations were said to be represented by the patients expressions of anxiety, mood, and pain.

In summary, it is clear that Rogers' concept of field is designed to be a means of perceiving or conceptualizing human beings and their environments as irreducible regions or wholes—hence the claim that "human beings *are* energy fields, they do not *have* them" (Rogers, 1986). Rogers's fields are also dynamic or in continuous motion and this quality is denoted by the term energy. It is important to keep these notions firmly in mind during the examination of the TT literature, to which we now turn.

By examining how these key Rogerian concepts are used in the context of the TT literature, it is possible to gain an understanding of the meanings given to them by TT practitioners and advocates. The linking of TT energy and the energy fields of Rogers is given explicitly in Keller and Bzedek, who also misrepresent Rogers's idea of Unitary Man—later refined to Unitary Human Being by Rogers—by confusing it with holism:

> Holism is represented in nursing science by Rogers' (1970) theory of unitary man. According to this theory, all persons are highly complex fields of various forms of life energy. (1986, p. 101)

Neither is Rogers's SUBH in any way synonymous with holism—in fact she claims the opposite (Rogers, 1986)—nor do her "energy fields" in any way whatsoever contain a "life energy." But these are the fields of life energy claimed, in the TT literature, to be manipulated by TT practitioners. For example, Meehan describes a patient's nurse assuming that, ". . . in a state of health the energy field as it extended beyond Mr. Cullen's [the patient's] body would move in an open and symmetrical flow" and with respect to the patient's energy field, the nurse could, "through the natural sensitivity of her hands, perceive the pattern of the energy flow as subtle cues in her hands" (1990, p. 75).

This flow of a palpable energy is given further clarification: "Thus, it is posited that human beings are open systems of energy, and exchange of energy is the underlying dynamic of all human and environmental interaction" (Meehan, 1990, p. 201). Recently, this view was also propounded by Turner:

> Central to the practice [of TT] is the assumption of a human energy field and an environment filled with life energy which is also present in all living organisms. During TT, this energy is replenished and balanced through a mutual human and environmental field process facilitated by the practitioner. Support for this view comes from the nursing theory of Martha Rogers (1970, 1990) which is based entirely on a field world view. (1994, p. 40)

More recently still, we find that this view has not changed. For example, in Daley: "The TT perspective postulates that a healthy person has a balance between inward and outward energy flow, with illness being the result of an imbalance or disruption in this energy field or flow" (1997, p. 1125). Here both Turner (1994) and Daley (1997) link Rogers's human "energy field" with TT by filling it with the "life energy" of Krieger. But this field world view of Rogers's does not contain the notion of "field" as an area or region throughout which Krieger's life energy, and the TTers conscious willpower or "conscious intent," exert their influence. Neither is this "field," according to Rogers, something that human beings possess as an adjunct to their bodies. However, this appears to be the case according to Turner et al. (1998), where it is stated that this human energy field extends beyond the skin and therefore, by implication, the body. But, according to Rogers, it is not something that human beings have—it does not extend beyond the skin, it does not extend beyond the body. Turner then goes on to reiterate: "The idea behind TT is that the human energy field is abundant and flows in balanced patterns in health, but is depleted, blocked, and/or unbalanced in injury or illness. During TT, the practitioner replenishes depleted energy and clears and rebalances the energy flow in the injured person through conscious intent and hand movements which repattern the energy flow" (1998, p.12).

Now Rogers's field is said, by Turner, to flow as if it were a physical phenomenon—a field of flowing energy that is capable of being manipulated at will via the practitioners hands. This is similarly described in Samarel et al.: "The practitioners hands are used to pattern accumulated areas of tension in the human energy field" by "focusing intent on the specific direction of the patient's energy field pattern manifestation; and using the hands to pattern energy with the intent of facilitating positive experiences" (1998, p. 1370). Similarly, Meehan (1998) also states that "the nurse notes the overall pattern of energy flow and any area of imbalance or impeded flow."

From this review of the TT literature regarding Rogers's fields, it is clear that TT's "energy field" and Rogers's "field" are incongruous. For example, examination of the excerpt above from Turner et al. (1998), reveals a fundamental misunderstanding of Rogers's concepts. Her abstract fields are not abundant nor depleted or blocked or unbalanced with energy; in fact, they are incapable of being so. Neither can her abstract patterns be assigned to Krieger's life energy and so be repatterned as Turner describes. Rogers's fields are not fields of energy and they are not reducible to component parts, such as energy for example. Further, as noted above, nowhere in Rogers's framework of the SUHB is there an inherent universal healing energy, as Meehan (1998) correctly notes. Nor is there an energy field that human beings have or their environments have that extends beyond the skin, and therefore their body, as a region in which healing energy exists and is experienced and manipulated through and by the hands.

This incongruity with Rogers's ideas appears to be recognized by Meehan. In response to the way the Science of Unitary Human Beings was presented in a TT research proposal, she notes that "the definitions of the [TT] interventions and the explanation of the theoretical rationale for them are not always congruent with the Science of Unitary Human Beings as it is most currently stated." Furthermore, "the statement that 'energy exchange is the underlying dynamic of all human and environmental interaction' should be changed to 'mutual human-environmental process is the underlying dynamic of all human and environmental fields' ... 'energy transfer' should be changed to 'mutual process' and 'energy exchange' should be changed to 'energy process' " (Meehan, 1990, p. 202). With reference to a description of a TT intervention this restatement became:

> The nurse is viewed as being integral with the patient's environmental energy field patterning, and therapeutic touch treatment is viewed as a purposive patterning of energy field mutual process in which the nurse uses his or her hands as a mediating focus in the continuing pat-

terning of the mutual patient-environmental energy field process.
(Meehan, 1990, p. 74)

Now of course, the TT advocate's incongruous notion of a manipulable universal life energy has disappeared, to be replaced with another equal incongruity—a purposive patterning of energy field mutual process. This is incongruous because pattern, according to Rogers, is an abstraction incapable of manipulation and is only inferred from observable phenomena, her pattern manifestations. In the absence of any evidence in accord with a relevant background scientific knowledge, this restatement of the TT process in Rogerian terminology could be interpreted as no more than a TT practitioner attempting to effect a positive outcome from the patient by engaging in wishful thinking and hand movements.

In summary, these references to energy and energy fields in TT literature are not the concepts of Rogers. According to Rogers, energy signifies the dynamic nature of a field and field is a unifying concept (Malinski, 1986). For Rogers, her terms represent abstract concepts that are an attempt to provide a way of perceiving an individual, his or her environment, and the relationship between the two. She does not describe them as physical phenomena capable of being perceived, manipulated or exchanged by a TT practitioner's hands.

TT practitioners' confusion about Rogers's terminology could have arisen for a number of reasons. Rogers often used vague language when precision was required or used vague language that seems precise. It is no surprise for example, that in Malinski's (1986) discussions of Rogers's metaphysics, misinterpretation and then misrepresentation of her key concepts occurs and as a consequence ambiguity is created. Thus, following a discussion of TT, Malinski (1986) states, in language probably derived from Krieger, that the nurse assesses and unruffles the field and balances the flow of energy. In the following paragraph Malinski then encapsulates this term in what appears to be a misrepresentation of Rogers's ideas: "Given that people and environment are integral, that all is related within a dynamic flow of energy patterning" (Malinski, 1986, p. 26). This could lead the reader to incorrectly equate flow of energy in the preceding paragraph with flow of energy patterning in the subsequent paragraph to which, from the analysis of Rogers above, it bears no similarity. Rogers's notion of "pattern" does not refer to life energy. In other words, "pattern" refers explicitly to an "energy field" not, as Malinski misinterprets, to some imposed "life energy" within it, that is, not to a "field of life energy."

Further, carelessly juxtaposing language from popular works on quantum mechanics against similar language of Rogers when attempting to draw parallels between the two can lead to error. For example, "Capra points out that relativity theory tells us that mass is a form of energy. Although the definition of *field* varies between Rogers and Capra, the idea that underlying everything is energy patterning seems consistent" (Malinski, 1986, p. 21). Here, the reader could be forgiven for interpreting the concept of energy, as defined in physics, to be synonymous with that in Rogers's framework—which it clearly is not. Whatever the cause, TT practitioners and advocates with reference to the TT literature *reify* Rogers's metaphysical concepts, that is, they treat them as though they are physical, albeit nonempirical, phenomena.

In conclusion, the abstract energy fields of Rogers and the energy fields of TT practitioners and advocates are not the same. Neither is the energy that TT practitioners claim they manipulate to be found anywhere in Martha Rogers's SUHB. This energy is also incongruent with Rogers's notions of energy, pattern, and energy field. As a consequence, TT theorists and practitioners cannot appeal to Rogers with reference to these two concepts in particular as if they were identifying specific concrete interconnections and processes of change, and so neither can they claim that Rogers provides a theoretical foundation on which to base TT.

Thus, the claim that there is an actual connection between patients and nurses that permits the process of TT is not made more credible, intelligible, or precise by the abstract metaphysical postulates that objects and their environments in some way or another form irreducible and indivisible wholes ("fields") that are dynamic or energetic ("energy") *in some way or another*. The theoretical work required by TT remains to be done, including that of rendering its claims consistent with a background scientific knowledge untouched and unchanged by Rogers's belief that the world is organized in a certain way.

REFERENCES

Benor, R. 1996. "Therapeutic Touch." *British Journal of Community Health Nursing* 1 (4): 203–208.

Daley, B. 1997. "Therapeutic Touch, Nursing Practice, and Contemporary Cutaneous Wound Healing Research." *Journal of Advanced Nursing* 25: 1123–32.

Keller, E., and V. Bzedek. 1986. "Effects of Therapeutic Touch on Tension Headache Pain." *Nursing Research* 35 (2): 101–106.

Malinski, V. M. 1986. *Explorations on Martha Rogers Science of Unitary Human Beings*. Norwalk, Conn.: Appleton-Century-Crofts.

Meehan, M. T. C. 1985. *The Effect of Therapeutic Touch on the Experience of Acute Pain in Postoperative Patients*. New York University, University Microfilms #DA85-10765.

———. 1990. "The Science of Unitary Human Beings and Theory-Based Practice: Therapeutic Touch." In *Visions of Rogers' Science-Based Nursing*. Edited by E. A. M. Barrett. New York: National League of Nursing.

———. 1998. "Therapeutic Touch as a Nursing Intervention." *Journal of Advanced Nursing*, 28 (1): 117–25.

Quinn, J. 1989. "Therapeutic Touch as Energy Exchange: Replication and Extension." *Nursing Science Quarterly* 2 (2): 79–87.

Rogers, M. 1970. *An Introduction to the Theoretical Basis of Nursing*. Philadelphia, Pa: F. A: Davis Co.

———. 1986. "Science of Unitary Human Beings." In *Explorations on Martha Rogers Science Of Unitary Human Beings*. Edited by V. M. Malinski. Nowalk, Conn.: Appleton-Century-Crofts.

———. 1990. "Nursing: Science of Unitary, Irreducible, Human Beings: Update 1990." In *Visions of Rogers' Science-Based Nursing*. Edited by E. A. M. Barrett. New York: National League of Nursing.

———. 1992. "Nursing Science and the Space Age." *Nursing Science Quarterly* 5 (1): 27–34.

Samarel, N., J. Fawcett, M. M. Davis, and R. M. Francisca. 1998. "Effects of Dialogue and Therapeutic Touch on Preoperative and Postoperative Experiences of Breast Cancer Surgery: An Exploratory Study." *Oncology Nursing Forum* 25 (8): 1369–76.

Turner, J. G. 1994. *The Effect of Therapeutic Touch on Pain and Infection in Burn Patients*. Tri-Service Nursing Research Grant Application N94-020

Turner, J. G., A. J. Clark, D. K. Gauthier, and M. Williams. 1998. "The Effect of Therapeutic Touch on Pain and Anxiety in Burn Patients." *Journal of Advanced Nursing* 28 (1): 10–20.

6.

Touch of Mysticism

Robert Glickman
with an introduction by James Randi

INTRODUCTION

Therapeutic Touch or TT is a disturbing phenomenon that has spread rapidly throughout the medical community, specifically among those in the nursing profession.

Bob Glickman is a registered nurse in Philadelphia. He is proud of his honorable profession and dismayed at how many people in the nursing community, including the principal professional associations, have uncritically embraced TT and use it regularly even though there has never been any proven therapeutic value.

Glickman tried for months to coax practitioners of Therapeutic Touch to submit to a simple, inexpensive test of their claims here at the Foundation. His report will give you some idea of just how they wriggle when confronted with a legitimate challenge of their claims.

TT has been used increasingly in hospitals over the past twenty years. It consists of a practitioner running his or her hands over the body of the patient, about six inches away from the person. It is claimed that the practitioner can detect what is called the "human energy field" (HEF) and that it can be felt as distinctly as if it were a layer of sponge rubber. The practitioner can then adjust this field to the advantage of the patient, we're told.

Tests of cures claimed to have been attained through TT would be extraordinarily expensive, subject to many variables, and liable to produce endless discussion and argument. Bob Glickman and I decided it

Originally published in *Swift* 1, no. 2 (1997). Copyright © 1997 James Randi Education Foundation. Reprinted with permission from authors and publisher. The author would like to thank James Randi for his guidance and Chip Denman for his superior editing skills.

seemed best to test the basic claim: that the HEF could be detected by an experienced practitioner and that it could be detected with an accuracy that would establish its existence.

What follows is an interesting dialogue between Bob and some folks on an Internet e-mail discussion group devoted to Therapeutic Touch.

—James Randi

DISSCUSSION

The single test of N.W. [see chapter 16 in this volume] was deemed a good start into the investigation of TT. Obviously, more TTPs [Therapeutic Touch Practitioners] would have to be tested before a true picture on the ability of TTPs to feel HEFs would emerge. A second test was to be conducted at the James Randi Educational Foundation in Ft. Lauderdale, Florida on June 2, 3, and 4, 1997. The judge for the test would have been PBS's *Scientific American Frontiers* TV program. Since it was feared that TTPs would decline taking the test stating that Randi would use his magician skills to prevent them from passing the test, this arrangement was made with the producers of the program. By placing the supervision and judging of the test under the authority of SAF, we hoped to circumvent this claim.

The test would use a fiberglass construct with two sleeves to allow for the insertion of a subject's arms. The TT practitioner (TTP) would assess the energy emanating from the construct to determine whether the right or left sleeve was occupied as determined by a randomizing coin flip. Following some preliminary trials, a score of fifteen or greater out of twenty would be considered a positive result and would allow that practitioner to advance to the final test. This final test would be done the following day and a score of twenty out of twenty would win the $1,100,000 award.

One of the many places to look for potential TT practitioners is on the Internet. I submitted the challenge to the Nurse Rogers e-mail service where devotees of Martha Rogers discuss her many theories and Therapeutic Touch. For the most part, the invitation wasn't well received.

Francis C. Biley, R.N., Ph.D., of the University of Wales College of Medicine is a contributing author of *The Theory and Practice of Therapeutic Touch* published by Churchill Livingstone (1995) and coordinator of the International Region of the Society of Rogerian Scholars. She is also the listowner of the Nurse Rogers e-mail discussion group. "After spending some time on formulating a critique of the methodology for the following quasiexperiment, I have decided that it really isn't worth doing," said Biley. "Although I applaud Glickman and his associates for spending time on the subject, it is quite obvious that they need to expand their methodological understanding beyond 'if you can't measure it, it doesn't exist.' "

Ana Cris da Sal is an R.N. and a nursing researcher in Brazil. "I am getting skeptic [*sic*] by the skeptic methods," said Cris da Sal. "They seem to be so . . . hmmm . . . antique?! A researcher, a real one, before accepting or not the phenomenon, should study it (by modern methods, of course). TT, for instance, should be tested beside quantum physics and physiology. I'll be pleased to win the prize proving—or not, as a real researcher must think—the existence of the human energetic field."

Joanne Griffin is a TT researcher at New York University. "I almost treat messages like the one from Mr. Glickman like the jokes which I usually enjoy enormously and often forward to my friends," said Griffin. "It seems obvious to me that he does not understand the basic definition of energy field as Rogers used the term, and it isn't worth the time to respond."

I responded to these rather negative outlooks. "I thought this was an open [Internet] board with people open to new ideas," I replied. "I thought TT proponents would appreciate the chance to prove to the waiting world that TT's HEF exists."

One of the main problems with Rogerian Science is the duality and elusiveness of simple meanings. All too often, much discussion on these postings was devoted to the defining of concepts. The term "human energy field" sometimes referred to the TT HEF in a Rogerian context and sometimes it didn't. However, most of the writers in this service seemed to accept the notion of the TT concept and its HEF.

The "not-worth-doing" argument didn't make sense to me. The test doesn't need extremely large sample groups, complicated procedures, extreme methodological strategies and statistics, or even quantum mechanics. It's not an "if-you-can't-measure-it, it-doesn't-exist" notion. TT practitioners have made the claim that they feel energy fields. We simply designed a test to see if they can.

"I feel that this is important research in spite of the fact that it may seem too simplistic to some," I explained, in the course of my ongoing online dialogue. "Had research such as this been done in the infancy of TT and Rogerian Science, maybe this challenge wouldn't be necessary now."

Biley, at this point, encouraged me to keep on posting. She also agreed about the duality and elusiveness of simple meanings, and the fact that Rogerians spend a lot of time defining concepts. "I sometimes wish that they could just get on with it," she said, "but then I think it's the beginning of an evolving science and there is much we don't yet understand."

At this point, I thought I had my foot in the door. "I am glad you see my point about the elusiveness of definitive meanings for terms in Rogerian Science and that there is much that is not yet understood," I wrote. "This is why I'm sure that you know that it is important to follow the scientific method. In an evolving science, the scientific method is even more important. It prevents confusion and the contradiction of terms."

"Let me state for the record that the I am not a Therapeutic Touch practitioner," wrote Martha H. Bramlett R.N., Ph.D. "While I've taken classes and have used it on occasion (and my recipients have reported positive results), I certainly do not place myself in the class with some of the experts that have participated in this discussion.

"The crux of this issue seems to be one in which sciences are clashing," she continued. "Mr. Glickman is making a sincere effort to try to understand a purported phenomenon. Yet when presented to the Rogerian Science nursing community, the effort has met with great consternation. Several things contribute to this. First, the term Therapeutic Touch is somewhat imprecise since Rogerian Therapeutic Touch as pioneered by Dr. Krieger has a very different theoretical base than that presented by many of those who report themselves to be Therapeutic Touch practitioners. Thus, when Mr. Glickman says Therapeutic Touch, we don't even know if we're talking about the same thing, and in fact, from the discourse, I feel sure we're probably not.

"Many have tried to explain this difference; however, if each of us remember [sic] back to when we first started working with Rogerian Science, we will probably all remember the struggle we endured to hone the conceptual picture involved. Our conceptual perspective dictates what we see, and sometimes limits our abilities to see through another perspective. Science is replete with examples of this. Einstein altered his formulas because his belief in a static universe was so compelling, he couldn't believe his own calculations, and he later admitted this.

"The question arises as to what constitutes scientific investigation. I think many of the Therapeutic Touch practitioners and Rogerian scientists have tried to explain to Mr. Glickman that his tests are inappropriate for the phenomenon to be tested. The energy field he is trying to measure is not the one we're saying we feel. Perhaps at some point such a measure will exist, but not right now. I would ask Mr. Glickman to be patient with our science and our methodologies. I do not ask him to accept what we say, only to allow for the possibility that it may exist, and at some point of evolution our methods may provide him with the proof he so desires."

I responded that we weren't interested in investigating a purported phenomenon. "We are not sure there is one," I wrote. "What we are trying to investigate is a legitimate claim. That claim is that TTPs are able to feel HEFs. The water is definitely muddied as to how to define these fields. That is not my fault. I am more or less stumbling into a work in progress and am trying to sort things out. You say that you had taken TT classes and used the technique. Did you feel an HEF? Were the TT courses Rogerian-based or the other type? These aren't my terms. I am willing to test any TTP who states they can feel an energy field, be they Rogerian or not. I see nothing in the test we have devised that could be considered inappropriate. TTPs of all stripes claim to feel HEFs. What is so complicated about that? Why wouldn't anyone want this to be tested?"

They really lost me with the statement that "the energy field he is trying to measure is not the one we're saying we feel." The energy field I was trying to measure was exactly the one the Rogerians were saying they felt!

"I think a Rogerian would say that they 'perceive' a field manifestation, rather than feel a field, i.e., we chose to call what ever [*sic*] is going on a perception of an energy field rather than say that it is an energy field or is energy," Biley wrote.

The debate continued. "Last time the test was offered, I said all that I had to say about the matter," said Richard Cowling, R.N., referring to several e-mail exchanges he and I had prior to a November 1996 TT test in Philadelphia, in which one rather maverick TTP came from Los Angeles and tried the test. She scored chance results. "I think that the dialogue spawned by this test has done a great deal of good by allowing people to openly describe various vantage points. I do not share Mr. Glickman's philosophy of science, but respect his right, as I hope he does mine, to advocate for a specific world view."

I had been writing all along in the simplest and clearest terms possible to avoid any misunderstanding. I had also studied the evidence for TT. From Krieger's initial hemoglobin study to the present, supporting evidence is virtually nonexistent. TT studies have suffered from poor design, poor methodology, poor controls, improper or absent double-blinding measures, and improper statistics.

The healing effects noted by many TT practitioners can too easily be attributed to the placebo effect. This is the prime source of static and false positives in healing studies. To make any definitive statement about any healing modality, it must be effectively ruled out in any study. The TT scientific research was groundless. In Rogerian Science, speculation is mounted on more speculation, creating newer and grander ideas, but no actual specific testing is done. If anything, many of these ideas are beyond testing. Without this vital testing, upon which factual and useful data can be built, statements like "I believe that [an] energy field is not emanating and physically palpable, but rather manifest as pattern" are virtually devoid of meaning.

Richard Cowling wrote to me, encouraging my attendance at a conference in Los Angeles sponsored by the University of Southern California, University of California at Los Angeles, and University of California at Irvine called "Reclaiming Voice: Ethnographic Inquiry and Qualitative Research in a Post-Modern Age." He quoted the introductory description, which began: "At a time when the pressure for change in the academy is increasingly linked to the resurgence of conservative and neoliberal discourses and practices, researchers need to be more direct in countering the attacks in the public space against alternative methodologies. While the need for research to be theoretically rigorous and ethically accountable is vital, we must be clear that rigor and accountability are not the sole provinces of conservative and neoliberal educational discourses and practices.

This became the last bit of actual dialogue that I was going to receive from the Rogerians. So I ended with this parting shot:

> Richard, my words here are meant to be a constructive criticism and not an attack or a lack of respect for you and your efforts and the efforts of others. As a nurse, I am interested in what effects Rogerian Science and TT will have on my profession. I have examined the TT research thoroughly. I have only begun looking into Rogerian Science, but the combined TT/Rogerian research I have reviewed is poor. Wishful thinking is the engine that drives science, but it can't be the science by itself. There are all kinds of "sciences" out there that are actually pseudosciences. Many have the rubber stamp of approval of apparent scientific boards and Universities. TT is also considered by many to be "scientific" and this has been expressed in volumes of literature and support. It is also featured and promoted by many universities and nursing organizations such as the ANA and NLN. This support still doesn't make TT scientific. With TT, the science has been totally ignored. The scientific literature on TT is baseless. Although accepted by too many in nursing, no one has yet been able to prove the most basic tenet of TT: Can anyone actually feel a field?
>
> There are several gurus today who have attracted a large following by mixing mainstream medicine with a multitude of fantasy ideas. Not knowing the difference between fantasy and reality is dangerous. People who don't know the difference but should and have a "scientific" background are perhaps among the most dangerous of all.

POSTSCRIPT

The fallout from the SRAM and JAMA articles challenging the ability of TTPs to feel the HEF has been interesting. Proponents of TT have placed their efforts in criticizing the research and intentions of the skeptical investigators. Such criticism is a legitimate and important part of the scientific process. However, it would also be expected that when a challenge is made to an area of legitimate scientific study that its supporters would respond with research and study addressing the questions raised and providing experimental confirmation of their contending claims. If TTPs truly have the ability to feel energy fields, it would be advantageous to both sides of the debate for TT proponents to work with skeptical TT investigators to develop a mutually agreed-upon test that would establish the ability of a TTP to feel a HEF, while dealing with the limitations TTPs perceive in skeptical research.

TT promoters fail to acknowledge the obvious fact they have yet to prove that an HEF can be felt, much less manipulated, via the human hands. It is an ominous and staggering notion to consider that over 40,000 professional nurses may have tricked themselves into thinking they can feel an energy field. Yet until they can demonstrate their ability to sense an HEF, the assumption stands that they simply cannot.

This leads to the next predictable response from TT proponents: that an ability to sense the HEF is not critical to the efficacy of TT. Proponents of TT now claim that the intention to heal is the only necessary factor when dealing with TT. If that is the case, then the North American Nursing Diagnosis Association should remove "Energy Field Disturbance" from the official nursing diagnosis list.

7.

Therapeutic Touch in Mass Media, Specialized Media, and on the Internet: Content, Community, and Controversy*

William Evans

Alternative medicine in general and Therapeutic Touch in particular have entered a new era of respectability—and profitability. Approximately 42 percent of United States adults utilized one or more alternative medical therapies in 1997 (Eisenberg et al., 1998). Roughly 43 percent of those who used alternative therapies in 1997 also visited an alternative medical practitioner. Eisenberg (1998) estimates that Americans spent $21.2 billion on visits to alternative medical practitioners in 1997. Moreover, the percentage of adults who utilized alternative medicine increased substantially between 1990 and 1997 (Eisenberg et al., 1993, 1998), suggesting that the 1990s will likely be remembered as the decade in which alternative medicine went mainstream.

TT is often classified as a form of "energy healing," along with *Reiki* and magnet therapy. According to Eisenberg et al. (1998), visits to energy healers increased more than 500 percent between 1990 and 1997. Roughly 1.9 million Americans visited an energy healer of one sort or another at least once in 1997.

TT is among the most commonly utilized and most commonly talked about forms of energy healing. Indeed, it is one of the most visible of all alternative therapies. The success of TT in attracting consumer attention—and consumer dollars—is due in no small part to its success in the nursing community. It has been championed by many nurses, and it is practiced by nurses in many hospitals in the United States and around the world (Rosa et al., 1998). As a result, Therapeutic Touch enjoys much media attention in both specialized medical publications as well as popular news media.

Which is not to say that the efficacy of TT has been established via

*The author offers his thanks to Rebecca Long, Béla Scheiber, and Stanley Verhoeven for their advice and assistance in the preparation of this chapter.

empirical research. Most mainstream nurses and physicians remain skeptical regarding the claims of its proponents and practitioners. It remains one of the most controversial of alternative therapies. This chapter examines the role of mass media, specialized media, and the Internet in the dissemination of information regarding TT. This includes information regarding TT that is aimed at nurses, physicians, and alternative health advocates, as well as its popular news coverage that reaches more general audiences. An analysis of texts targeted at various audiences can help us understand the popular appeal of TT and the role of media in public understanding (and misunderstanding) of it.

THERAPEUTIC TOUCH IN SOCIAL AND HISTORICAL CONTEXT

Dolores Krieger is typically credited as the founder of TT. Her book, *The Therapeutic Touch: How to Use Your Hands to Help or to Heal* was published in 1979 and remains one of the most frequently cited publications regarding TT. Krieger's article "Therapeutic Touch: The Imprimatur of Nursing" was published in the *American Journal of Nursing* in 1975 and represents the first extended account of TT to appear in a nursing journal.

But one must look back well beyond 1975 if one is to understand the origin and evolution of TT. Both critics and advocates of TT have claimed that it can be viewed as a contemporary version of healing via the "laying-on of hands," a folk- and religious-healing practice used in various forms in many cultures for many centuries. In fact, Krieger writes that "Therapeutic Touch derives from a mode of healing that persons of all cultures since the dawn of documented history have been able to use" (1979, p. 17). When asked about predecessors of TT, one of its practitioners responded:

> The predecessor is the laying-on of hands. That's probably the oldest and most basic healing technique. You'll find laying-on of hands in the Bible, and you can find references to some type of laying-on of hands in the earliest recorded histories. The difference is that the laying-on of hands is typically done within some kind of religious framework. It's linked with faith. The hands are laid on, and (supposedly) the faith of the recipient is what allows the healing to happen. In Therapeutic Touch there's no assumption that the recipient must believe anything. They don't even have to know that it's happening for there to be an effect. It need not take place in a religious or spiritual framework. It may, if that is the belief system held by the practitioner, but it need not, which makes it applicable across the board. (Horrigan, 1996, p.70)

Indeed, TT can be viewed as a secular or at least nonsectarian version of an ancient faith healing practice. It promises healing to everyone regardless of religious belief or affiliation. As such, TT is particularly well-positioned for growth in the emerging era of religious pluralism in the United States and in many other nations. As Goldstein (1999) notes, many alternative medical therapies are essentially religious practices currently in the process of reinventing themselves as scientific practices, hoping for assimilation into contemporary culture and mainstream medicine.

But the religious roots of TT makes it suspect to many medical professionals who rely primarily on scientific reasoning when they assess the likely efficacy of a medical therapy. TT proponents must convince a wary medical profession that the practice is amenable to scientific assessment, and that it is not merely faith healing cleverly disguised to survive in an era of scientific method in nations where health care is dominated by secular professions and institutions.

Therapeutic Touch is noteworthy (and newsworthy) because it is advocated by a group of professionals who are affiliated with mainstream health organizations and who work in traditional medical institutions: nurses. As we will see, it has not been welcome by all or even most nurses. But many of its most successful advocates have been nurses! The TT movement in nursing has provided an occasion for nurses to assert their independence from physicians and to stake out a distinctive realm of expertise. Arguments regarding TT often implicitly invoke a distinction between allegedly feminine ways of knowing and allegedly masculine ways of knowing commonly associated with science. Controversies surrounding it cannot be fully understood unless one keeps in mind the authoritative yet also subordinate role that nurses have played in medical care and medical research.

TT has made perhaps more inroads into traditional medical settings than any other alternative therapy. As such, debates regarding it would seem to provide a glimpse of a future in which proponents of various alternative therapies push for mainstream acceptance. The outcome of ongoing debates regarding Therapeutic Touch will likely tell us much regarding if and how alternative therapies will be accommodated by traditional medicine.

IDENTIFYING THERAPEUTIC TOUCH AUDIENCES AND COMMUNITIES

News and information regarding TT is disseminated by a variety of sources, in a variety of media, and consumed by a variety of audiences.

The research reported in this chapter seeks to better understand the various audiences for TT information and to assess the TT-related content consumed (and in some cases created) by communities interested in it.

The Medline database was used to assess the dissemination of TT in the medical literature and among medical communities. Medline is maintained by the National Library of Medicine and indexes more than 3,900 journals in medicine, nursing, and related fields.

The Alt-HealthWatch database was used to access TT literature targeted at readers interested in alternative health and medicine. Alt-HealthWatch is maintained by SoftLine Information, Inc. and provides the full text of articles from 171 journals, magazines, and newsletters that focus on alternative health issues. Publications available via this database include the *American Journal of Natural Medicine*, *Homeopathy Today*, and *Reiki News*.

The Dialog database was used to access coverage of TT in U.S. daily newspapers. A product of the Dialog Corporation, the Dialog newspaper database provides the full text of stories from fifty-eight U.S. daily newspapers, including large-circulation newspapers such as *USA Today* and the *Los Angeles Times* as well as smaller-circulation newspapers such as the *Akron Beacon Journal* and the *Palm Beach Post*.

To identify the most important websites that focus on TT, I relied on Internet search engines (e.g., *Google, HotBot*) that permit users to discover how many and which websites are linked to a particular page, a procedure that can provide an estimate of the centrality or authoritativeness of specific websites. This procedure for identifying "central" or particularly authoritative sites—that is, websites to which many other websites offer links—has been recommend by computer and information scientists (Chakrabati et al., 1999; Chen et al., 1998) and utilized, for example, by Sandvik (1999) to identify the most important websites that focused on a specific medical topic (in this case, female urinary incontinence).

In addition to websites, Internet discussion groups or newsgroups are important areas of TT-related activity on the Internet. The *Deja.com* search engine was used to identify USENET discussion groups that most commonly discuss TT. The *Liszt* search engine was used to identify mailing lists whose participants commonly discuss TT.

TT IN THE MEDICAL LITERATURE

The Medline database includes 242 items published between 1975 and 1998 that include the phrase "Therapeutic Touch" in their titles or in their subject fields. Of these 242 publications, 48 are letters to journal

Figure 1: Medline Articles on Therapeutic Touch, 1975-1998

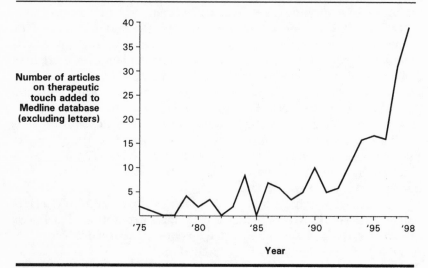

Number of articles on therapeutic touch added to Medline database (excluding letters)

Year

editors rather than articles per se. These letters are excluded from the numerical analysis that follows, which is based on 194 articles that focus on TT.

Figure 1 shows the distribution of these 194 articles over time, from 1975 through 1998. Articles on TT have become far more common in the past several years, beginning with 1993. The years 1997 and 1998 saw a particularly dramatic increase. Indeed, there were more TT-related articles published in 1997 and 1998 (n = 70) than during the eighteen years following the publication of Krieger's seminal 1975 article (n = 64). Although TT is now twenty-five years old, it has only in recent years attained substantial attention in the medical literature.

Not every area of medicine has been attentive to TT, at least to judge by publication patterns manifested in Medline. Of the 194 TT-related articles listed in Medline, 164 (or 84.5 percent) were published in nursing journals. Medical journals accounted for only sixteen articles, or 8.2 percent. Eleven articles (or 5.7 percent) were published in alternative medical journals (e.g., *Journal of Complementary and Alternative Medicine*). Three articles (1.5 percent) were published in social science journals (e.g., *Psychological Reports*).

In sum, nursing journals have been by far the most common source of TT-related publications included in the Medline database, while medical journals have remained relatively uninterested in the subject. This disparity underscores the role of TT as an occasion for nurses to assert their autonomy from physicians, to develop their own therapeutic interventions, and to develop their own procedures for assessing these therapies. However, physicians have seemingly not yet accorded TT standing as a topic worthy of serious consideration. The medical literature remains segregated in terms of attention to it. If TT is to become assimilated into contemporary medicine, it will likely need to receive more serious and more frequent attention in the medical research literature.

No single journal dominates coverage of TT in the nursing literature. Articles on it have appeared in journals targeted at a general nursing audience (e.g., *American Journal of Nursing*), at nurses interested in alternative therapies (e.g., *Holistic Nursing Practice*), and at nurses who work in or study particular nursing contexts (e.g., *Oncology Nursing Forum*). The nursing journals that most frequently published TT-related articles were the following, each of which published seven articles between 1975 and 1998: *Complementary Therapies in Nurse-Midwifery*, *Journal of Advanced Nursing*, *Journal of Christian Nursing*, and *Journal of Holistic Nursing*.

It is not possible to reliably categorize articles as offering favorable or unfavorable coverage of TT based only on abstracts provided in the Medline database. However, a close reading of Medline abstracts suggests that most coverage of TT in the nursing literature has been favorable, a point made by previous researchers who have reviewed this literature (Meehan, 1998). The *Journal of Christian Nursing* is unusual in that most of its coverage of TT has been negative. As Huebscher (1999) notes, contributors to this journal seem to object to TT not because it may be inefficacious or at least insufficiently investigated. Rather, they fear that it is too closely tied to new age spirituality, which is seen as threatening to Christianity. *Journal of Christian Nursing* contributors seem to sense and fear that TT is a harbinger of a trend that will see sectarian health care superseded by nonsectarian, if still religious, health care.

It should be noted that not all of the 194 TT-related articles indexed in Medline offer original research reports. In fact, many of the articles provide only commentary, instructions, or literature reviews. Scheiber (1997) reviews several studies that find that while there is much attention to TT in both mass and specialized media, the extant literature includes relatively few empirical research reports regarding TT. Nonetheless, Scheiber notes, proponents often claim that a large number of scientific studies have been published regarding TT [see chapter 21 in this volulme]. Although it is generally risky to draw such conclusions based only on Medline abstracts, in this case it seems safe to say that TT proponents who may claim (as they often do) that there are "hundreds" or even "dozens" of published scientific studies regarding its efficacy are guilty of exaggeration. Even in the medical literature proper, one will find far more arguments than evidence regarding TT.

TT IN THE ALTERNATIVE HEALTH LITERATURE

The Alt-HealthWatch full text database begins coverage of the publications it offers with 1992. This database includes forty-three articles published between 1992 and 1998 that include the phrase "Therapeutic Touch" in their titles. The most common publication outlet for articles about TT was *Massage Magazine*, which ran nine articles on the subject. *Massage Magazine* is a bimonthly trade publication targeted at massage therapists and bodyworkers; its masthead features the slogan "Keeping Those Who Touch In Touch." This magazine's treatment of TT is typical of coverage in the publications offered via the Alt-HealthWatch service. A close look at *Massage Magazine* coverage of TT can tell us much about the ways in which the practice is covered in publications targeted at readers interested in alternative health issues.

Coverage of TT in *Massage Magazine* was almost entirely favorable. There was no trace of skepticism in eight of the magazine's nine articles on the subject. The sole article that included negative coverage of TT focused on a particularly high-profile *JAMA* report regarding research that found that its practitioners could not detect a "human energy field" that, according to its proponents, surrounds human bodies and is sensed and manipulated by the practitioners (this *JAMA* article, by Rosa et al., 1998, is discussed in more detail below). Although the *Massage Magazine* coverage of the *JAMA* report took care to summarize the findings of the *JAMA* report, the article featured quotes from TT proponents who reassured readers that the *JAMA* study should be discounted. Dolores Krieger is quoted as saying that the Rosa et al. study was "terribly flawed" and that its conclusions were "slightly ridiculous." Another practitioner is quoted as saying that *JAMA* had published a "very silly study."

Although *Massage Magazine* readers were told mostly good things regarding TT, only one of the nine articles explicitly encouraged readers to practice it. More common was high but nonspecific praise for TT as a professional pursuit and as an area of scientific inquiry. *Massage Magazine* contributors portrayed TT as relevant because it provided evidence that massage therapy and bodywork, broadly defined, can improve human health.

Massage Magazine seemed particularly eager to feature stories suggesting that TT was winning the attention and respect of mainstream medicine. Some of the magazines' headlines included: "Army Gives Grant for Therapeutic Touch"; "NIH Awards Grants for Massage, Therapeutic Touch"; and "NIH-Funded Study Measured Less Stress in Those Who Had Therapeutic Touch." These articles focused on the prestige of the funding agencies, the relatively large dollar amounts of the grants, and the credentials of the researchers who received the grants, most of whom worked in reputable universities and medical colleges. In this way, TT was offered as an example of the growing scientific legitimacy of practices related to bodywork, practices that were once excluded from science.

The imprimatur of the NIH in particular and mainstream science in general lends credibility to TT and to related bodywork and energy healing practices. Ultimately, the results of government-funded studies may not be as important as the fact that the government funded the studies in the first place. As *Massage Magazine* coverage of TT suggests, the mere fact that the practice has received attention from mainstream medicine is an important victory for proponents of alternative health and medicine. There may be little evidence in the mainstream medical literature to suggest that TT is efficacious. But the fact that controversies regarding it have engaged the NIH and mainstream medical researchers has allowed its proponents to argue that TT has earned a place in mainstream medicine.

TT IN THE NEWS

The Dialog newspaper database includes 487 stories that included the phrase "Therapeutic Touch" and that were published between 1980 and 1998. But these stories were not evenly distributed across the years. There was little newspaper attention to TT before 1993. Numerical reports risk misleading us here, since Dialog coverage of the newspapers it indexes does not uniformly extend back to 1980. Coverage for most of the newspapers in the database extends back only to the late 1980s to early 1990s. And several newspapers were added to the Dialog database in each of the past few years. Still, it seems safe to say that newspaper coverage of TT was relatively uncommon prior to 1993. Of the 487 newspaper stories mentioning TT, 425 (or 87.3 percent) were published since 1993. And 179 stories (or 36.8 percent) were published in 1998—TT's most newsworthy year to date.

More than one-half of the 179 TT-related stories published in 1998 dealt with a single news event: the publication in *JAMA*'s April 1 issue of research by Rosa et al. which reported that TT practitioners had failed to perform at better-than-chance rates when asked to detect the presence of a nearby but unseen and untouched human hand. This article put TT on the national media agenda. The *JAMA* report was covered by almost one-half of the 108 newspapers in the Dialog database, including *USA Today*, the *Washington Post*, and the *Los Angeles Times*. It was covered by the *New York Times* and in the evening television newscasts of ABC, CBS, and NBC. No other TT-related story has yet garnered such widespread media attention. This one *JAMA* report was among the biggest health-related stories of 1998. Indeed, it was one of the biggest stories regarding alternative medicine that has yet to appear in U.S. news media.

The Rosa et al. research was deemed newsworthy by journalists for three reasons. First, the research began as the fourth-grade science-fair project of Emily Rosa, an eleven-year-old (when published in *JAMA*) who was also the second author of the *JAMA* report. Emily was nine-years old when her data collection began. The fact that a child had conducted research that was published by one of the world's most prestigious medical journals was irresistible to journalists. This fact alone would guarantee widespread media coverage. Many newspaper headlines were careful to stress the age (and often gender) of the report's second author (even if there seemed to be some confusion regarding her age). Headlines included:

9-Year-Old's Therapy Study Lands in Medical Journal (*Seattle Times*).

Journal Publishes Medical-Validity Study by Girl, 11 (*Rocky Mountain News*).

4th-Grader's Study Rebuts Touch Therapy (*Los Angeles Times*).

Healing Touch? Girl, 9, Debunks Idea in Study (*Sacramento Bee*).

A Child's Paper Poses a Medical Challenge (*New York Times*).

Kid Stuff (*USA Today*).

The second reason that the Rosa et al. report generated a large amount of media attention is that the report was published in *JAMA*, the *Journal of the American Medical Association*. Along with the *New England Journal of Medicine*, *JAMA* dominates U.S. news coverage of medical research (Evans, 1995). *JAMA* has developed an extensive media relations operation to help insure that it remains trusted and often utilized by journalists hungry for medical news, a staple of U.S. news media. The imprimatur of *JAMA* promises that the research it reports will be both important and of the highest quality.

Many newspapers framed the Rosa et al. report as important primarily because it was published in *JAMA*. For example, the *Boston Herald* used the headline "AMA Says Touch Healers Debunked by Girl's Study." Many articles on the study specified in the lead paragraph that the study had been published in *JAMA*. The *USA Today* article began:

> A Colorado student's science fair study questioning the validity of "Therapeutic Touch," in which a healer supposedly manipulates a patient's energy field, has made its way into today's *Journal of the American Medical Association*.

This particular study was deemed important in part because it carried the imprimatur of *JAMA*, and by extension, the American Medical Association.

The third reason that the Rosa et al. report generated great media attention is that it was timely, arriving at the end of an eighteen-month period that saw increasing news coverage of NIH's controversial Office of Alternative Medicine (now the National Center for Complementary and Alternative Medicine) as well as increasing news coverage of alternative health and medicine in general. Journalists seemed primed to carry the Rosa et al. report in that it resonated with growing media and public attention to research in alternative medicine.

TT proponents were not dissuaded by the *JAMA* article. They launched a campaign of sorts to challenge the study, and, by extension *JAMA* and the AMA. The *New York Times* ran an editorial headlined "Touch Therapy Wasn't Disproved." The *Sacramento Bee* ran a story about the many nurses and other TT proponents who had criticized the Rosa et al. report, headlined "Study Attacking Therapeutic Touch Called Unfair." By September of 1998, the *Omaha World-Herald* could report that "Bad Publicity Has Little Effect on Touch Therapy Followers."

Indeed, media coverage of TT in the year following the *JAMA* report suggests that journalists and the public may have a short memory. The Rosa et al. report was quickly all but forgotten in the many subsequent stories that mention TT. Curiously, this *JAMA* report may have augmented rather than diminished the standing of TT among journalists and laypersons. The fact that *JAMA* and the AMA entered the debate regarding TT may ultimately be more significant than the findings reported.

It should be noted that TT is typically only mentioned rather than discussed in detail in news coverage of alternative health. Stories that focus on TT remain uncommon, but it is commonly mentioned in the many stories that focus on alternative health issues that cut across more than one technique or practice, especially stories that discuss public utilization of massage therapies, energy healing, and relaxation techniques. TT is typically mentioned in these stories as an example of such therapies.

Moreover, it is depicted in these stories as a therapy that is used by many nurses and that enjoys the attention of government-funded researchers. The *Seattle Times* reported that Therapeutic Touch, a technique new to the Pacific Northwest, is using relaxation to help ill and injured people recover. The University of Washington Medical Center has recently joined nursing schools and hospitals such as New York University and Johns Hopkins Hospital in introducing Therapeutic-Touch treatment to patients and health professionals (Cronin, 1997).

An *Atlanta Journal-Constitution* story on alternative medicine included this passage:

> The healing nature of auras is being aggressively studied across the nation. It has been estimated that more than 40,000 nurses and therapists are practicing what is called "Therapeutic Touch," a little-understood treatment that has to do with manipulating the aura of a person in pain or in need of healing. Practitioners believe that by finding "hot spots" or "cold spots" in a person's aura they can detect disease or injury. Healing can be promoted by massaging the injured part of the aura. (Parham, 1997)

As this rather confused account of TT suggests, the public receives surprisingly little accurate information regarding TT via the mass media, despite the fact that TT is often mentioned in stories regarding alternative medicine. Relatively few stories mention any specific conditions for which TT is said to be an appropriate treatment. Instead, TT has become for journalists an often utilized if seldom explained example of an alternative medical treatment that enjoys widespread use and at least grudging acceptance by mainstream medical institutions.

TT ON THE INTERNET

At the time this chapter was being written, in July 1999, there were at least 12 websites that focused primarily on TT and at least another 250 sites that focused on alternative health and medicine and that included substantial material regarding it (e.g., journal articles, news stories). Internet portals *Yahoo, Infoseek,* and *Snap* maintained a dedicated category for TT-related sites within their alternative health directories.

Three TT-related websites were especially popular in terms of the number of other sites that provided links to them. By this measure, the most "central" website was "Therapeutic Touch: Is it Valid?" (www. voicenet.com/~eric/tt), a site created and maintained by Eric Krieg, an electrical engineer and a member of the Philadelphia Association for Critical Thinking (PhACT). Sixty-six websites provided links to Krieg's site, which in turn consisted primarily of links to other sites pertaining to TT. Krieg's links were categorized as "Sites skeptical of TT" and "Sites favorable to TT." Krieg's site did indeed offer resources likely to be interesting to both believers and skeptics. It seemed designed to be a clearinghouse of sorts for Internet resources regarding Therapeutic Touch.

The second most "central" website, again in terms of the number of links to it elsewhere on the web, was the document "Therapeutic Touch," created by Stephen Barrett, M.D., and included in *Quackwatch* (www.quackwatch.com), a website offering skeptical resources regarding alternative health and medicine. Thirty-three websites provided links to this document, which provided a brief, encyclopedia-style account of TT as well as links to sites that provide skeptical perspectives regarding it. Barrett's document included this statement: "There is no scientific evidence that the 'energy transfer' postulated by [TT] proponents actually occurs. It is safe to assume that any reactions to the procedure are psychological responses to the 'laying-on of hands.' " Barrett went on to request that "if you are on the staff of a hospital in which TT is practiced, please lodge a protest."

The third most "central" site was maintained by the Nurse Healers —Professional Associates International (NH-PAI), based in Reston, Virginia. This organization billed itself as "The Official Organization of Therapeutic Touch" (www.therapeutic-touch.org/html/touch.html). Eleven websites featured links to this site, which offered information on NH-PAI training programs and a membership form with which visitors could submit credit card information to secure a NH-PAI membership, at a cost of $75. The top or home page of the NH-PAI site claimed that:

In 1992, the National Institute of Health (NIH) created the Office of Alternative Medicine. The experts in this office found that Therapeutic Touch has one of the strongest research bases of any of the alternative/complimentary modalities. There are over two dozen doctoral dissertations, dozens of masters theses, and many post-doctoral studies, several of which have been funded by NIH. Research continues at a rigorous pace in institutions of higher learning throughout the country. TT is accepted in a growing number of hospitals and universities throughout the U.S., Canada, and around the world.

This passage is typical of attempts by proponents to establish credibility by invoking the NIH and claiming that much scientific research exists to support the efficacy of TT. As noted above, the later claim is misleading—it functions as a convenient legend of sorts. Still, to judge by the commonality of such appeals in the pro-TT literature, this claim is thought to be highly persuasive. Certainly, the fact that such claims are common in the TT literature suggests that the imprimatur of mainstream medicine can be valuable for those who would hope to move alternative medical treatments into the mainstream.

In terms of Internet newsgroups and discussion lists, discussions of TT have been most common in Usenet newsgroups *misc.health.alternative* and *alt.healing.reiki*. The *Deja.news* database archives contained 239 messages posted to *misc.health.alternative* between January 1, 1996, and July 15, 1999, that included the phrase "Therapeutic Touch." This phrase was included in 137 messages posted during the same period by *alt.healing.reiki* participants.

Most *misc.health.alternative* posts regarding TT fall into one of the following two categories: (1) posts that offered evidence, pro and con, regarding the efficacy of TT, and (2) posts that discussed what sorts of people were qualified to assess TT and why. Although this framework might suggest that sophisticated, enlightened discussion was common, *misc.health.alternative* discussions often took the form of nasty exchanges between believers and skeptics, exchanges that featured more insults than evidence of careful deliberation.

One *misc.health.alternative* post recommended to participants a book titled *Spiritual Healing—Does it Work? Research Says Yes!*, claiming that "This book contains 'excellent' information to refute the claims that skeptics and other may confront you with. . . . It contains over 117 studies (scientific) as well as double-blind studies. It received reviews from many M.D.s and Ph.D.s (some with both degrees) who highly praise the work!"

This post brought engendered only two responses, one that read, "This great resource should be used by anyone who is being pestered to cite studies, etc. by skeptics and others trying to disprove the validity of alternative and spiritual healing modalities." A skeptic responded, "For those too stupid to search the peer-reviewed literature for themselves, huh? Okay, we'll bite. You post the 'proof' of Therapeutic Touch, citing placebo-controlled double-blind peer-reviewed studies, showing significant and replicatable results," a challenge that was not taken up by any *misc.health.alternative* participants.

The lengthiest and most acrimonious *misc.health.alternative* thread regarding TT concerned allegations that a TT proponent who participated in the list claimed to have Ph.D. degree that he or she did not in fact possess.

In sum, the *misc.health.alternative* debates regarding TT are intractable. Believers and skeptics repeatedly marshal a small number of what are now time-honored arguments, always failing to persuade one another. This impasse stems not from a lack of available evidence regarding TT, but from the fact believers and skeptics have markedly different views regarding what the scientific evidence tells us.

In *alt.healing.reiki*, the participation of skeptics was far less common. *Alt.healing.reiki* participants seldom expressed any doubts regarding the efficacy of TT. For *alt.healing.reiki* participants, TT was simply one of many forms of energy healing that could be effectively utilized by bodyworkers. Most TT-related posts to *alt.healing.reiki* either asked for or provided information regarding how and where one could receive training in it, or how one could use TT as an energy healing "modality." Strikingly, *alt.healing.reiki* participants engaged in almost no discussion of the scientific evidence regarding TT, either pro or con. Even the Rosa et al. report in *JAMA* went largely unnoticed, being quickly dismissed as a flawed study produced by skeptics inherently hostile to alternative healing practices. *Alt.healing.reiki* participants were primarily believers for whom it made little sense to concern themselves with others who may not believe.

The most focused Internet discussions of TT to date have occurred on the mailing list *tt*. This list is operated by Eric Krieg who began it in May of 1998 with the goal of providing a TT-related discussion forum in which both believers and skeptics would be welcome and where debate would remain civil. By July of 1999, *tt* had grown to sixty-two subscribers. This is a small community, but it is one in which participants have so far adhered to Krieg's mission statement. Which is not to say that tensions between believers and skeptics have not already threatened to disrupt the list. One *tt* subscriber recently complained about what he perceived to be a preponderance of skepticism on the list. This subscriber suggested that the list be renamed *tt-skeptic* and that a new list titled *tt-active* be created, thereby segregating the believers and skeptics. The suggestion was made perhaps half in jest, but it does illustrate how rapidly and seemingly inevitably conflict between believers and skeptics emerges on the Internet.

Kreig's *tt* list may prove to be an exception, just as his "Therapeutic Touch: Is it Valid?" website seems to have succeeded in part because of its neutrality. But for the most part, TT on the Internet has been characterized by segregation of believers and skeptics. What small amount of interaction has occurred between believers and skeptics has tended to become acrimonious. Websites that feature TT-related information have tended to be designed primarily by and for either believers or skeptics. The Internet seems to have cultivated rather narrowly defined communities that have little opportunity or desire to talk to one another about TT even though they may share an interest in the practice.

CONCLUSIONS

Ultimately, the evidence that emerges from scientific studies of Therapeutic Touch may be less important than the fact that science and scientists have taken it seriously. There is ample evidence in the debates between believers and skeptics to suggest that believers are unlikely to accept any evidence that would seem to conclusively falsify the basic premises of TT. Therefore, the subject will likely remain controversial for many years to come.

While debate rages on, proponents can continue to say that TT is taken seriously by many nurses, medical researchers, universities and medical schools, and by the NIH and the AMA. As noted above, this in itself is a victory. TT proponents have succeeded in reinventing an essentially religious practice as a medical practice. This framing of TT as a medical issue has been aided and abetted by journalists. Knowing that their readers and viewers are keenly interested in alternative medicine, journalists eagerly report on government-funded research into alternative medicine even if they are also unprepared to understand the complex issues of scientific method and human physiology that make research on alternative medicine difficult to communicate to lay audiences. The media framing of TT as a medical topic is as important to the public perception of Therapeutic Touch as the outcome of scientific investigations of its efficacy.

Of course, the results of scientific studies will have an impact on this debate. If and when TT is more conclusively shown to be inefficacious, nurses who have embraced it, and perhaps the entire nursing profession, would risk losing credibility. This, in turn, could sacrifice some of the gains nurses have made in cultivating their own autonomous journals, in developing nursing curricula, in setting professional standards, and in attaining government funding for their research efforts. Indeed, nurses would seem to have both the most to gain and the most to lose in the contest related to TT.

TT enjoys widespread media coverage, but this coverage is seldom substantial. Newspaper readers are unlikely to find much information regarding practices specific to TT or the scientific evidence regarding its efficacy. It is seldom and only vaguely defined in newspaper stories. Extended accounts of TT practices and the claims of its proponents are rare. TT is typically mentioned in newspapers only in passing, as an example of an alternative medical therapy that has been used by many people, embraced by many nursing professionals, and taught in mainstream medical schools. The large amount of superficial media coverage of the subject makes it easier for proponents to suggest that it is already supported by a vast body of scientific evidence. Such claims may seem plausible to lay readers unfamiliar with the scientific literature regarding TT but who nonetheless often see it mentioned in the health and medicine sections of their newspapers.

The Internet offers more substantial information regarding TT than do newspapers, but information may seldom be sought on the Internet by those who haven't already made up their minds regarding it. Websites and discussion groups seem to be segregated. Believers and skeptics seldom interact. When interaction occurs it is seldom constructive or even polite. The Internet seems likely to exacerbate rather than resolve TT-related conflicts between believers and skeptics.

Debates regarding TT will be reflected in popular media but not resolved by popular media. Debates regarding it will be resolved, if at all, only after much scientific evidence is published and the medical community successfully persuades TT advocates to accept this evidence. This would seem to be a difficult or even impossible task. We can expect that for many years to come TT advocates will continue to dismiss scientific evidence that challenges its efficacy.

In the meantime, the strategies of TT proponents will likely be adopted by proponents of other alternative healing practices who wish to establish a foothold in mainstream medicine. TT will likely be remembered as one of the earliest alternative healing practices to make a successful transition from a religious practice to a medical practice. Those who would hope to understand the rise of alternative medicine would do well to study the dynamics of the TT controversy. The TT movement and its reception in mass and specialized media reveal a great deal about where medicine is headed and why.

REFERENCES

Chakrabarti, S., B. Dom, D. Gibson, J. Kleinberg, et al. 1999. "Hypersearching the Web." *Scientific American* (June): 54–60.

Chen, C., J. Newman, R. Newman, and R. Rada. 1998. "How Did University Departments Interweave the Web: A Study of Connectivity and Underlying Factors." *Interacting with Computers* 10: 353–73.

Cronin, M. E. 1997. "Healing Hands." *Seattle Times* (January 1): D1.

Eisenberg, D. M., R. B. Davis, S. L. Ettner, S. Appel, et al. 1998. "Trends in Alternative Medicine use in the United States, 1990–1997: Results of a Follow-Up National Survey." *JAMA* 280: 1569–75.

Eisenberg, D. M., R. C. Kessler, C. Foster, F. E. Norlock, et al. 1993. "Unconventional Medicine in the United States. Prevalence, Costs, and Patterns of Use." *New England Journal of Medicine* 328: 246–52.

Evans, W. 1995. "The Mundane and the Arcane: Prestige Media Coverage of Social and Natural Science." *Journalism and Mass Communication Quarterly*, 72:168-177.

Goldstein, M. S. 1999. *Alternative Health Care: Medicine, Miracle, or Mirage?* Philadelphia: Temple University Press.

Horrigan, B. 1996. "Janet Quinn, RN, PhD: Therapeutic Touch and a Healing Way." *Alternative Therapies in Health and Medicine* (July 2): 69–75.

Huebscher, R. 1999. "Therapeutic Touch: What is the Controversy and Why Does Controversy Exist?" *Nurse Practitioner Forum* 10: 43–46.

Krieger, D. 1975. "Therapeutic Touch: The Imprimatur of Nursing." *American Journal of Nursing* 75: 784–87.

———. 1979. *The Therapeutic Touch: How to Use Your Hands to Help or to Heal.* Englewood Cliffs, N.J.: Prentice-Hall.

Meehan, T. C. 1998. "Therapeutic Touch as a Nursing Intervention." *Journal of Advanced Nursing* 28: 117–25.

Parham, B. 1997. "Spiritual Healing." *Atlanta Journal-Constitution* (May 10): 4F.

Rosa, L., E. Rosa, L. Sarner, S. Barrett. 1998. "A Close Look at Therapeutic Touch." *JAMA* 279: 1005–10.

Sandvik, H. 1999. "Health Information and Interaction on the Internet: A Survey of Female Urinary Incompetence." *BMJ: British Medical Journal* 319: 29–32.

Scheiber, B. 1997. "Therapeutic Touch: Evaluating the 'Growing Body of Evidence' Claim." *Scientific Review of Alternative Medicine* 1: 13–15.

8.

Skeptics Confront Therapeutic Touch: A Case Study*

Béla Scheiber

"The Therapeutic Touch (TT) movement is the greatest scientific scandal ever to disrupt and befuddle our nation's admirable but naïve nurses. Colorado's Rocky Mountain Skeptics deserve unbounded praise for leading the fight against this recent New Age nonsense—a pseudotherapy with no more validity than benevolent witchcraft."

—Martin Gardner

The Boulder, Colorado based Rocky Mountain Skeptics (RMS)—founded in 1983—only became aware of TT in 1988. It is not understating the case to say that, prior to that year, TT had received little notice in the public press and even less criticism in the professional nursing journals. From the appearance of Grad in 1961 until RMS got involved, only three critical papers of any significance had been published: Walike et al., 1975; Sandroff, 1980; and Clark and Clark, 1984. The ever growing number of skeptical organizations at that time, when listing pseudosciences, never mentioned TT. That is until 1988 when skeptics, and those opposing health fraud, first got a sneak preview of events to come.

The event that would forever place TT in the lexicon of skeptics occurred in October 1988 when the founder of RMS, Béla Scheiber, received a letter from the Director of the Denver Veterans Administration Hospital's Pain Clinic, psychologist Bertram Rothschild, Ph.D. The letter sought information about an unusual subject in connection with a request by a nurse working at the hospital. As was explained in the letter, she approached Dr. Rothschild seeking his permission to administer TT to patients under his jurisdiction. Not being aware of what TT was, he asked her for an explanation of the practice. She gave the "party line" that there indeed was a corpus of scientific experiments to

---

*The author is greatly indebted to the members of the Rocky Mountain Skeptics, who not only gave financial support in its TT efforts, but who also donated their time and effort to make the project a success.

support the efficacy of TT. Since he was a member of RMS, Dr. Rothschild turned to the organization for assistance in evaluating her claim.

Scheiber did some research and produced the 1984 Clark and Clark paper. He then sought the help of Mr. James Randi, the noted critic of pseudoscience, who said that he had not heard of TT directly but did have some related literature—mostly on Kirlian photography. Other skeptics throughout the United States were contacted. All expressed ignorance on the subject.

After receiving the Clark and Clark article and the Kirlian photography information, Dr. Rothschild determined that TT would not be used in his clinic. In an official VA Memorandum dated October 21, 1988, Dr. Rothschild wrote to Scheiber: "Thanks for the leads, they were quite productive. Considering the shabby state-of-the-art of therapeutic touch. I certainly won't permit it to occur in the Pain Clinic here. Thanks again."

This single event was the beginning of what may be characterized as the most intense, long-term confrontation between the skeptic community and those who practice or promote TT.

Three years later, in October 1991, a simple full-page flyer promoting a class in TT arrived in the mail for Scheiber from Carol Galipeau, R.N., who was working at Denver's Swedish Medical Center when she spotted it. The leaflet promoted classes in TT for which nurses, upon completion, would be awarded continuing education units (CEUs). The flyer also proudly proclaimed the launching of a "Department of Energy" (DOE) at the hospital's Employee Health and Fitness center [see appendix 6]. The thought that, within the community in which RMS members resided, hospitals were treating patients with an unproven therapy, setting up DOEs, awarding CEU credits—and all this happening quietly, stealthily—provided the impetus for an RMS fact-finding project.

When Scheiber presented the flyer to Linda Rosa (Rojas), an RMS member with a B.A. in Anthropology and a B.S. in nursing (*Skeptic*, 1994, p. 107) she was appalled that her chosen profession was losing sight of its scientific roots. They both recognized that this would provide an opportunity for RMS to act as a group on a project that could make a difference.

At the next general meeting of RMS, Scheiber presented the TT flyer and formed an ad hoc committee to discuss options. They were chiefly curious about why the Colorado Board of Nursing (CBN) would allow CEU credits for a practice with such poor professional credentials. Sue Houck, Bill Aldorfer, and Randy Bancroft offered to help (Rojas, 1992, p. 5).

In reviewing nursing newsletters, school of nursing publications, and professional journals, they discovered that CEUs were not just being awarded for TT but for neurolinguistic programming, refexology, applied kinesiology, crystal healing, and acupressure. They found that a second Denver hospital, St. Luke/Presbyterian, was also training nurses in TT and had already established a DOE. The nursing situation in Colorado was worse than they had thought.

The committee invited Colorado Board of Nursing (CBN) administrator Karen Brumley to give a talk about the TT and other pseudosciences; she firmly declined. The ad hoc committee was undaunted by this response. In fact, it just encouraged them to dig deeper. They decided that if CBN wouldn't come to RMS, RMS would go to the CBN.

Having a nurse, Rojas, in the group soon proved to be an unanticipated benefit. The committee quickly discovered that TT was not just a pseudoscience issue but a highly charged social one involving misguided feminism. Most, if not all, of the key TT proponents in Colorado at the CBN and the University of Colorado Nursing School were female. Furthermore, most of the key figures in TT history were females. Never the less, to those on the ad hoc RMS committee, gender was not the issue—it was science. Linda Rojas was the logical one to present our concerns to the CBN since she was a member of the nursing establishment and could not be dismissed as an outsider.

A strategy soon evolved: Bill Aldorfer would draft the first version of a brief statement that was to be read by Rojas to the CBN at their January 30, 1992 meeting. That first draft was harsh and critical and demanded that CBN remove all CEUs from a list of nonsense courses. Scheiber modified the tone from one of confrontation to one of inquiry. The statement asked: "What evidence has persuaded the Board of Nursing to lend their tacit endorsement to these practices through the continuing education and relicensing process? Who is accountable? . . . How can Board-recognized, credentializing organizations be made responsible and accountable for the content of continuing education classes?" (*Rocky Mountain Skeptic*, 1992, 1993a, 1998). The committee believed that the Board would have to respond specifically to their inquiry. The Board did indeed form a task force to investigate RMS's concerns.

The "Task Force to Colorado State Board of Nursing Regarding Therapeutic Touch" met April 8, 1992 at the University of Colorado Health Science Center, School of Nursing for not longer than one and a half hours. Even though the minutes [see appendix 7] of that meeting mention the Rocky Mountain Skeptics, they were not called to testify. In fact, RMS only found out in a letter from CBN dated June 8, 1992, that, at their May 28–29 meeting, they accepted and approved the recommendations made by the Task Force on April 8. The RMS committee was simply told that the Task Force had met and that the CBN would continue its support of CEUs for TT.

In response to this blatant disregard of public concern, Rojas (then Vice-President of RMS), acting with approval from Scheiber (then President of RMS), wrote a response back which said, in part: "We therefore request a bibliography of the studies reviewed by the Board. We also request a copy of the Subcommittee's report to the Board, as well as a copy of the minutes and other proceedings of the Board when it ruled on this matter in May 1992." What RMS received was a single page document, "Recommendations from a State Board of Nursing Sub-committee to Investigate the Awarding of Continuing Education Units to Nurses for the Study of Therapeutic Touch and Other Non-traditional and Complementary Healing Modalities" [see appendix 4] and a multi-page document submitted to the CBN Task Force by Janet Quinn listing 200 publications on TT [see chapter 21 in this volume for a skeptical discussion of this list]. Other documents requested by RMS were not included.

A hand-delivered letter dated February 23, 1993, made a second request under the Colorado Open Records Act provision CRS 24-72-203 (Colorado's version of the Federal Freedom of Information Act) to the CBN to obtain the minutes of the Task Force's meeting with names of those who participated.

RMS people were confused. The presentation to the Board had not singled out the practice of TT but, rather, had asked about the accountability process for awarding CEUs for a list of fringe practices. It was clear from the minutes that the Task Force was empowered only to investigate TT: "The goal of this meeting is to submit a summary on Therapeutic Touch as continuing education for nurses and compile research and writings on the modalities" [see appendix 7].

The participants at the Task Force meeting read like a who's who in Colorado TT: Sally Phillips—Chair of CBN and coauthor of a favorable TT paper with Jean Watson (Watson, Phillips, 1992) who is herself a major proponent of TT worldwide as well as the Director of the Center for Human Caring; Coleen Whalens—member of Swedish Hospital's Planning Committee for TT; Fran Reeder—approved the thesis, *A Phenomenological Inquiry On the Child's Lived Experience of Perceiving the Human Energy Field Using Therapeutic Touch*, for her Ph.D. in 1991; and Janet Quinn—leading practitioner and proponent of TT as well as an Associate Professor within Jean Watson's Center for Human Caring.

It was evident that serious discussion of our concerns had not taken place. Moreover, it was clear to those involved in the previous episode that a further visit to the CBN was required. Soon after receiving the June 8 letter from CBN another general meeting of RMS took place. Scheiber made the case that RMS should continue its TT activity, and, in fact, to enlarge its scope. Many new people offered to help, including, but not limited to, Carla Selby, Martin Tobias, Meg Hedgecock, and Bob Attwood.

Bill Aldorfer (1993) enrolled in a class advertised in the Colorado Free University catalogue as an "easily learned healing technique . . . to alleviate pain in yourself and others. . . . [TT] is currently being used successfully to help with PMS, migraine, chronic back pain, and depression." The course, "Therapeutic Touch: Healing at Your Fingertips," was conducted in three hour sessions, one day of the week, over a four-week period at a cost of $59. "For an additional $5, I could have requested and received certification for twelve Continuing Education Units (CEU) toward the twenty CEU biannual requirement needed to maintain registration as an RN or LPN" (Aldorfer, 1993, p. 2).

On January 28, 1993, RMS got a second chance to testify in front of the CBN. As part of her statement, Selby said: "The subcommittee recommended to this board, and you accepted, a definition of nursing that redefined the profession by stating: 'Because Nursing is both a science and an art, nurses require access to and familiarity with many belief systems and knowledge bases, including, but not limited to, the traditional sciences' [see appendix 4]. That is not what the law says. In defining the 'practice of professional nursing' [the Colorado Nursing Practice Act of July 1, 1985, p. 2] declares it to be: '. . . the performance of both independent nursing functions and delegated medical . . . functions . . . which [require] such specialized knowledge, judgment, and skill involving the application of principles of biological, physical, social, and behavioral sciences as are required for licensing as a professional nurse [from CRS 12-38-103(10)]" (*Rocky Mountain Skeptic*, 1993b, p. 5).

Later, Selby conveyed the philosophy which RMS has held since its inception: "No one is denying that new discoveries may come from any quarter. No one is advocating a closed-mindedness in the investigation into techniques for 'easing human suffering and the stimulation of healing.' But there is only one reliable means known for making a determination about the validity of such claims—that is the scientific method" (p. 7).

Aldorfer described the TT class he attended. He described the training in great detail; he spoke about "chakras," "sky-energy," "energy fields," and how to store "energy" from the healer into cotton for later use on a patient. In his concluding remarks he said, "The Board is obligated to document its support of the 'no-harm' claim with valid, replicated, unequivocal clinical data. The Board is likewise obligated to document its support of the 'energy field' claim with valid, replicated, unequivocal clinical data. To date, no valid, replicated, unequivocal clinical data have been produced by any advocate of the TT ceremony"

(*Rocky Mountain Skeptic*, 1993c, p. 9). Aldorfer then continued with what can only be described as the ultimate indictment:

> The Board must know that the most damning indictment of all came from the Registered Nurse who trained me in the ceremony of Therapeutic Touch. She advised me that it could take time for me to "feel" the "energy field" of a subject, and told me that it was entirely appropriate to fake the manipulation. The registered nurse told me that, while she was rehearsing her technique, she lettered a sign and attached it to her refrigerator door. The sign said: "FAKE IT 'TILL YOU MAKE IT."

After the presentations, several hours of discussion ensued among the Board members. What made the process intriguing is that this time a member of the Colorado Attorney General's office was present. It was clear that his role was to advise the Board so that they would avoid any legal trouble. They finally "voted to reaffirm the decision made at the May, 1992 Board meeting to approve Therapeutic Touch as acceptable content for continuing education. The vote was 8 members in favor, 1 opposed (Thomas Haga), and one abstaining" (letter dated February 10, 1993, from CBN to RMS) [see appendix 8].

After the vote, and while the TV news crew was still present, one of the Board members stated that Mr. Aldorfer was the one who must have been duped because the course he took was not one for which CEU credits could have been awarded. Therefore it did not represent those kinds of classes. With the last word from the Board criticizing the RMS investigation the TV crew left. One phone call determined that, in fact, the course was an authorized one that could be awarded CEUs. The Board was wrong! The TV crew was gone and RMS's last word—the truth—was not heard.

Nearly a half dozen RMS members had been present at this second hearing. They were dismayed at what had just happened and discussed the possibility of further action.

Soon after this second encounter with the CBN, the skeptic group realized that TT was more than just an insignificant practice that had no scientific basis. They figured that TT was in some yet to be discovered way "sacred" to those who had influence over the nursing profession in Colorado. For some reason TT was not just being taught but actively advocated and promoted out of proportion to its stature within the alternative medical community. RMS decided to investigate further; the Nursing Practice Task Force (NPTF) was formed to methodically research the connection between CBN, the University of Colorado Health Sciences Center (UCHSC), and the Nursing School within UCHSC.

At the first official meeting of the NPTF of RMS in downtown Denver most of those who had contributed up to that point were present. The first objective would be to establish the roles of those within the University of Colorado School of Nursing who were in leadership positions and actively engaged in promoting TT. Second, would it be productive to bring the CBN's willful disregard of the evidence to the attention of the state legislature? The NPTF believed that they had provided ample opportunities for the CBN to take steps to correct the CEU process without loosing political face. The Board had declined the opportunity and the NPTF thought that a wider dissemination of information was warranted.

Carla Selby was appointed to head up a task force to investigate the University of Colorado's involvement with TT, and Larry Sarner would lead an effort to inform the Colorado State Legislature. Both groups would explore options for education and action.

These two individuals were well qualified to take on their appointed tasks: Selby was very knowledgeable and comfortable dealing with the University and had had previous discussions with some of the Regents on other subjects; Sarner had a personal relationship with the State Senator from his district, Jim Roberts, and had previous experience within the political arena.

Sarner soon discovered that the terms for several of the sitting CBN members were to expire that year, 1993. Since each member of the CBN was appointed "pro forma" by the State Senate's committee on Health, Environment, Welfare, and Institutions (HEWI) based on recommendations by the Chair of the CBN and then rubber-stamped by the Governor, Sarner advised NPTF that they could intercede in this process by testifying in front of the HEWI committee during the reappointment hearings of the CBN members. He arranged for Senator Roberts to act as RMS's sponsor.

Before the HEWI committee could place the NPTF concerns on the agenda, Senator Roberts voiced them in front of the full Senate. He said specifically that nurses were receiving poor training in satisfying their continuing education requirements and that the CBN, when presented with the facts, chose to endorse the status quo and thus placed in jeopardy the health care of the citizens of Colorado. Senator Roberts discussed the NPTF issues with the Chair of HEWI, Senator Sally Hopper. He said further that RMS would like to go on record as not approving the reappointment of those whose terms were to expire. A date when HEWI would listen to an NPTF presentation was set for April 29, 1993.

Linda Rojas, a nurse, was the logical choice for presenter; Sarner prepared a fifteen minute presentation. The night before the scheduled appearance, Sarner told Selby that some political mischief had occurred. He had been notified that day that the fifteen minutes would be reduced to only two; some quick editing was required.

In the afternoon of April 29 Senator Roberts introduced Rojas to the HEWI committee. She did the best anyone could do—given only two minutes. Many members of RMS were present, as well as the Chair of the CBN, Sally Phillips, surrounded by those CBN members whose new terms were being questioned and other nurses. Several members of HEWI seemed clearly puzzled by the entire proceeding and the concept of Therapeutic Touch. One quipped that he saw nothing wrong with being touched. Another looked thoroughly bored.

One senator did finally ask if anyone in the room could demonstrate this thing called Therapeutic Touch. The silence in the room spoke more to the legitimacy of our concern than the two minute speech. The same people who had written that TT was acceptable, who had held a sub-committee meeting with Sally Phillips present, who had seen Aldorfer demonstrate TT, were silent. RMS did not volunteer to demonstrate TT to the senators thinking that those who promote and allow it to be taught had the burden of proof. The silence seemed to be relentless. Sally Phillips, the Chair of the CBN, who coauthored a paper with Jean Watson (Watson, Phillips, 1992) which stated, "Diverse efforts are underway to introduce (or reintroduce) specific caring and healing modalities, including basic message [*sic*], therapeutic touch, essential oils, visualization, imagery, aroma therapy, relaxation, meditation, and reflexology" (p. 20), had nothing to say. Yet she was there to speak on behalf of those Board members whose terms were to be considered for reappointment by HEWI. Why she did not choose that moment to demonstrate TT to the senators remains speculative. Finally, the votes were cast. All those whose terms on the CBN were up were reappointed to the Board.

Sally Phillips and the rest of the CBN members did not leave that hearing with total vindication. Nor would the status quo be preserved much longer. In a letter dated May 7, 1993, Senator Sally Hopper wrote to the Board of Nursing:

> The Senate Health, Environment, Welfare, and Institutions (HEWI) Committee members are concerned that the continuing education courses on nontraditional healing practices being approved by the Colorado Board of Nursing are not receiving sufficient review.
>
> Since continuing education is a condition for renewing licensure for the various nursing professions under the jurisdiction of the board, the review and approval of appropriate courses closely concerns the health and safety of the citizens of this state. As such, the Senate HEWI Committee expects board members to thoroughly review alternative healing practices, such as Therapeutic Touch, neurolinguistic programming, and crystal healing, prior to approving the study

of these healing methods for continuing education. Please send copies of future board meeting agendas listing hearings of the above courses, and any other courses based on nontraditional healing practices to the Senate HEWI committee members [see appendix 9 for full text].

The demands placed upon the CBN seemed daunting. How would they respond? Certainly it would require a great amount of effort and expense for the board to educate themselves on all the strange techniques being taught that were receiving CEUs. They chose a simple solution. They voted unanimously on January 26, 1994—after considerable discussion at their September 23, 1993 meeting—to repeal the requirement of continuing education as a mandatory requirement for license renewal. The letter [see appendix 10] explaining their decision went out in February, 1994. It takes great pains to rationalize their action. CBN's history with RMS is not mentioned anywhere in the letter. Perhaps it was nothing more than coincidence that the demands placed on them by the HEWI committee had occurred just a few months prior.

Meanwhile, Carla Selby was formulating an approach to the University of Colorado's Board of Regents and faculty. The apparent problem was in the School of Nursing. Dr. Jean Watson was both the dean of the school and head of an entity within it, the Center for Human Caring (CFHC) which had been started in 1986. Its original mission statement read, in part: "The development of a theory of flexible health care relating to the importance of human responses with scientific and technological aspects of such care" (Academic Relevance Committee [ARC], November 17, 1983, p. 1) [see appendix 11]. In 1989 the mission statement was revised and now stated, in part: "The art and science of human caring is a framework for nursing, health care and health policy" (ARC, 1983, p. 1). This change may seem minor; in fact it was significant as an indicator of future endeavors. The *art* of nursing now had equal standing with science. It was also significant that Janet Quinn, Ph.D., R.N., FAAN, a vocal and prominent proponent of TT, was hired by the center at approximately this time as a Senior Scholar. Quinn had published several research papers in nursing journals and thus added the veneer of scientific respectability to the Center.

CFHC was ostensibly a separate entity within the School of Nursing: "Initially, there seems to have been no clear delineation between the functions of these two units, possibly because the position of Director and Dean were held jointly by Dr. Watson. The Visiting Board minutes for 1988 and 1989 reflect the blending of the goals and interests of the School of Nursing and the Center for Human Caring without clear separation of missions or activities" (ARC, 1993, p. 2). And while this cozy relationship between the School of Nursing and CFHC came to a technical end in 1991 when Dr. Watson relinquished the Deanship, given her position of regional, national, and growing international influence, it appeared likely that she was able to influence the selection of the incoming dean, Clair Martin. This was also the period when doctor of philosophy candidates within the School of Nursing began submitting theses and getting them accepted with such titles as *A Phenomenological Inquiry On the Child's Lived Experience of Perceiving the Human Energy Field Using Therapeutic Touch* (France, 1991).

Carla Selby proposed to the RMS task force that they investigate the relationship between the CBN and the Nursing School within the UCHSC. RMS discovered: (1) At a lecture on March 31, 1993, entitled *A Frog, A Rock, A Ritual: Myths, Mysteries and Metaphors for an Eco-Caring Cosmology* by Dr. Watson, the author made such comments as, "Desperate Earthlings of the past, those afflicted with . . . commercial and machine entrophy are being scattered to the universe and being replaced by guardians, angels in fact, of esthetic, mystic and spiritual unification, of human and planetary evolution." (2) A colorful promotional brochure for TT videos costing $675 and featuring Janet Quinn was produced and distributed at CFHC and promoted by the National League for Nursing; (3) TT Courses for credit were taught by Janet Quinn at CU.

At Selby's recommendation, the members of RMS were informed of our efforts and were asked to contribute. Members who had had personal contact with one or more of the Regents informed them about RMS's efforts and concerns that: The University of Colorado Health Science Center risked tarnishing their excellent national standing as research institution if individuals used it as a cloak of credibility to advocate, promote, and capitalize on the *ritual* of TT. It took a considerable amount of effort by many individuals to educate the Regents, one at a time, about TT and its infiltration into the University of Colorado, and the possible, indeed likely, impact on the institution's credibility. RMS's efforts paid off.

The Academic Relevance Committee (ARC) had at that time been established by CU to investigate the myriad of quasiaffiliated groups and centers that had proliferated within it. The Center for Human Caring went to the top of the list; it became one of the first centers to be investigated. The ARC was charged with investigating CFHC and presenting its findings to the Chancellor of UCHSC and the Regents.

On December 16, 1993, the Regents, at a regular meeting, made public the report dated November 17, 1993, which contained the findings and recommendations of the ARC [see appendix 11]. Not only were RMS's concerns found to have merit but also one of the Regents, Jim Martin, publicly declared, "I do think the Rocky Mountain Skeptics do serve a useful purpose in monitoring this scientific accountability. I think it does keep the process open and people focused on what is scientific and what isn't."

While the complete seven page document can be found in appendix 11, a few excerpts are appropriate:

> The Center [for Human Caring] Directors should realize that they do themselves, their concepts and the School harm by the use of jargon that cannot clearly be understood, and by the espousal of theoretical constructs which appear devoid of proof. Course titles such as Emerging Otologies, Developing Resources of the Inner Self-in-Context, and Existential Advocacy: An Ethic of Embodiment do not encourage widespread appeal or understanding. The criticism of Therapeutic Touch has cast suspicion over the entire Center. If it is good therapy, it should be validated and encouraged. If not, it should be terminated. The sense of our Committee is that the scientific basis for Therapeutic Touch has not been validated and that efforts at this Center to do so have been inadequate. . . . Finally, if and when the administrative relationships of the Center are clarified, the Center mission more focused, a frequent review mechanism established, the role of Therapeutic Touch investigated, and jargon and mysticism eliminated from course work, then seed money for a variety of programs, of which the Denver Nursing Project in Human Caring is the best example, might flow appropriately to the Center. Unless these issues are dealt with, the good ideas with which the Center started may be overlooked in a tide of mounting criticism of unorthodox and unproven or untestable viewpoints and hypotheses.

The Academic Relevance Committee instructed the Chancellor and the Dean of the School of Nursing to empanel an independent committee and charged it to investigate TT thoroughly and objectively. The outcome of this process has become known as "The Claman Report." The following were the ARC's precise instructions:

> Our Committee believes that the following should be done with regard to Therapeutic Touch. The Chancellor and the Dean of the School of Nursing should appoint a special committee of investigators to carefully read the very extensive literature on this subject, to view all the videos and relevant course material, and to witness actual demonstrations of this technique. It should solicit testimony from both critics and advocates. The members of the committee should be investigators well-versed in the scientific method and should come from several disciplines on the Health Sciences Center campus *with the exception of the School of Nursing* [emphasis in original]. Nurses should be represented on the committee but it would be appropriate if they came from other

nursing schools to avoid the appearance of conflict of interest. Our Committee cannot feasibly take on this time consuming and important task because of our charge to review approximately thirty-five other Centers on this campus, because two members of the Committee are faculty of the School of Nursing, and because not all members possess the background needed to fairly critique this program. Rather than superficially review this most contentious area, we feel that it should be done once and for all in depth, and in a *thorough scientific manner* [emphasis added]. We believe that a focused committee with this single charge could come up with a useful report in a short time frame. If Therapeutic Touch is not recognized as a bonafide activity with academic relevance, then no further course work should be offered under the aegis of the University. (pp. 6, 7)

With the above directive firmly in place, Chancellor Fulginiti, who was aware of RMS's involvement at every stage of the investigation, contacted us for our recommendations of people to serve on this new TT committee. The RMS list was composed of nearly a dozen scientists and members of the skeptic community. All were rejected. The final list of committee members included: Henry N. Claman, M.D., Distinguished Professor of Medicine and Immunology, UCHSC, Denver, Chair of the "Chancellor's Committee on Therapeutic Touch (CCTT)"; Robert Freedman, M.D., Professor of Psychiatry, UCHSC, Denver; David Quissell, Ph.D., Professor and Chair, Dept. of Basic Sciences and Oral Research, School of Dentistry, UCHSC, Denver; Joan Fowler-Shaver, Ph.D., R.N., Professor and Chairperson, Dept. of Physiological Nursing, University of Washington, Seattle; and Ora Lea Strickland, Ph.D., Independence Foundation Research Chair and Professor, Nell Hodgson Woodruff School of Nursing, Emory University, Atlanta.

The Rocky Mountain Skeptics immediately began a lengthy correspondence with both Chancellor Fulginiti and Dr. Claman. With a file of material supporting our position, we called for a serious investigation into the claimed efficacy of TT. Selby and Scheiber met with Chancellor Fulginiti in his office to convey the seriousness of our concerns.

On March 21, 1994, three members of RMS met with Dr. Claman and several members of his committee. The skeptics prepared for this important opportunity for several days. George Lawrence, Ph.D., Senior Research Associate at the University of Colorado Laboratory for Atmospheric and Space Physics, prepared a ten minute statement which described the misuse of quantum physics by proponents of TT; Carla Selby gave a presentation that contrasted the philosophy and practice of science with the mischaracterizations that TT proponents made; and Béla Scheiber summarized RMS's work with state institutions involved with TT. One item he considered noteworthy was the interrelationship between the CBN, which used Janet Quinn's work to justify its position on TT, and the Center for Human Caring, which benefited from CBN decisions.

Toward the end of the meeting, two other critics of TT came to testify. Larry Sarner and Linda Rosa (she had resumed her maiden name) had resigned from RMS a few months earlier but still had an interest in TT. They provided the committee with copies of their *Survey of "Research" on Therapeutic Touch* (Rosa, 1994) that summarized their objections to many of the published studies.

Finally, the CCTT held a public meeting on April 25, 1994, where many nurses supportive of TT spoke. A couple of individuals gave testimony about the "healing" they had received for various ailments. RMS members Martin Tobias and Béla Scheiber both addressed the committee at this time. Scheiber summarized RMS' concerns:

> The Rocky Mountain Skeptics is first and foremost a watchdog group which monitors activities and claims made in the name of science. We are part of a number of independent groups throughout the world united by our concerns for activities masquerading as science.
>
> For the last several years we have been pursuing the trail of shadowy evidence used to defend a highly promoted ritual called Therapeutic Touch.
>
> Yes!—we strongly support academic freedom. At the same time we strongly support the right—in fact the duty—of a scientific researcher to conduct research on topics she or he view as having merit. For we all benefit from such activity. However, we, the leadership of the Rocky Mountain Skeptics, would be in conflict with the goals of our organization if we did not speak up and bring to the attention of others our concerns for the indefensible and unethical practice of individuals within an institution of science promoting a product or procedure before appropriate scientific protocol has been satisfied.
>
> A researcher has the obligation not to exaggerate and certainly not to benefit financially from a procedure not shown to be effective or for that matter safe. Certainly, researchers at the University of Colorado's Health Science Center have an additional burden of ensuring that new procedures not be prematurely advocated or promoted because the institution's hard earned credibility is also at stake. The wholesale promotion—financial and academic—of Therapeutic Touch is not supported by the evidence. It may be in the future—we do not claim psychic powers—but it does not today. Do the research; publish the findings, but do not jeopardize the credibility of research being pursued at this institution." [The content of this brief statement was through the cooperative efforts of Ms. Carla Selby and Mr. Béla Scheiber.] (*Rocky Mountain Skeptic*, 1994, p. 1)

The Report of the *Chancellor's Committee on Therapeutic Touch* (*CCTT*) dated July 6, 1994, was delivered to Chancellor Fuginiti from Henry N. Claman, Chair, and then made public. The report can be read in its entirety in appendix 3.

A memorandum prepared by the Dean of the Nursing School, Clair Martin, to the Chancellor directly responds to the final report issued by the CCTT [see appendix 12]. It is a curious memorandum since the following is written in "Recommendation 1. The need for external impact":

> The School of Nursing is preparing its Self-Study Report for a site visit and reaccreditation by the National League for Nursing. This process will critically explore the integrity and quality of all courses offered by the School in its baccalaureate, nursing doctorate and master's degree programs. The site visit is scheduled for 1995 and will provide external review and the critical reflection of School faculty. Therapeutic Touch courses are included in this review.

While this recommendation gives an impression of an objective, external effort to evaluate the Nursing School, it in fact represents more of the same "clever" obfuscation that RMS had encountered in the early days in front of the CBN. What the memorandum did not say was that Dr. Jean Watson was the president-elect of the National League for Nursing from 1993 until 1995 and then its president until some unknown event terminated it prematurely in 1997.

In a final parting letter to Chancellor Fulginiti (September 18, 1994) RMS noted this serious conflict of interest (not mentioned anywhere in the ARC report or the CCTT) [see appendix 13]. After receiving our letter, the Chair of the Board of Regents, Guy J. Kelley, wrote to us on April 24, 1995, that:

> I received the copy of the letter you sent 18 September 1994 to Chancellor Fulginiti about the report on Therapeutic Touch (TT). I appreciate your watchful eye over activities like TT. The University of Colorado is an academic and research institution.
>
> Activities at CU must be academically relevant and follow rational thought and investigation. CU is not a church. There is *academic* freedom not total freedom to engage in any activity with any process. Even if there is little hope of demonstrating the validity of a hypothesis, the validity of the process should not be in question.
>
> Academicians need the freedom to explore, but the discipline to use processes of investigations which are reliable and valid. Academic freedom shouldn't lead to scientific anarchy.
>
> I appreciate your concern and your efforts. (Emphasis in original. See appendix 14)

Three years after initiating what was thought would be a short investigation of TT, RMS found itself embroiled in a national controversy. The efforts of RMS, detailed by many newspaper and magazine articles, became well known within the skeptic and TT communities throughout the world.

And what about those individuals who were the center of much of the controversy? Dean Clair Martin of the School of Nursing was no longer the Dean by sometime in 1995, Sally Phillips left her post as Chair of the CBN in 1993, and Dr. Janet Quinn is still with CFHC but keeps a low profile in Colorado (she was invited to contribute to this book but the request went unanswered). Even "Therapeutic Touch" underwent a schism with a new group no longer referring to TT, and its early founders, directly; they call it "Healing Touch." Meanwhile, the Rocky Mountain Skeptics have gone on to other areas of interest but they always keep an eye on the strange world of Therapeutic Touch and its "interesting" players.

REFERENCES

Aldorfer, W. 1993. "RMS Attends a Class for Credit." *Rocky Mountain Skeptic* 11 (2): 2, 3

Clark, P. O., and M. J. Clark. 1984. "Therapeutic Touch: Is There a Scientific Basis for the Practice?" *Nursing Research* 33 (1): 37–41.

France, N. E. M. 1991. *A Phenomenological Inquiry On the Child's Lived Experience of Perceiving the Human Energy Field Using Therapeutic Touch.* Thesis submitted to the Faculty of the Graduate School of the University of Colorado in partial fulfillment of the requirements for the degree of Doctor of Philosophy School of Nursing.

Grad, B., R. Cadoret, and G. Paul. 1961. "An Unorthodox Method of Treatment of Wound Healing in Mice." *International Journal of Parapsychology* 3: 5–24.

Rocky Mountain Skeptics. 1992. "RMS Address to the Colorado Board of Nursing." 9 (6):7.

———. 1993a. "RMS Address CBN." 10 (6): 2.

———. 1993b. "Oral Presentation to the State Board of Nursing by the Rocky Mountain Skeptics (Part 1)." 11 (2).

———. 1993c. "Oral Presentation to the State Board of Nursing by the Rocky Mountain Skeptics (Part 2)." 11 (2).

———. 1994. "RMS Testifies at University TT Hearing." 12 (1): 1.

———. 1998. "Skeptics Meet the Board of Nursing." 16 (1, 2): 12.

Rojas, L. 1992. "Touchy Subject." *Rocky Mountain Skeptic* 9 (6).

Rosa, L. March 21, 1994. Survey of "Research on Therapeutic Touch." Report to the Therapeutic Touch Review Committee, Health Sciences Center, University of Colorado Health Sciences Center, Dr. Henry Claman, Chairman.

Sandroff, R. 1980. "A Skeptic's Guide to Therapeutic Touch." *RN* (January): 25–30, 82–83.

Skeptic. 1994. "About the Authors." 3 (1): 107.

Walike, B., P. Bruno, S. Donaldson, R. Erickson, et al. 1975. ". . . attempts to embellish a totally unscientific process with the aura of science . . ." in Letters, *American Journal of Nursing* 75 (August): 1275, 1278, 1282.

Watson, J., and S. Phillips. 1992. "A Call for Educational Reform: Colorado Nursing Doctorate Model as Exemplar." *Nursing Outlook* 40 (1): 20–25.

9

Getting in Touch with TT Experimenters*

Dale Beyerstein

Proponents of alternative or complementary medicine often accuse skeptics of having closed minds and of being unwilling to look at the evidence for their various new—or very old—therapies. This charge deflects attention away from evaluating the evidence for the unconventional therapies and allows the proponents to get away with three things: First, they switch the burden of proof from the proponent of the claim, where it belongs, onto the critic. Second, proponents can hide the fact that they have presented virtually no evidence for their claims by making it *seem* that they have *already* presented great quantities of evidence that have been ignored. Third, they poison the well against skeptics, who are portrayed as having a vested interest in suppressing or discounting unconventional therapies, and so nothing they might say needs to be answered.

The idea of the closed-minded skeptic has risen to the status of myth, but the facts tell a very different story. Skeptics often go to extraordinary lengths to evaluate data on unusual claims, only to be met with a lack of cooperation from the True Believers. This chapter describes my repeated attempts over more than a two-year period to contact Dr. Daniel Wirth (he holds a J.D. degree in law) in hopes of obtaining more information about his published research suggesting that Therapeutic Touch can help heal wounds.

A second myth common in paranormal circles is that these researchers can establish the validity of paranormal claims on their own, in isolation from the scientific community. Then, when their final report is published, they hold the scientific community to be closed minded if the results are not immediately accepted without any questions regarding how they were obtained—about the design of the experiment,

---

*The author would like to thank and acknowledge the valuable technical assistance provided by Rececca Long.

the conditions under which it was done, and so on. Yet the scientific community asks these questions of its own members when they present surprising results; scientists do not assume that just because an experiment is published it is therefore without errors which might in some way account for the results.

My attempts to get information from Daniel Wirth began when I noticed a very favorable article (Breckinridge, 1994) on TT published in Canada's national newspaper, the *Globe and Mail*. Until that time it was my understanding that there were no placebo-controlled studies without major flaws offering positive evidence for TT. The article suggested that the *Globe and Mail* had found one:

> One of the best studies [of TT] to date is a randomized, double-blind experiment that involved forty-four men who had undergone identical surgical biopsies on their arms. The men were asked to put their arms through an opening in a wall. Twenty-three received Therapeutic Touch; the others didn't.

The results showed that by the eighth day the average wound size was one-tenth the size in the treated group (Wirth, 1990). By the sixteenth day, thirteen of the twenty-three treated subjects were completely healed, but none were fully healed in the untreated group.

No citation was given within the article, so my first job would be to identify the article referred to by the *Globe and Mail*. Networking among Skeptics would prove helpful. I remembered seeing articles on TT by Bullough and Bullough (1993) and Scheiber (1993) in the *Skeptical Inquirer*. I called Béla Scheiber at the Rocky Mountain Skeptics in Boulder, Colorado. After hearing a couple of sentences from the newspaper article, he identified the source; within the hour he had faxed me the article, Wirth (1990), which has been cited by many proponents of TT.

As described by Wirth (1990), the experimental protocol sounded even better than the *Globe* had led me to believe, and the results appeared even more dramatic than the newspaper had reported. A full description of Wirth's study is given by me in "Replication of TT Research: A Case Study" [see chapter 17 in this volume]. The experiment was indeed double-blind, placebo-controlled, and the protocol, as described in the article, was just what was needed to demonstrate the effect of TT on wound healing.

Yet I had a number of questions for Daniel Wirth. First, why was this article published in an obscure new age journal rather than in a mainstream medical journal? It was very well written and appeared to have such good experimental design. If substantiated, Wirth's results would have extraordinary theoretical implications for mainstream medicine and could ease the suffering of millions of people if they became widely known. Yet this article was published in *Subtle Energies*, out of Golden, Colorado, rather than in a journal such as the *New England Journal of Medicine*.

I wondered if Wirth had even submitted the article to any of the major medical journals. Practitioners of alternative medicine regularly criticize mainstream medicine for not paying attention to their discoveries, but this criticism is not fair when the alternative practitioners will not meet their opponents halfway by submitting their results to the journals read by those they criticize. Publication in a mainstream journal would provide doctors and scientists the opportunity to critique, and perhaps replicate, studies with results that seem contrary to the existing body of scientific knowledge.

Proponents of TT who believe the myth about skeptics being closed minded might assume that a mainstream medical journal would reject an article with positive results for a non-science-based therapy out of hand. However, history has shown that this is not a valid assumption. To cite just a few examples, clinical studies reporting positive results for *moxibustion*, which involves the burning of herbs at acupuncture points (Cardini, 1998); *reflexology*, which is a method of diagnosing illness by examining the soles of the feet (Oleson, 1993); and *homeopathy*, which consists of treatment with solutions so diluted that none of the original substance remains (Davenas, 1988; Jacobs, 1994), have been published in the *Journal of the American Medical Association*, *Obstetrics and Gynecology*, and in *Nature* and *Pediatrics*, respectively. Barnes et al. (1999) performed a MEDLINE search and found an increasing level of published research on complementary medicine. Further, a study by Ernst et al. (1999) found no evidence of peer-reviewer bias against an unconventional drug treatment. It cannot, therefore, be assumed that mainstream medical journals would automatically reject an article such as Wirth's.

Even the submission of a controversial article to a major medical journal, let alone publication, provides peer-review in accordance with the scientific process. Wirth's results, since they are so robust and so inconsistent with what is presently known about wound healing, would certainly be very surprising to the editors of any mainstream journal of scientific medicine. The editors would probably want to see Wirth's raw data and would ask, at the very least, questions about the experiment such as those I pose below.

On occasion, the editor of a major medical journal will arrange for a replication of an experiment that has yielded extraordinary results. A case analogous to the Wirth study is the experiment reported in Davenas et al. (1988). This experiment presented positive evidence for homeopathy. Jacques Benveniste, a respected scientist at INSERM 200 outside of Paris, France, along with senior author Elisabeth Davenas, published the study in *Nature* which presented results no less unexpected than those reported in Wirth (1990) and equally inconsistent with currently held beliefs in the medical community. They reported that a protein, IgE, diluted to as little as 10^{-120} of its original strength (so diluted that it is extremely unlikely that any of the protein remains), can granulate basophil in a test tube. Since the results were extraordinary, *Nature* agreed to publish them with the proviso that its then editor, John Maddox, along with a team of people well versed in detecting fraud, self-deception, or experimental error, could visit the lab and participate with the group in a replication of the experiment. The test conditions would not allow the kinds of experimental error that Maddox's team had hypothesized to explain Davinas's and Benveniste's original results. The results of the second experiment (Maddox, Randi and Stewart, 1988) failed to confirm those of the first and the results were published in the next issue of *Nature*. But, since Wirth's experiment involved human subjects being willing to undergo tests over a sixteen-day period, it would be understandable that such an agreement would not work in his case. Nevertheless, alternative arrangements could have been made, perhaps involving an independent team replicating the results. The analysis of the raw data and a discussion of Wirth's protocol could well have been sufficient to allow publication of the article, and attempts at replication would certainly have followed.

My second question was why these results had not been widely replicated by the TT community, since Wirth's protocol is relatively simple. I knew from Scheiber (1993) [see also chapter 21 in this volume] that other experimental data submitted by TT practitioners were either not derived from experiments as well controlled as Wirth's or had results that were not nearly so dramatic. The best studies concentrated on pain relief, a notoriously vague and subjective result. Only Wirth himself has tried to replicate his wound-healing experiments.

The third question that troubled me was why the purported wound-healing effects of TT were not widely known already. Wirth's results indicated an effect so strong that one would expect it to have been discovered centuries ago, long before our era of double-blind placebo-controlled studies. Consider an analogy: Willow bark has long been known in folk medicine to be an analgesic, or pain reliever, and to reduce fever. People would chew on it or boil it and drink the resulting brew. The effect is so strong that modern scientific studies were not needed to prove its effectiveness. Of course, isolating its active ingredient, *salicylic acid*, allowed us not only to synthesize *acetylsalicylic acid* (aspirin), but also to standardize concentrations, determine the optimum dosage and the levels for overdosage, and minimize some of the harmful side effects. Nevertheless, willow bark was known to *be* effective long before this was done.

One of the strongest supposed advantages of TT is the simplicity of its practice. For centuries, healers have engaged in similar rituals. Wirth et al. (1993a) points out that TT "was derived from the ancient healing practice of laying on of hands." If such therapies are indeed efficacious for healing wounds, surely some of the practitioners would have noticed such effects. As with the example of willow bark and modern aspirin, perhaps the effects of earlier rituals were not as pronounced or as systematic as those reported by modern proponents of TT; but all the same, there should be much more anecdotal evidence for these effects than there currently is. This, however, was not a question I needed to put to Daniel Wirth since the most important issue was the results of his experiment. Experimental results speak for themselves; no matter how improbable they might seem a priori, if they can be replicated then explaining them is the first order of business. Why the effects hadn't been discovered earlier is a later question to be answered by sociologists of science.

My fourth question was why Wirth's 1990 article did not identify the other individuals with critical roles in conducting the study. A "Dr. M." made a significant contribution by incising and measuring the wounds of all the subjects. An individual referred to as "EI" had a major role in greeting each subject, putting them at ease, ensuring that the routine was completed in the allotted time, and so forth. Normal academic practice would be to have identified these individuals, and perhaps to have accorded them coauthorship; however, they are not so much as acknowledged in a footnote. I also found it somewhat surprising that the name of the TT practitioner was not provided in the paper, at least in the form of an acknowledgement for her contribution.

The more I thought about it, the more convinced I became that this experiment needed to be replicated. Our British Columbia Skeptics organization consists of several professionals I could call on to join with me to do the replication. We could do it at one of the universities in Vancouver with which our members are affiliated. I resolved to contact Wirth and discuss my questions. I also intended to tell him that my group would be doing a replication in Vancouver and ask for his cooperation. There are always details that do not make their way into a published paper, given the space limitations. A group replicating another group's research wants to be sure that they are replicating the experiment as originally done in order to assure that differences in the results of the two experiments are not the result of a different methodology. To be sure that this will not be a problem, many details not discussed in the original paper must be ironed out in advance of the second experiment. Further, anyone replicating another group's results will be saved untold delays and problems by consulting the original experimenters for methodological details. Another reason for close communication between the two groups from the beginning is that such discussions will sometimes suggest alternative explanations that were not thought of by the original experimenters, and the design of the second experiment can be modified to test them and rule them out. I had several such questions I wished to ask Wirth; these are listed by me in chapter 17 in this volume.

Yet another question for Daniel Wirth came to mind. Because his experiment involved inflicting surgical wounds on test subjects, I presumed that Wirth had obtained and documented appropriate review and approval for his use of human subjects. Perhaps Wirth had done the experiment at his own institute, Healing Sciences Research International, but I knew from his article that he had recruited his subjects through advertising on bulletin boards at a local university. If so, he would have had to present his proposal to a committee at that university to gain approval for this research involving human subjects. I wanted practical advice from Wirth on how to get the protocol for these experiments accepted by the human subjects committees at either of the two universities where we could be doing our replication.

I anticipated no trouble contacting Daniel Wirth. Nor did I anticipate any difficulty in getting my questions answered, for three reasons: First, the points raised in the previous paragraphs are well understood in the scientific community, and scientists understand the importance of having other groups replicate their experiments. Therefore, scientists do not normally view questions about experimental design as hostile even if they are skeptical in nature, especially when research results go against currently held views. Second, recognition of their work is a powerful incentive for scientists and other academics to cooperate; as Carl Sagan pointed out, there is no better road to fame in science than to present results that are novel but survive critical examination. Third, most academics are also teachers and the chance to share their knowledge with others, even those less well-informed, is part of what makes someone disposed to teaching. What follows is the story of my failed attempt to get my questions answered.

I first thought I would introduce myself to Wirth by telephone. Wirth's paper included a mailing address in Orinda, California, but, as is common, no telephone number. I called Directory Assistance. There was no listing in Orinda for Daniel Wirth (or D. Wirth for that matter) or for the Healing Sciences Research International, of which he identifies himself as president and research director. I consulted Daniel

Sabsay, of the East Bay Skeptics, who determined that the address provided in Wirth's paper is the address of the Orinda Post Office where, presumably, Wirth or his organization rents a box. A call to the San Francisco Public Library in August 1994 failed to turn up any information on Healing Sciences Research International in any of the directories they consulted. The Business Licenses office of Conta Costa County, the county in which Orinda is located, had never issued a business license to this organization or to anyone named Daniel Wirth.

Prior to discovering that Wirth's mailing address was the post office, I thought that my difficulties might be due to him having moved since the article was published. I tried contacting the International Society of the Study of Subtle Energies, publisher of the *Subtle Energies* journal in which Wirth's paper had appeared. A very helpful person took my call, but she returned from her files with the same address that appeared in the article and she had no phone number for Wirth. My last desperate attempt at tracking Wirth's telephone number was on July 16, 1995, when Béla Scheiber supplied me from his CD-ROM listings with all the D. Wirths in the area around Orinda, as far away as San Jose. Again I struck out.

If I couldn't phone, I could write. I sent Wirth a letter on October 15, 1994, asking questions about his experimental design and for his assistance in replicating the experiment. That letter was never answered. Ten months later, on August 15, 1995, I sent a second letter by registered mail. The post office confirmed that my registered letter was picked up; again, this letter was never answered.

Knowing that the Orinda address for Wirth's office is close to John F. Kennedy University, a school that used to have a program in parapsychology, I thought that Wirth might at one time have had a connection with the institution, either as a student or faculty member. A phone call to that institution confirmed that Daniel Wirth received an M.S. in Parapsychology (a division of the Graduate School of Consciousness Studies) in 1989. I telephoned the JFK Alumni Association, on January 11, 1995, but Greg Newton of that organization couldn't give me a telephone number for Wirth because of confidentiality provisions.

The reason that Daniel Wirth refers to himself as "Dr." is that he has a J.D. degree. However, Wirth is not a member of the California Bar Association. This organization assured me that Wirth has never been registered in California, which explains why he is not cited in the *California Legal Directory*. Further, he is not listed in the *Martin Hubbell Directory* (a national listing of lawyers). From this I conclude that he is not (and probably has never been) a member of any state bar association in the United States. Thus another potential avenue for locating Wirth proved a dead end.

Being unsuccessful in my attempts to contact Wirth directly, I thought that I might be able to reach him through one of his colleagues. Perhaps Wirth would talk with me if one of his colleagues first put in a good word on my behalf. Once again the Skeptics network paid off. Wilma Russell and Earl Hautala of the Bay Area Skeptics located Wirth's M.S. thesis at the JFK library and sent me the abstract, introduction, and other interesting excerpts. Janet Quinn, one of the most important proponents of TT, was the external examiner. This may explain how Wirth originally became interested in the subject. More significant, however, was the discovery that his thesis supervisor was Jerry Soifin. Although Dr. Soifin had since left JFK because the School of Consciousness Studies had been disbanded, I did locate him by telephone on June 1, 1995. He informed me that he had nothing to do with Wirth's current research and could not comment on it. Moreover, he told me that he could not give me a current telephone number for Wirth and did not know anyone else who could. Dr. Soifin gave me the impression that Daniel Wirth did not wish to be contacted by people interested in his research.

My next thought was to try to contact Wirth's collaborators. By this time the Skeptic network had sent me some other papers from Healing Sciences Research International which listed coauthors. I thought that I might be able to track some of these people down. The address on the papers was always that of Healing Sciences Research International, which had already proven a dead end, but I hoped to locate some of the coauthors through their professional associations. There were people listed with Ph.D.s but their disciplines were not given, so that would not be a fruitful avenue. There were R.N.s listed, but their names were common and there are so many R.N.s that I thought it would be impractical to attempt to pursue this approach. But there was a dentist, D. R. Brenlan, D.D.S., who had collaborated with Wirth on a paper on postoperative pain after removal of molars (Wirth et al., 1993b). A call to the California Board of Dental Examiners, however, didn't yield anything useful; no David R. Brenlan had ever been eligible to practice in California. The California Dental Association had no record of him either.

Another study (Wirth et al., 1993a) was a replication of Wirth (1990) with twenty-four subjects receiving punch biopsies to their arms. Similarly dramatic results were reported. One author was W. S. Eidelman, M.D. On the remote chance that Dr. Eidelman might have been the mysterious "Dr. M." who performed the biopsies and evaluated the subjects in the original study, I attempted to track him down. Perhaps he could answer my questions about that study or help me locate Daniel Wirth. The San Francisco Public Library was obliging, as always, and reported that there was no one by that name listed in the *ABMS Directory of Board Certified Practitioners*. Reasoning that he may not be a specialist, I contacted the California Medical Board. Imagine my joy in discovering that they had found a William S. Eidelman registered since 1976. His address was in Santa Monica but researchers often collaborate over large distances. What was the upshot of this? Directory Assistance had no telephone number for a Dr. Eidelman at the address provided by the Board, and no forwarding address. Once again my investigation ground to a halt.

The reader who has persevered with my tale thus far might assume that Daniel Wirth is a hermit, but this inference would be premature. "Selective" would seem to be the more accurate term. In the acknowledgements of his M.S. thesis, he thanks twenty-six noted parapsychologists and people involved in alternative medicine from all over the world, including D. Scott Rogo, Charles Tart, William Roll, Erlendur Haaraldsson, Brenda Dunne, Stanley Krippner, Bernie Siegel, Charles Lea, and Herbert Benson. In addition to having Janet Quinn as his thesis external examiner, he cites Dolores Krieger for helpful comments. Not only this, but Wirth's TT research was the subject of a BBC documentary, rebroadcast on the Discovery Channel in the United States. Michael Stanwyk of East Sussex, UK, who is an author of nursing-journal articles critical of TT, contacted the producer of this documentary to try to find out how to contact Wirth. Stanwyck ran into a brick wall, just as I had.

In this modern day, no attempt to track information is complete without using the Internet. I posted messages in many places asking anyone who had ever collaborated with Wirth, or been a subject in one of his experiments, or who even *knew* of anyone who was, to contact me. I left these on the bulletin boards of the Microsoft Network and CompuServe that related to either nursing or the paranormal. Messages were also posted by others on my behalf on the following newsgroups: *alt.paranet.abduct*, *alt.paranet.metaphysics*, *alt.paranet.science*, *alt.paranet.skeptic*, *alt.paranet.ufo*, *alt.paranormal.channeling*, and *alt.paranormal.forteania*. All I received were a couple of messages with more suggestions on how to contact the mysterious Daniel Wirth. Not a single person wrote to tell of even a "friend of a friend" who had participated in one of Wirth's experiments.

When my efforts to locate Wirth through the Internet proved unsuccessful, I tried once again to reach him by mail. This time I tried a new tack. I sent him a registered letter (dated September 17, 1996) with a version of this chapter up to this point. It described my difficulties with getting my questions answered. I wanted to give Wirth the opportunity to explain why he hadn't answered any of my previous letters or to correct any mistakes I might have made. He wrote back on September 27, 1996. He didn't explain his failure to answer my earlier letters nor did he answer any of the questions I had posed about his research. He mentioned nothing about my intention to replicate his research and made no offer to provide me with any assistance. Nor did he identify any mistakes in my article requiring correction. He merely pointed out that he had published other work besides the article I was interested in. The last paragraph of his response appears to reflect his law background more than a desire to support scientific inquiry:

> Let me recommend that before you publish your article, you clearly delineate areas of opinion from areas of fact. In this respect, as a licensed practicing attorney, I would suggest that you contact legal counsel in order to distinguish the difference between opinion and libelous comments.

At least I can now say that I have heard from Dr. Wirth, even though none of my questions about his experiment have been answered. Without his cooperation, I conclude that there is no point in our group attempting to replicate his experiment.

REFERENCES

Barnes, J., N. C. Abbot, E. F. Harkness, and E. Ernst. 1990. "Articles on Complementary Medicine in the Mainstream Medical Literature." *Arch Intern Med* 159: 1721–25.

Breckenridge, J. 1994. "Hands-off Treatment Moves In." *Globe and Mail,* July 9, p. A1.

Bullough, V. L., and B. Bullough. 1993. "Therapeutic Touch: Why Do Nurses Believe?" *Skeptical Inquirer* 17 (2): 169–74.

Cardini, F., and H. Weixin. 1998. "Moxibustion for Correction of Breech Presentation." *JAMA* 280: 1580–84.

Davenas, E., F. Beauvais, and J. Amara et al. 1988. "Human Bashophil Dengranulation Triggered by Very Dilute Antiserum Against IgE." *Nature* 333: 816–18.

Ernst, E. et al. 1999 "Reviewer Bias Against the Unconventional? A Randomized Double-blind Study of Peer Review." *Complementary Therapies in Medicine* 7 (1): 19–23.

Jacobs, J. et al. 1994. "Treatment of Childhood Diarrhea with Homeopathic Medicine: A Randomized Controlled Trial In Nicarauga." *Pediatrics* 93 (5): 719–25.

Maddox, J., J. Randi, and W. Stewart. 1988. " 'High-dilution' Experiments a Delusion." *Nature* 334: 287–90.

Oleson, T., and W. Flocco. 1993. "Randomized Controlled Study of Premenstrual

Symptoms Treated with Ear, Hand, and Foot Reflexology." *Obstetrics and Gynecology* 82: 906–11.

Scheiber, B. 1993. "Colorado Board of Nursing Support Therapeutic Touch, Skeptics Continue Challenge." *Skeptical Inquirer* 17 (3): 327–30.

Wirth, D. P. 1990. "The Effect of Noncontact Therapeutic Touch on the Healing Rate of Full Thickness Dermal Wounds." *Subtle Energies* 1 (1): 1–20.

Wirth, D. P., J. T. Richardson, W. S. Eidelman, and A. C. O'Malley. 1993a. "Full Thickness Dermal Wounds Treated With Noncontact Therapeutic Touch: A Replication and Extension." *Complementary Therapies in Medicine* 1: 127–32.

Wirth, D. P., D. R. Brenlan, R. J. Levine, and C. M. Rodriguez. 1993b. "The Effect of Complementary Healing Therapy on Postoperative Pain after Surgical Removal of Impacted Third Molar Teeth." *Complementary Therapies in Medicine* 1: 133–38.

10.

Therapeutic Touch: Is There a Scientific Basis for the Practice?

Philip E. Clark and Mary Jo Clark

Therapeutic Touch, the art of interpersonal energy transfer for the purpose of healing (Krieger, Peper, and Ancoli, 1979), is an intervention that is believed by some to have potential for nursing. Workshops are being held across the country and there is at least one graduate course in the art of Therapeutic Touch (Krieger, 1979). Indeed, there are nurses who use the practice as a therapeutic modality (Sandroff, 1980). What empirical support exists for such practice?

Nursing literature covers several aspects of Therapeutic Touch. Selected articles relate the history of the laying-on of hands (Zefron, 1975), describe a theoretical framework in which to interpret the phenomenon of Therapeutic Touch (Miller, 1979), and map the human field (Boguslawski, 1979). The literature also suggests ailments that Therapeutic Touch may ameliorate (Boguslawski, 1979), and even describes a format for charting the effects of the intervention (Krieger, 1979). Sandroff (1980) presents an overview by three prominent nurse researchers on the subject of Therapeutic Touch.

Although such contributions to the literature are interesting, they do not provide empirical support for practice. To determine the validity of Therapeutic Touch as a treatment modality, reports of research investigating its effects must be examined. Such an examination is the intent of this article.

One of the earlier examples of research on Therapeutic Touch (Grad, Cadoret, and Paul, 1961) examined wound healing in mice. After wounding and wound measurement, each of 300 mice were randomly assigned to one experimental or one of two control groups. The experimental group was treated by a healer. One control group was treated by medical students who claimed no paranormal healing abilities; the other received no treatment.

Prior to wounding, the mice were observed and weighed periodically for one to two weeks to eliminate unhealthy mice. During this time, the mice were also subjected to frequent handling similar to that they would experience during treatment. The mice were anesthetized and hair was removed from a 0.8 × 1.6 inch area on the back. Oval wounds of about 0.4 × 0.8 inches were cut with scissors in such a way that the wound lay with its long axis along the spine and with the wound center 1.2 inches from the base of the tail. Wound size was measured immediately after wounding and the mice rank-ordered according to the precise wound size. The three mice with the largest wounds were randomly assigned, one to each of the three treatment groups. Random assignment continued with each of the succeeding groups of three mice. This procedure assured an equal distribution of wound sizes to the three treatment groups.

Treatment occurred in two conditions: open and closed bag (Grad et al., 1961). The open bag condition permitted the healer or medical student to place his hands in a paper bag that contained a mouse in a cage. Handling of the cage only was permitted; the mice were not handled directly. The closed bag condition permitted handling of the paper bag only. The control group receiving no treatment was also exposed to both bag conditions.

The mice were housed in ten rooms with thirty mice per room. Of the thirty mice in a particular room, ten mice were treated by the healer, ten by medical students, and ten received no treatment. All of the mice in any one room were treated under the same condition. Mice in five of the rooms were treated in the open bag condition; mice in the other rooms were treated in the closed bag condition.

Differences in wound size were assessed by a two-way analysis of variance. The investigators reported adjusting wound measurements due to moderate skewing of distribution. It was tested using the adjusted data. Homogeneity of variance was established only within each bag condition. Separate factorial analyses were applied to the means of wound measurements of mice in the open bag condition and closed bag condition.

On the fifteenth and sixteenth days of the study, the investigators found significantly smaller wound sizes for the mice treated by the healer in the open bag condition. On subsequent days, the difference in wound size was not significant. Nor was there ever a significant difference between mice treated by the healer in the closed bag condition and the mice in the control groups.

This investigation of one healer's ability by Grad et al. (1961) appears to have been well controlled. The findings, though statistically significant in the open bag condition, were transient. One must question, then, the utility of the healer, since the other groups of mice achieved a similar degree of healing by the end of the study.

A second investigation by Grad (1963) dealt with a healer's influence on the growth of barley seeds. Twenty-four peat pots, each containing twenty barley seeds, were randomly assigned to two groups of equal size. The experimental group of seeds was watered initially with a 1 percent saline solution from an open beaker held for fifteen minutes by the healer with his hand tended over the beaker.

The rationale for using a 1 percent saline solution in the manner described, rather than having the healer touch the plants or their pots directly, derived from a number of previous exploratory experiments conducted by Grad. He stated that "best results were obtained under conditions of an inhibition of the normal growth of seeds" (1963, p. 118). Salt was considered an inhibiting factor and a 1 percent saline solution was considered optimal for the purpose of inhibiting growth without killing the plants.

With respect to the treatment of the watering solution as opposed to direct treatment of the plants, Grad stated: "Experiments soon demonstrated that significant differences could readily be *obtained without* the need for Mr. E. to treat the plants with his hands, but it was enough simply to add water, water which he had previously treated" (1963, p. 121). Speculation that heat from the healer's hands influenced the growth of experimental plants is eliminated by the use of a treated watering solution. The maintenance of double-blind conditions was simplified as the healer was not aware of which group of plants had been treated at the time he measured them.

The dependent variables were the number of plants per pot, the average height of plants per pot, and plant yield per pot. Yield was defined as "the total of all the *heights* of each plant in a given pot" (Grad, 1963, p. 125). Plants were counted and measured by the healer on the eighth through thirteenth days after treatment.

Grad reported specific measurements of the three dependent variables. Data analysis by means of a t test indicated that on one day only, the experimental group contained a significantly greater number of plants. In addition, the experimental plants were reported as significantly taller and to have had a significantly greater yield for a period of five days (Grad, 1963).

The use of the healer to prepare all pots and seeds and to measure all plants might have contributed to some bias in the study. Grad (1963) explained that the double-blind aspects of the study prevented the healer from becoming aware of which were the treated plants. Also, any additional influence due to healer contact with the pots, seeds, or plants should have been reflected in both groups and would not have contributed to the significant differences found. Grad's rationale for the use of the healer in this capacity was simply the lack of other personnel to carry out the task. Employment of another person would have eliminated this threat to internal validity. The reported results of this study seem more stable over time and, therefore, may be considered somewhat more convincing than those of the previous study.

A similar study examined the effects of two healers on rye grass seeds (MacDonald, Hickman, and Dakin, 1977). For one healer, the plant heights in the experimental group were significantly smaller than those of the control group. For the other healer, the plant heights in the experimental group were significantly greater. Although the investigators viewed the results as supporting those of Grad, such an equivocal report must be questioned.

Grad replicated his previous work with barley seeds in a series of four experiments. In the original work with barley seeds, the saline solution treated by the healer was contained in an open beaker. In this series of four experiments, the saline solution treated by the healer was contained in a stoppered bottle or in a stoppered bottle in a stapled paper bag.

The use of the paper bag was introduced as an additional measure to assure double-blind conditions. The stoppered container was used to prevent contamination of the solution by the healer's perspiration or respiration, which would have been possible in the previous experiment. Significant results in the stoppered condition would support the conclusion that something, perhaps a healing energy, had passed from the healer's hands, through the glass, to the solution.

The previous measures of mean number, height, and yield of plants were also used in these four experiments. The results were essentially mixed. The measures of plant number, height, and yield reported were only occasionally significant. At other times, no differences between groups were noted. None of the results in this series of experiments was as stable over time as those of the original work with barley seeds. For an excellent review of these studies with mice and plants, see Grad (1965).

Smith (1972) examined the potential effects of a healer and a magnetic field on the enzyme trypsin. The rationale for enzyme activity as a measure of the effects of a healer's performance is derived from biochemical evidence that cellular metabolism involves specific enzyme activity and from the supposition that illness is a result of absence of or dysfunction in enzyme activity. As stated by Smith: "if enzyme failure is the ultimate physical cause of disease, any therapeutic effect should be detectable at the same level, that is, with enzyme activity" (1972, p. 15).

The investigator used four solutions of the enzyme trypsin—a control solution, a solution exposed to ultraviolet light and treated by the healer, a solution held by the healer, and a solution exposed to a magnetic field. Using a series of graphs, Smith (1972) reported means and standard deviations of the activity levels of the various solutions. No statistical tests for the significance of the findings were reported. Smith concluded that the healer and magnetic field exerted similar effects, as those two solutions displayed increased enzyme activity.

Smith (1972) also reported two replications of this study, one using the same healer and one using three other self-proclaimed healers. The results of the initial experiment were not reproduced. Smith reported a third replication with three healers and claimed an increase in enzyme activity. Very few details with respect to any of the replications are discussed.

There was no report of statistical testing for significance of differences between activity levels of the treated and control groups. It is unknown whether the reported increases in enzyme activity demonstrated in the initial study were statistically significant or due to chance. The absence of increased enzyme activity during two of the three replication studies suggests that the initial results may have been due to chance.

The efforts of Dr. Delores Krieger merit consideration as some of the first attempts by nurses at scientific inquiry into this treatment modality. Krieger (1976) reported a significant increase in hemoglobin levels in response to the efforts of a healer. However, there are a number of questions raised by the rationale for hemoglobin as the dependent variable and by the methods used in the study.

Krieger (1976) postulated that the healer facilitates the flow of a healing energy and that this energy is bound to oxygen. Hemoglobin was chosen as a measure of this energy flow because "hemoglobin . . . is one of the body's most sensitive indicators of oxygen uptake" (Krieger, 1976, p. 123). Hemoglobin is not, however, a measure of oxygen uptake, but a measure of oxygen capacity (Selkurt, 1975). An appropriate measure of oxygen uptake is oxygen saturation of the blood.

Krieger also stated that another reason for the selection of hemoglobin was the similarity of hemoglobin to chlorophyll. She reported that "Grad found that the treated seeds . . . had a greater net weight and significantly more chlorophyll content than the control group" (Krieger, 1976, p. 122). Based on reports of Grad's studies, it is difficult to determine how this conclusion was reached. The dependent measures in Grad's research (1963, 1964, 1967) were mean number, height, and yield of plants. There are no reports of measurement of chlorophyll content. Greater chlorophyll levels could be assumed to coincide with greater yield but without specific measurement and comparison, it is not known if significant differences in chlorophyll levels between groups were present.

Krieger's final rationale for the selection of hemoglobin as the dependent variable was that the production of hemoglobin was dependent upon the functioning of several enzymes and that "Smith's study indicated that enzyme systems responded to the laying-on of hands" (1976, p. 124). While Smith (1972) did report an increase in trypsin activity, she did not report testing for statistical significance between pre- and posttreatment measures of enzyme activity or between the four solutions tested; nor was the increased activity reproduced in two of three replications. Therefore, Krieger's assumptions based on Smith's study are questionable.

Several methodological considerations also weakened Krieger's (1976) study. Krieger does not report the manner in which subjects for the experimental and control groups were selected. She does report using a t-test on the variable of hemoglobin to establish the comparability of both groups. The t-test, a test for differences in means, does not convey any information with regard to the distribution of a particular trait within groups (Huck, Cormier, and Bounds, 1974). A stronger method for assuring homogeneity of the experimental and control groups, in terms of age, sex, and hemoglobin values, would have been random assignment.

Another methodological problem was the use of meditation by some subjects, allowing for meditation as a rival hypothesis. When a healing ability or energy force, which cannot be objectively defined, demonstrated, or controlled, is an independent variable in a field study, any possible threat to internal validity should be eliminated. Control for extraneous variables is much better research methodology than the use of a chi-square to rule out any possible effects of meditation on hemoglobin.

The final methodological problem concerns the inappropriate use of multiple t-tests. A more suitable method of analysis would have been an analysis of covariance, which would have adjusted posttest means to account for differences in pretest means. This test would be used provided the underlying assumptions could be met (Huck et al., 1974). The appropriate statistical analysis is critical to a correct interpretation of the data, since Hurt (1976) reported in a critique of Krieger's study (1976) that hemoglobin values of the control group also increased. This increase was significant at a probability of less than

0.05. The statistical tests as employed by Krieger do not account for the simultaneous pin in hemoglobin levels by both experimental and control groups, thus resulting in possibly erroneous conclusions.

This study conducted in 1976 is a replication of previous work by the same investigator (Krieger, 1973). It purported to correct several criticisms of the original study (Schlotfeldt, 1973). Similar significant increases in hemoglobin levels were reported for the experimental subjects in the previous study (Krieger, 1973).

Further work by Krieger et al. (1979) reported the objective verification of clients' relaxation during Therapeutic Touch. Measured physiologic variables, presumed from the text to be galvanic skin resistance, pulse, temperature, and others, indicated that the patients were relaxed. The status of these measures pretreatment, during treatment, and posttreatment were not reported. It is unknown what changes occurred in these variables during the Therapeutic Touch or if these changes were significant. It is unfortunate that the actual measures were not reported, because the work seems to serve as a bridge between the relaxation response and Therapeutic Touch for at least one subsequent investigator (Heidt, 1981).

Heidt (1981) attempted to examine the possible effects of Therapeutic Touch on anxiety. Pre- and posttreatment anxiety levels were assessed by questionnaire for three groups—a Therapeutic Touch group, a casual touch group, and a no-touch group. The investigator reported that the Therapeutic Touch group had significantly lower levels of anxiety than either of the other two groups. However, due to problems in research design, one must question whether or not Therapeutic Touch was the major factor in the anxiety reduction.

It is difficult to substantiate the validity of a questionnaire as the sole, measure of an emotional response. A corroborating physiologic variable such as pulse rate, respiratory rate, or galvanic skin resistance would have provided a more explicit measure of anxiety. That the investigator did not include such a measure is surprising, in light of her review of the literature that discusses the relaxation response, a phenomenon manifested by changes in respiratory rate, pulse rate, blood pressure, and so on (Wallace, Benson, and Wilson, 1971; Beary, Benson, and Klemchuk, 1974; Benson, Beary, and Carol, 1974).

The comparison of two types of Touch-Therapeutic touch and casual touch with no-touch does not answer the question of whether or not Therapeutic Touch itself can affect anxiety. To test for the hypothesized energy transfer between client and healer, one must control for the unusual nature of the therapy and for client expectations, in short for the placebo effect.

Heidt's (1981) experimental design compared two distinct treatments. The casual-touch group in Heidt's study did not control for the possible placebo effect because this group did not receive the behavioral stimulation of the Therapeutic Touch routine. Therefore, it is impossible to determine if the anxiety reduction reported was due to an hypothesized transfer of energy or to placebo effect.

A more appropriate control group would be one that received a sham Therapeutic Touch procedure (i.e., the passing of the hands over the body with no energy transfer). This should be possible since Therapeutic Touch is defined as a purposeful act (Heidt, 1981; Krieger, 1973). Such a control group would allow the possibility of a double-blind procedure, therefore controlling more effectively for the placebo effect. Should both the actual and sham Therapeutic Touch procedures produce similar effects on subjects, one could conclude that some form of placebo effect was in operation. However, if only the Therapeutic Touch group showed significant effects, the possibility of a placebo effect would be eliminated.

A second study examining the possible effects of Therapeutic Touch on anxiety (Randolph, 1980) used muscle tension, galvanic skin resistance, and temperature as measures of anxiety. The experimental and control groups were exposed to a stressful movie while receiving Therapeutic Touch or casual touch, respectively. The observable treatment in both groups was the placement of the practitioner's hands on the subject's abdomen and back. The investigator reported no significant differences in the posttreatment measures employed to assess anxiety.

Randolph's study (1980) is the first published nursing investigation of Therapeutic Touch that is double-blind. It is also the first to expose two groups to what appeared to be the same procedure except, of course, that the experimental group was presumed to have received the hypothesized energy transfer involved in Therapeutic Touch. Finally, the research design and statistical analysis were appropriate to the question of whether or not Therapeutic Touch can affect anxiety.

Randolph (1980) suggested at least two possible mitigating factors that could have produced the nonsignificant results. The Therapeutic Touch practitioners were not allowed to apply their art in the usual way (i.e., they were not allowed to perform an assessment prior to treatment). It may be that something in the assessment phase is essential to the effects of Therapeutic Touch (Randolph, 1980).

Another possible mitigating effect may have been the level of health of the subjects (Randolph, 1980). Randolph dealt with healthy subjects, while previous research employed subjects, human, animal, or plant, with a natural or induced illness. Randolph's conjecture is supported by Grad (1963), who also suggested that statistically significant results were more easily obtained if the subjects were to some degree unhealthy.

The advantage with animal or plant subjects is that "illness" of relatively short course can be induced. The short duration of such induced illness would strengthen the internal validity of a study by eliminating the threat of history. Two interesting studies in psychic healing (Graham and Watkins, 1971; Wells and Klein, 1972) illustrate this methodology. The subjects were ether-anesthetized pairs of mice and the dependent variable was arousal time. Anesthesia was considered a state of "illness" and the interventions of the healers were designed to speed arousal time of the mice treated.

If the subjects are human, it is necessary to control for the placebo effect. Future studies should be double-blind. Also, exposure of control and experimental groups to the behavioral stimulation of Therapeutic Touch may help to control for this effect.

Since there has been at least one replicative failure with a report of mood change in the healer (Smith, 1972), and since research results have been reported consistent with the mood of the healer (Grad, 1967), some control of the healer may be necessary. To protect against mood change, the healer should live a fairly regulated life during the experimental period. Consistent meal, sleep, recreational, and exercise patterns may enhance the results of the original study and increase the chances of a replicative success, if the healer maintains a similar lifestyle for the subsequent studies.

In the final analysis, the current research base supporting continued nursing practice of Therapeutic Touch is, at best, weak. Well-designed, double-blind studies have thus far shown transient results (Grad, 1961), no significant results (Randolph, 1980), or are in need of independent replication (Grad, 1963). Therapeutic Touch as a modality does excite interest. However, without a broader research base, it may be presumptuous to teach the art or seriously discuss the use of this practice in the treatment of illness. The practice of Therapeutic Touch by nurses will never gain professional credibility without clear, objective evidence to support it. Without this evidence, the nurse practitioners of Therapeutic Touch will be relegated to the practice of "placebo mumbo jumbo."

REFERENCES

Beary, J., H. Benson, and H. Klemchuk. 1974. "A Simple Psychophysiologic Technique which Elicits the Hypometabolic Changes of the Relaxation Response." *Psychosomatic Medicine* 36: 115–20.

Benson, H., J. Beaty, and M. Carol. 1974. "The Relaxation Response." *Psychiatry* 37: 37–46.

Boguslawski, M. 1979. "The Use of Therapeutic Touch in Nursing." *Journal of Continuing Education in Nursing* 10: 9–15.

Grad, B. 1963. "A Telekinetic Effect on Plant Growth." *International Journal of Parapsychology* 5: 117–33.

———. 1964. "A Telekinetic Effect on Plant Growth. Part 2. Experiments Involving Treatment of Saline in Stoppered Bottles." *International Journal of Parapsychology* 6: 473–98.

———. 1965. "Some Biological Effects of the 'Laying-on-of-hands': A Review of Experiments with Animals and Plants." *Journal of the American Society for Psychical Research* 59: 95–127.

———. 1967. "The 'Laying-on-of-hands': Implications for Psychotherapy, Gentling, and the Placebo Effect." *Journal of the American Society for Psychical Research* 61: 286–305.

Grad, B., R. Cadoret, and G. Paul. 1961. "An Unorthodox Method of Treatment of Wound Healing in Mice." *International Journal of Parapsychology* 3: 5–24.

Graham, K., and A. Watkins. 1971. "Possible Pk Influence on the Resuscitation of Anesthetized Mice." *The Journal of Parapsychology* 35: 257–72.

Heidt, P. 1980. "Effect of Therapeutic Touch on Anxiety Level of Hospitalized Patients." *Nursing Research* 30: 32–37.

Huck, S., W. Cormier, and W. Bounds. 1974. *Reading Statistics and Research.* New York: Harper & Row.

Hurt, S. 1976. "A Comment." *Psychoenergetic Systems* 1: 129–30.

Krieger, D. (21–23 March 1973) "The Relationship of Touch with Intent to Help or Heal to Subjects' In-vivo Hemoglobin Values: A Study in Personalized Interaction." Paper presented at the American Nurses' Association, Ninth Nursing Research Conference, San Antonio, Texas.

———. 1976. "Healing by the 'Laying-on' of Hands as a Facilitator of Bioenergetic Change: The Response of In-vivo Human Hemoglobin." *Psychoenergetic Systems* 1: 121–29.

———. (1979) *The Therapeutic Touch: How to Use Your Hands to Help or Heal.* Englewood Cliffs, N.J.: Prentice-Hall.

Krieger, D., E. Peper, and S. Ancoli. 1979. "Therapeutic Touch, Searching for Evidence of Physiological Change." *American Nurses' Association* 79: 660–62.

MacDonald, R. G., J. L. Hickman, and H. S. Dakin. 1977. "Preliminary Physical Measurements of Psychophysical Effects Associated with Three Alleged Psychic Healers." In *Research in Parapsychology.* Edited by J. D. Morris, W. G. Roll, and R. L. Morris.Metuchen, N.J.: Scarecrow Press.

Miller, L. 1979. "An Explanation of Therapeutic Touch Using the Science of Unitary Man." *Nursing Forum* 18: 278–87.

Randolph, G. 1980. "The Difference in Physiologic Response of Female College Students Exposed to Stressful Stimulus, When Simultaneously Treated by either Therapeutic or Casual Touch." Ph.D. diss., New York University. *Dissertation Abstracts International.* University Microfilms No. 8017522 41:523B.

Sandroff, R. 1980. "A Skeptic's Guide to Therapeutic Touch." *RN* 43: 25–30, 82ff.

Schlotfeldt, R. 21–23 March 1973. "Critique of the Relationship of Touch with Intent to Help or Heal to Subjects' In-vivo Hemoglobin Values: A Study in Personalized Internation." Paper presented at the American Nurses' Association, Ninth Nursing Research Conference, San Antonio, Texas.

Selkurt, E. 1975. "Respiratory Gas Exchange and Its Transport." In *Basic Physiology for the Health Sciences*. Edited by E. Selkurt. Boston: Little, Brown & Co.

Smith, J. 1972. "Paranormal Effects on Enzyme Activity." *Human Dimensions* 1: 15–19.

Wallace, R., H. Benson, and A. Wilson. 1971. "A Wakeful Hypometabolic State." *American Journal of Physiology* 221: 795–99.

Wells, R., and J. Klein. 1972. "A Replication of a Psychic Healing Paradigm." *Journal of Parapsychology* 36: 144–49.

Zefron, L. 1975. "The History of the Laying-on of Hands in Nursing." *Nursing Forum* 15: 350–63.

11

The International TT Picture*

Steven Pryjmachuk and Stephen James Colgan

Although founded in the United States, the practice of Therapeutic Touch has spread abroad, and TT is now taught in more than one hundred colleges and universities in at least seventy-five countries (Krieger, 1993). This chapter describes the history and the current status of TT in the United Kingdom and in Australia, and the response of skeptics in those nations.

TT IN THE UNITED KINGDOM
(Steven Pryjmachuk)

In comparison to the United States, TT has made little impact in the healthcare professions in the United Kingdom. However, there are signs that interest in TT as well as skepticism of the practice are on the increase. A general interest in complementary therapies is certainly evident in the UK, both among the public and among health professions, but by-and-large this interest tends to lie in more widely known therapies such as *acupuncture*, *aromatherapy*, and *homeopathy*.

The two most well-known TT proponents in the UK are Jean Sayre-Adams, a nurse and former pupil of TT cofounder Dolores Krieger, and Stephen Wright, a nurse with a distinguished career who is currently Professor of Nursing and Holistic Studies at St. Martin's College in Lancaster. Sayre-Adams and Wright are the authors of the only UK text on the subject (Sayre-Adams and Wright, 1995a). They have also pub-

---

*Mr. Colgan wishes to thank Dr. Rhelma Price for supporting his skepticism while he was an undergraduate nursing student, and for his previous collaborations. Appreciation is expressed to Rebecca Long for her assistance in editing this chapter.

lished a significant article on TT in *Nursing Times* (Sayre-Adams and Wright, 1995b). Both are major players in the *Sacred Space Foundation*, a "spiritual" venture based in Cumbria in the North of England which plays a significant role in promoting TT. The *Sacred Space Foundation* launched its "journal of spirituality," unsurprisingly entitled *Sacred Space*, in autumn 1999 (Sacred Space Foundation, 1999).

The British Association of TT (BATT) is another pool of support for the practice of TT. A UK journal, *Complementary Therapies in Nursing and Midwifery*, is also sympathetic to the cause, having published a number of TT articles since its inception a few years ago. In addition, there are a number of practitioners who hold academic posts in UK universities. This may well add legitimacy to the practice, but it is likely that these post-holders were appointed, not because of their expertise in TT, but because of expertise in more mainstream aspects of nursing.

The Road to Credibility?

It is important to note that a registered TT practitioner differs from a registered nurse, midwife, or health visitor in that there is no legal or statutory value attached to the term "registered." "Registered" simply means that the TT practitioner has satisfied the demands of the BATT and that the practitioner is eligible to be entered onto the Association's register.

In the United Kingdom, nursing, midwifery, and health visiting are three separate, though closely related, professions. That is, the UK authorities recognize, under statute, the titles Registered Nurse (R.N.), Registered Midwife (R.M.) and Registered Health Visitor (R.H.V.). Entry into these three professions is via programs provided by the Higher Education (HE) institutions, the majority of which are universities. It has only been during the past decade that the responsibility for nurse, midwife and health visitor education has shifted from the National Health Service (NHS) to HE; thus there has recently been a large-scale and complete transfer of the hospital-based schools of nursing and midwifery into HE establishments. The move from NHS to HE has meant that nursing, midwifery, and health visiting have achieved some status as academic subjects, although the relatively recent nature of the move means that these subjects are in their infancy.

Nurses are trained via a program that leads to professional registration and to an academic award. The type of award depends on the number of credits awarded. A diploma is awarded when 240 total credits (120 "level 1" and 120 "level 2" credits) have been attained; a degree requires a further 120 credits at "level 3." Most students opt for a three-year diploma program, though demand for and commissioning of degree places is on the increase. Midwifery follows a similar pattern, except those entrants who are already registered adult nurses can obtain R.M. status in eighteen months instead of the usual three years. Health Visitors are the UK's public health nurses. There is no direct entry into health visiting; entrants are required to already hold R.N. status.

Each country of the UK—England, Scotland, Wales, and Northern Ireland—has its own national board charged with maintaining standards in nurse, midwife, and health visitor education. The UK's supreme regulatory body for the three professions, and the body that maintains the Register, is the United Kingdom Central Council (UKCC). The national boards are obliged to work in partnership with the UKCC.

There is little formal acceptance of TT in the HE sector. The *Sacred Space Foundation* is a primary contributor to the training of TT practitioners by way of a loose association with the University of Manchester's School of Nursing, Midwifery, and Health Visiting. Given that the Manchester School is one of the top nursing schools in the UK, it might seem that TT has pulled off a major coup. Fortunately, this is not the case. Although the Foundation's publicity material refers to "university accredited courses" in TT (Sacred Space Foundation, 1999), in reality there is only a single level 2 continuing education module (worth only 40 credits), led by Sayre-Adams and "hosted" by the University's School of Nursing, Midwifery, and Health Visiting (University of Manchester, 1999).

The Manchester University School of Nursing, Midwifery, and Health Visiting was formed in 1996 by a merger of the University's School of Nursing Studies and an NHS college, the Manchester College of Midwifery and Nursing. The Manchester College was itself formed as a result of mergers between a number of hospital-based schools of nursing and midwifery in the Manchester area, amongst them "STAG" College of Nursing, a college with which TT-proponent Stephen Wright had some association. The current level 2 TT module, and a level 3 module that also existed at the time, originated at Manchester College and were simply transferred over to the University upon integration. Soon after integration, the University decided to revalidate all of the former Manchester College's continuing education courses to ensure that they were in line with its own academic standards. Although the level 2 module was, indeed, validated by the University, the level 3 module was not revalidated and no longer operates.

The Manchester level 2 module is covalidated by the English National Board (ENB), which works in partnership with the UKCC. However, the UKCC's attitude to complementary and alternative therapies is cautionary. In its *Guidelines for Professional Practice*, the UKCC states:

> If a complaint is made against you, we can call on you to account for
> any activities carried out outside conventional practice. You should

carefully consider the content and status of any courses which you undertake and how you promote yourself. (United Kingdom Central Council, 1996)

Although validation of the level 2 module by the University and the ENB add some credibility to the practice of TT, the most valuable aspect of the course for TT practitioners lies in the fact that it confers them "registered" status (Lewis, 1999).

Lewis, a member of the BATT, reports that there are approximately fifty known TT practitioners in the UK, the overwhelming majority being nurses. This contrasts sharply with his observation that there are around 85,000 practitioners in the United States. Moreover, despite the BATT requirement that completion of a level 2 course is a prerequisite for registration as a practitioner, Lewis's figures suggest that the majority of known TT practitioners in the UK lack this qualification. In other words, the majority of the UK's TT practitioners do not fulfill the BATT's own criteria for registration (Lewis, 1999).

A Heated Debate

The appearance of Lewis's (1999) article in the *Nursing Standard* (a large circulation, but low impact UK journal) provoked some heated comments from Claire Rayner, a well-known, well-respected journalist and broadcaster, and a former nurse (Rayner, 1999). Rayner's piece, entitled "Stuff and Nonsense," was a scathing attack on TT and other "new age" complementary therapies. She writes:

> Gobbledegook about this sort of "new age" stuff is appearing all over the place nowadays and is, indeed, high fashion. However, most sensible people would expect nurses . . . to be at the forefront of efforts to protect a gullible public from such charlatanism. . . . And when they tell their clients they are trained nurses as well as practitioners of this esoteric nonsense, they do real nursing a disservice since their qualification lends an air of respectability to totally unproven techniques. (pp. 2, 22)

Over the following weeks, numerous letters appeared in the *Standard*—the majority condemning Rayner. Amongst them were one from N. Mellon, the BATT Chair, and one from Professor Stephen Wright himself. Mellon claimed that Rayner's "anti-Therapeutic Touch tirade was based on scepticism and ignorance" (Mellon, 1999), and Wright asked, "Can this be the same Claire Rayner?" (Wright, 1999). Wright's question related to perhaps the most ironic point in this whole debate: Rayner had been one of the original patrons of the *Didsbury Trust*, a body that was set up specifically to introduce TT to the UK and which later metamorphosed into the *Sacred Space Foundation*. Rayner did not respond to any of these letters.

Because most of the letters to the *Standard* were supportive of TT and/or complementary therapies, a passing observer might assume that UK nurses are in general favorably disposed toward the practice. However, the letters pages of any periodical or newspaper are rarely representative of the views of the majority, particularly when a group of people are forced to defend their beliefs. The facts, on the other hand, speak for themselves: There is only one university-accredited TT course in the country, the practice is not widespread, and there are only a handful of practitioners. Though most nurses known to the writer seem to think there is nothing wrong with using touch therapeutically—indeed, most see touch as an *essential* part of nursing—there is often bemusement, even among supporters of complementary therapies, when they discover what the practice of TT is actually about.

Conclusion

In summary, there is no concerted anti-TT program or organisational activity in the UK, although the *Association for Skeptical Enquiry* has expressed some concerns. The lack of concerted opposition probably stems from the fact that TT has not permeated mainstream health care. There is only one university-accredited TT course in the country, the practice is not widespread, and there are only a handful of practitioners. Most nurses, midwives, and health visitors in the UK have little informed knowledge of TT; of those knowledgeable of the practice, it appears that few are actively interested in it.

THERAPEUTIC TOUCH IN AUSTRALIA
(Stephen Colgan)

In Australia, TT has not achieved the high media profile it has in the United States, nor has it been as widely practiced, promoted, or condemned. There have been no nurse academics such as Bullough and Bullough (1993, 1995) or editors of nursing journals such as Oberst (1995a, 1995b) publicly questioning the practice. No academic counterpart to the committee chartered by the University of Colorado Health Sciences Center (Claman et al., 1994) has been assigned to evaluate the evidence for TT, nor have any major Australian medical journals published clinical studies of TT. In contrast to the United States (Lemonick, 1998), Australia took little note if any of the publication in the *Journal of the American Medical Association* (*JAMA*) (Rosa et al., 1998) of an American schoolgirl's science fair project on TT. However, TT did make its way onto Australian television as part of a late night screening of *Unsolved Mysteries*.

One of a number of possible reasons for the low profile of TT in Australia may be its late introduction into the country. According to Debbie Smyth, an Australian TT practitioner and teacher, TT only began to be taught in Australia in 1989 (Smyth, 1995, p. 15). Its late introduction to Australia, combined with a lack of Australian TT teachers, led to many Australian nurses instead adopting *Reiki*, another related complementary therapy (McCabe, 1996b, p. 41).

Nevertheless, there are a number of high profile nurse academics and other nurses in Australia who are actively promoting and teaching TT and a range of other complementary therapies, through courses offered by universities, professional nursing organizations, and private companies. A number of articles in Australian nursing journals claim that complementary therapies such as TT are being increasingly used by nurses in palliative care, hospice care, aged care, and acute care facilities (Bettiens, 1998, p. 33; Hudson, 1998, p. 25, p. 29; Brown, 1999, p. 35).

Two major conferences promoting TT and other complementary therapies, one held in 1999 and the other scheduled for the year 2000, may also be taken as indications of the increasing presence of TT in Australia. At the First Intercontinental Conference of the Nurse Healers—Professional Associates International, Inc., held in Adelaide in February 1999, Dolores Krieger was a featured speaker and also conducted preconference workshops in advanced TT (Professional Associates International, 1998). The Fourth International Conference of the Australian College of Holistic Nursing, Inc., scheduled for the year 2000, will also feature prominent TT proponents such as Dr. Jean Watson, from the University of Colorado, and Professor Stephen Wright, from the UK (Royal College of Nursing Australia, 1999).

TT in Australian Nursing Education and Practice

The full extent to which TT and other complementary therapies are taught by Australian schools of nursing, or are taught within hospitals or other clinical practice settings in Australia, is very difficult to determine. As noted by Taylor (1996, p. 57), no comprehensive, readily accessible listing available of complementary therapy courses in Australia is available. However, reference to Therapeutic Touch can be found in the online course descriptions of a small number of Australian Schools of Nursing, in the online research and publication lists of some Australian nurse academics, and in articles published by Australian TT practitioners and Australian proponents of complementary therapies in general.

An appendix to Dolores Krieger's *Therapeutic Touch Inner Workbook: Ventures in Transpersonal Healing* (1997) lists schools around the world where TT is taught. Out of the eighty-eight locations listed in the appendix, the majority of which are in the United States and Canada, the School of Nursing at Flinders University in South Australia is listed (p.192) as the only school in Australia where TT is taught. In another appendix in Krieger's workbook (pp.176 ff.), there is a listing of seventy-seven healthcare facilities around the world where TT is practiced; within this list there is no entry for Australia.

The School of Nursing at Flinders University has a long history of association with TT. Courses in TT have been offered by the school since at least 1993, with advertisements for these courses appearing in Australian nursing journals as late as 1995 (Flinders University, 1995). Although not listed in Krieger's (1997) workbook, the School of Nursing at Monash University in Victoria has also offered a short course for nurses in TT (Monash University, 1995). Although Monash has since discontinued this short course, TT is still included within a course unit taught by the School of Nursing in 1999, "Therapeutic Communication" (Unit GHS1441). In this course unit, TT is "explored as an alternative form of therapeutic communication which can enhance clinical nursing practice" (Monash University, 1999). Similarly, in a course entitled "Health Education and Promotion in Midwifery" (Unit HHA1135) at the Victoria University of Technology in Victoria, TT is taught as one of a range of supportive pain reduction techniques for childbirth (Victoria University of Technology, 1999). TT and other complementary therapies have been introduced into the undergraduate nursing curriculum by the School of Nursing at Canberra University (Bettiens, 1998, p. 33; Bettiens, 1999).

Individuals and organizations outside the university-based schools of nursing also teach TT. For example, TT courses have been taught in Victoria by Healing Connections, an organization run by nurse TT practitioners Sue Dawson and Jane Abbott-Hall, and in New South Wales by Sirius Connections, a company which is associated with Healing Connections (Healing Connections, 1998). Dawson also teaches TT workshops in association with a professional nursing organization, the Victorian Branch of the Australian Nursing Federation (Australian Nursing Federation, 1999). Other known TT practitioners and teachers in Australia are: Monica Nebauer (Nebauer, 1994, p. 85), Rosanne Bettiens (Bettiens, 1999), and Debbie Smyth ("Therapeutic Touch Returns Nurture to Nursing," 1995, p. 24). Smyth was the first Australian nurse accredited to teach TT and studied it under Dolores Krieger at New York University in 1983. Since being accredited as a TT teacher, Smyth has taught the practice to nurses through university continuing education courses, a nurse degree program, and numerous workshops locally and nationally ("Therapeutic Touch Returns Nurture to Nursing," 1995, p. 24).

Australian TT Practitioners and Their Work

In 1994 Debbie Smyth received a Masters of Philosophy in Health and Behavioral Sciences from Queensland's Griffith University. Her thesis, "The Lived Experience of Healing—A Phenomenological Study of TT" (Smyth 1994), was later published in the *Australian Journal of Holistic Nursing* (Smyth, 1995; Smyth, 1996). Smyth describes her research as the only postgraduate research (to date) into the practice of TT in Australia. Smyth has also undertaken research, with Monica Nebauer, on the effects of TT on dental patients awaiting treatment. To date, this research has not been published (Smyth and Nebauer, 1989).

Other Australian nurses who have either presented conference papers on TT or undertaken research into TT include Amy Bartjes (1997a, 1997b), Lesley Cutherbertson (1996), and Elaine Davies (1996) at Flinders University; Monica Nebauer (1994) at the Australian Catholic University; Beth Nicols at Victoria University of Technology; Geraldine Milton (1996) at Monash University (coauthored with Susan Bermingham); and Mak, Bartjes, and Pillar (1996) at Flinders University.

Challenges to TT by Skeptics and Others

The inclusion of complementary therapies such as TT into nursing education and practice in Australia has mostly been unchallenged by the Australian nursing profession. The author, who would welcome being proved wrong, is unaware of any Australian nurse academic who has publicly and directly questioned the basis of these therapies and their inclusion into nursing practice, in any nursing journal or any professional nursing forum (or in any form of media at all). That is not to say that TT or the inclusion of complementary therapies into nursing education and practice in Australia has not gone totally unchallenged. As in the United States, the integration of complementary therapies such as TT into nursing education and practice in Australia has been questioned by Christian nursing associations, such as the Nurses Christian Fellowship (Hutchinson, 1997).

The Australian Skeptics have actively challenged the specific practice of TT as well as the integration of complementary therapies into the nursing education and practice. On a skeptical radio show in Victoria, members of the Australian Skeptics asked Lorraine Kelly (then a faculty member of the Flinders School of Nursing) how the university could offer short courses on a practice for which there is, at best, very weak scientific evidence. Butler (1993, p. 32) reports that Lorraine Kelly "seemed honestly unsettled that TT could be considered a questionable therapy. She did not feel that it was an inappropriate choice for nurses' further education, and that even if it was merely a placebo it was a worthwhile endeavour." Articles and letters published in *The Skeptic* (a publication of the Australian Skeptics) (Edwards, 1994; Williams, 1994; Rosa 1996), have also made the existence and work of U.S. Skeptics groups and academic committees known in Australia. These articles and letters were cited by the author and Dr. Rhelma Price in 1995 (Colgan and Price, 1995, pp. 18–19) as part of a critical response to the Royal College of Nursing Australia's 1995 discussion paper, "Complementary Therapies in Relation to Nursing Practice in Australia" (McCabe, Ramsay, and Taylor, 1995). Dr. Price is a scientist with a Ph.D. in reproductive immunology; at that time she taught anatomy and physiology to undergraduate nursing students at Deakin University, Warrnambool.

Conclusion

The practice and teaching of TT in Australia is nowhere near as widespread as it is in the United States. However, many nurse academics and nurse complementary therapy practitioners are actively promoting and teaching TT and a range of other complementary therapies within schools of nursing and through courses and conferences run by professional nursing organizations. Upcoming conferences featuring high profile nurse academics and TT practitioners may be taken as indications that proponents of TT and other complementary therapies are attempting to increase the acceptance and use of these therapies in Australia. To date, the promotion and inclusion of complementary therapies such as TT into nursing practice and education have mostly gone unchallenged by the nursing profession in Australia. Christian nurses in Australia and groups such as the Australian Skeptics have questioned these therapies and their integration in nursing education and practice, and have made American opposition to such practices better known in Australia. With the increasing scrutiny to which TT and other complementary therapies are being subjected worldwide, the integration of TT and other complementary therapies into nursing education and practice in Australia will probably become more widely and publicly questioned by the Australian nursing profession.

REFERENCES

Australian Nursing Federation. 1999. "ANF Education and Training—Complementary Therapies." *On the Record: ANF Victorian Branch Newsletter* (November): 17.

Bartjes, A. 1997a. "Therapeutic Touch Enhancement with Australian Bush Flower Essences." *Vision and Reality, Fourth Annual Conference* (November). The Therapeutic Touch Network in Ontario, Canada.

Bartjes, A. 1997b. "Therapeutic Touch: Compassionate Caring for Healing." *Conference Proceedings Seventh Asian Healing, Regional Conference: Carving a Path to Health and Healing* (November). Seventh Annual International Committee Catholic Nurses and Medico-social Assistants. Bangkok: St. Louis Hospital Press.

Bettiens, R. 1998. "Integrating Complementary Therapies in Mainstream Care." *Australian Nursing Journal* 6 (3): 33.

———. 1999. Home page. School of Nursing, Canberra University, Australia. http://wasp.canberra.edu.au/celts/about/fellows/rosanne.html (accessed 31 October 1999).

Brown, B. 1999. "Royal Hobart Hospital Embraces Therapeutic Care." *Australian Nursing Journal* 6 (8): 35.

Bullough, V. L., and B. Bullough. 1993. "Therapeutic Touch: Why Do Nurses Believe?" *Skeptical Inquirer* 17 (2): 169–74.

———. 1995. "More on Therapeutic Touch. Letter to the Editor." *Research in Nursing and Health* 18 (4): 377.

Butler K. 1993. "Therapeutic Touch—The Low Calorie Placebo." *The Skeptic* [Australian] 13 (4): 32.

Claman, H. N., R. Freeman, D. Quissel, J. Fowler-Shaver et al. 1994. *University of Colorado Report on Touch Therapy.* Denver: University of Colorado Health Sciences Center.

Colgan, S. J., and R. J. Price. 1995. "Response Document to Discussion Paper No. 2, 1995: Complementary Therapies in Relation to Nursing Practice in Australia." Unpublished paper submitted to the Royal College of Nursing Australia.

Cuthbertson, L. A. 1996. "The Effect of Complementary Therapy of Therapeutic Touch in Relieving Pain Experienced by Children." *International Conference of Paediatric Nursing: Down Under.* Brisbane, Australia.

Davies, E. 1996. "Complimentary Therapies—Therapeutic Touch for Living and Loving. Living, Loving, Remembering." *Proceedings of the SANDS Sixth National Biennial Conference 1996* (October): 111–12.

Edwards, H. 1994. "Therapeutic Touch." *The Skeptic* [Australian] 14 (2): 42–44.

Flinders University. 1995 "Therapeutic Touch Workshop." Advertisment. *Australian Nurses Journal* 2 (11): 17.

Healing Connections. 1998. *Therapeutic Touch: Using Hands to Help and to Heal,* Brochure for Therapeutic Touch Workshops. Victoria.

Hudson, S. 1998. "Natural Therapies and Oncology Nursing." *Australian Nursing Journal* 5 (9): 25.

Hutchinson, M. 1997. "Complementary Therapies in Nursing Practice." *Nurses Christian Fellowship* (July): 1–2, 5.

Krieger, D. 1993. *Accepting Your Power to Heal: The Personal Practice of Therapeutic Touch.* Santa Fe, N.Mex.: Bear & Company Publishing.

———. 1997. *Therapeutic Touch Inner Workbook: Ventures in Transpersonal Healing.* Santa Fe, N.Mex.: Bear & Company Publishing.

Lemonick, M. D. 1998. "Emily's Little Experiment." *Time* 151 (14): 67.

Lewis, D. 1999. "A Survey of Therapeutic Touch Practitioners." *Nursing Standard* 13 (30).

Mak, A., A. Bartjes, and N. Piller. 1996. "The Effects of Therapeutic Touch on Wound Healing of Patients with Venous Stasis Leg Ulcers." *Report Abstract—University 1996 Research Report, School of Nursing.* South Australia: Flinders University.

McCabe, P., L. Ramsay, and B. Taylor. 1995. *Discussion Paper no. 2, 1995: Complementary Therapies in Relation to Nursing Practice in Australia.* Deakin, ACT: Royal College of Nursing Australia.

Mellon, N. 1999. "Anti-Theraputic Touch tirade was based on scepticism and ignorance." Letter to the Editor. *Nursing Standard* 13 (42): 28.

Milton, G., and S. Bermingham. 1996. "Non-Pharmacologic Approaches to Pain Management: Therapeutic Touch." *Twenty-first Australian and New Zealand Scientific Meeting on Intensive Care* (October). http://anzics.herston.uq.edu. au/meetings/ASM/1996/TFMEET.HTM.

Monash University. 1995. "Courses for Registered Nurses." Advertisement. *Australian Nursing Journal* 3 (1): 39.

———. 1999. *Monash University Medicine Handbook.* Victoria: Monash University. http://www.monash.edu.au/pubs/1999handbooks/medicine/GHS1441.html (accessed 19 November 1999).

Nebauer, M. 1994. "Healing through Therapeutic Touch: One Person's Perspective." In *Caring as Healing: Renewal through Hope.* Edited by D. A. Gaut and A. Boykin. New York: National League for Nursing, pp. 85–101.

Nicols, B. 1995. "Therapeutic Touch a Power to Heal: a Research Analysis." *Proceedings of the Pathways to Healing Conference: Enhancing Life through Complementary Therapies* (September). Deakin, ACT: Royal College of Nursing Australia, pp. 100–107.

Oberst, M. T. 1995a. "Our Naked Emperor . . . Set Some Standards for Acceptable Practice." *Research in Nursing and Health* 18 (1): 1–2.

———. 1995b. "Our Naked Emperor Revisited." Research in *Nursing and Health* 18 (5): 382.

Professional Associates International, Inc. (1998) "First Intercontinental Conference of the Nurse Healers." Advertisement. *Australian Nursing Journal* 6 (3): 14.

Rayner, C. 1999. "Stuff and Nonsense." *Nursing Standard* 13 (39): 22–23.

Rosa, L. 1996. "Letters. Therapeutic Touch." *The Skeptic* [Australian] 16 (3): 66.

Royal College of Nursing Australia. 1999. 1999 Conference Listing. *Rhythm Flow and Synergy—Embracing the Spirit of Wholeness in Healing: Australian College of Holistic Nurses Inc. Fourth International Conference.* Webpage at http:// www.rcna.or.au/HolisticNsgConf.html (accessed 19 November 99).

Sacred Space Foundation. (1999) *Sacred Space* website. http://www.cumbria. org/sacredspace (accessed November 1999).

Sayre-Adams, J., and S. G. Wright. 1995a. *The Theory and Practice of Therapeutic Touch*. Edinburgh: Churchill Livingstone.

———. 1995b. "Change in Consciousness . . . Complementary Therapies are not Add-on Procedures but Windows Through Which the Healing Potential." *Nursing Times* 91 (41): 44–45.

Smyth, D. M. 1989. "Holistic Nursing." *Australian Nursing Journal* 5 (9): 29.

———. 1994. "The Lived Experience of Healing: A Phenomenological Study of Therapeutic Touch." Masters Thesis. Griffith University, Australia.

———. 1995. "Healing Through Nursing: The Lived Experience of Therapeutic Touch, Part 1." *The Australian Journal of Holistic Nursing* 2 (2): 15–25.

———. 1996. "Healing Through Nursing: The Lived Experience of Therapeutic Touch, Part 2." *The Australian Journal of Holistic Nursing* 3 (1): 18–25.

Smyth, D. M., and M. L. Nebauer. 1989. *Therapeutic Touch: Its Effects on Anxiety Levels of Patients Awaiting Dental Treatment*. Unpublished research.

Tattam, A. 1995. "Destiny or Dalliance." *Australian Nursing Journal* 3 (3): 18–21.

United Kingdom Central Council for Nursing, Midwifery, and Health Visiting. 1996. *Guidelines for Professional Practice*. London: UKCC, paragraph 81.

University of Manchester. 1999 Website of the School of Nursing, Midwifery, and Health Visiting Centre for the Study of Complementary Therapies. http://www.nursing.man.ac.uk/complementary/modules.htm (accessed November 1999).

Victoria University of Technology. 1999. *Postgraduate Course Handbook* (online pdf form). St Albans: Victoria University of Technology (webpage). Accessed 19 November 1999.

Williams, B. 1994. "News and Views." *The Skeptic* [Australian] 14 (3): 8.

Wright, S. 1999. "Letter to Editor." *Nursing Standard* 13 (42): 28.

Section II.

Physical Science of Therapeutic Touch

12

A Delineation of Facts about One Study of TT

Carla Selby and Béla Scheiber

These facts, which cannot be copyrighted, are extracted from articles published in the *Journal of the American Medical Association* (Rosa et al., 1998) and from *Skeptic* (1996). The coeditors of this volume had intended to reprint the entire *JAMA* article. Unfortunately, one of the authors, Larry Sarner, persuaded that publication to withhold the rights. We believe that the publication by *JAMA* was an interesting event in the history of TT and thus we are providing the facts contained therein. The article itself may be found in most medical, university, or municipal libraries; its complete citation is Rosa, Rosa, Sarner, and Barrett, "A Close Look at Therapeutic Touch," *Journal of the American Medical Association* 279, no. 3 (1998): 1005–10.

- The objective of the study was to "investigate whether TT practitioners can actually perceive a 'human energy field' " (p. 1007).
- Fifty-five percent of the text of the article (not counting abstract, figures, tables and references) is given to background information about Therapeutic Touch.
- Twenty-five self-identified TT practitioners were found by looking in advertisements and "by following other leads." Twenty-one agreed to participate in the proposed experiment (p. 1007).
- Of the twenty-one, nine said they were nurses, seven identified themselves as certified massage therapists, and the rest were from various professions or professed no particular expertise. Nineteen were women (p. 1007).
- Two series of tests were conducted, one in 1996 and one in 1997. The earlier tests of fifteen people were conducted in their homes or offices over a period of several months. The later series of tests was performed before a film crew at the request of its pro-

ducer. Excerpts from that taping were subsequently broadcast as part of the program, "Scientific American Frontiers" on or about November 19, 1997 (pp. 1007, 1009).

- The tests performed in 1996 were conducted by nine-year-old Emily Rosa. She "designed the experiment" (p. 1005) which was to be submitted as her fourth-grade science-fair project (p. 1007).
- Each participant sat behind a cardboard screen and placed his or her hands, with palms up, through holes "approximately 25 to 30 cm apart" at the base of the screen. A towel was fastened to the screen and placed over the subject's arms to cover the holes (p. 1007).
- "The experimenter flipped a coin to determine which of the subject's hands would be the target." At that point, the experimenter placed her hand 8 to 10 cm over the subject's randomly chosen hand. After the experimenter said, "okay," the test subject then stated whether it was her left or right hand that she believed was closer to the experimenter's hand. Seven to nineteen minutes usually comprised the time needed to complete ten tests (pp. 1007, 1008).
- In order to determine if such tactile cues as body heat transference or the movement of room air would influence the results, a "preliminary test" was conducted on seven people who had neither training nor belief in TT—four of these were children (p. 1008).
- Seven of the fifteen test subjects from the first test also participated in the second test (p. 1007).
- See figures 1 and 2 for a summary of the results of the two sets of tests.
- The conclusion reached by the authors is that "the mean correct score for the 28 sets of 10 tests was 4.4, which is close to what would be expected for random guessing" (p. 1009).

The above paragraphs (along with the two figures) comprise the bulk of the facts on which readers of the *JAMA* article can base any attempt to replicate this experiment or to judge the adequacy of the methodology. Upon reading the article, we have several questions that are unanswered by the study:

- No "formal ethics review committee" is described in the Methods section; this group would have ensured that the human subjects were treated humanely and ethically, as required by *JAMA*. Were the "World Medical Association Declaration of Helsinki" protocols observed? These protocols are:
  - **Informed Consent**. For experimental investigations of human

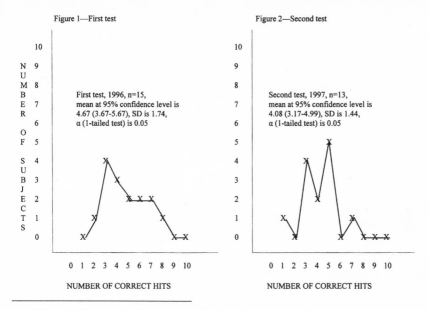

Figure 1—First test

First test, 1996, n=15, mean at 95% confidence level is 4.67 (3.67-5.67), SD is 1.74, α (1-tailed test) is 0.05

NUMBER OF CORRECT HITS

Figure 2—Second test

Second test, 1997, n=13, mean at 95% confidence level is 4.08 (3.17-4.99), SD is 1.44, α (1-tailed test) is 0.05

NUMBER OF CORRECT HITS

Figure 1 (first test) data points are from the graph in *Skeptic* 4, no. 4 (1996): 30. The statistical values are from *JAMA* 279, no. 13 (1996): 1008.

Figure 2 (second test) data points were calculated by subtracting the data points in the graph on page 30 of the *Skeptic* (figure 1 above) from the figure 2 graph in *JAMA* 279, no. 13 (1996): 1008. The statistical values are from *JAMA* 279, no. 13 (1996): 1008.

Our two figures above, when added together, give the results as a combined test as represented by figure 2 of the *JAMA* article.

or animal subjects, the authors are supposed to state in the Methods section of the manuscript that an appropriate institutional review board approved the project. For those investigators who do not have formal ethics review committees (institutional or regional), the principles outlined in the "Declaration of Helsinki" should be followed (*JAMA* Author Instructions, updated January 5, 2000, page 6).

- The design and performance of each experimental procedure involving human subjects should be clearly formulated in an experimental protocol which should be transmitted for consideration, comment, and guidance to a specially appointed committee independent of the investigator and the sponsor provided that this independent committee is in conformity with the laws and regulations of the country in which the research experiment is performed (*JAMA*, March 19, 1997, p. 925).

- What efforts were made by the experimenter to insure that conditions were substantially similar in the homes, offices, or other places in which the experiment was conducted?
- What, if any, impact did the film crew have on the general ambiance of the test area or the test subjects and the experimenter?
- Where are the "human subjects release forms?" Were these people fully informed about the risks, if any, they were undergoing as subjects for these experiments?
- Where are the data and the resulting statistics corresponding to the seven individuals (four of which were children) used as controls (p. 1008)? It would be valuable to compare those results with the experiment's results.
- Flipping a coin is not a particularly good way to obtain a random series. In fact, how was the coin flipped? Where did it come to rest? Was it allowed to come to rest naturally or was it stopped short of running out of rotary momentum? Who recorded which face of the coin was disclosed? Who monitored the recorder to insure that the correct face was noted and that the correct hand was targeted?
- Who recorded the spoken response of the subjects? How was this done?
- What was done to ensure that the experimenter's audible "Okay" did not in some manner convey information to the subject?

Readers of Rosa et al. or this article may have questions about other aspects of the methodology as published. Our list above is not meant to be exhaustive.

REFERENCES

Rosa L., E. Rosa, L. Sarner, and S. Barrett. 1998. "A Close Look at Therapeutic Touch." *JAMA* 279 (13): 1005–10.

"Detecting the 'Human Energy Field'—$742,000 Says Therapeutic Touch Is Bogus." *Skeptic* 4, no. 4 (1996): 30.

"World Medical Association Declaration of Helsinki." *JAMA* 277, no. 11 (March 19, 1997): 925–26.

"*JAMA* Author Instructions," from website: http://jama.ama-assn.org/info/auinst.html (updated January 5, 2000), downloaded February 8, 2000.

13.

The Effect of Therapeutic Touch on Pain and Anxiety in Burn Patients

Joan G. Turner, Ann J. Clark,
Dorothy K. Gauthier, and Monica Williams

The purpose of this single-blinded randomized clinical trial was to determine whether Therapeutic Touch versus sham TT could produce greater pain relief as an adjunct to narcotic analgesia, a greater reduction in anxiety, and alterations in plasma T-lymphocyte concentrations among burn patients. Therapeutic Touch is an intervention in which human energies are therapeutically manipulated, a practice conceptually supported by Rogers's (1970) theory of unitary human beings. Data were collected at a university burn center in the southeastern United States. The subjects were ninety-nine men and women between the ages of fifteen and sixty-eight hospitalized for severe burns, and they received either TT or sham TT once a day for five days. Baseline data were collected on day one, data were collected before and after treatment on day three, and postintervention data were collected on day six. Instruments included the McGill Pain Questionnaire, Visual Analogue Scales for Pain, Anxiety, and Satisfaction with Therapy, and an Effectiveness of Therapy Form. Blood was drawn on days one and six for lymphocyte subset analysis. Medication usage for pain in mean morphine equivalents, and mean doses per day of sleep, anxiety, and antidepressant medications were recorded. Subjects who received TT reported significantly greater reduction in pain on the McGill Pain Questionnaire Pain Rating Index and Number of Words Chosen and greater reduction in anxiety on the Visual Analogue Scale for Anxiety

Originally published in *Journal of Advanced Nursing* 28, no. 1 (1998): 10–20. Copyright © 1998 by Blackwell Science Ltd. Reprinted with permission. This research was supported by the U.S. Department of Defense, Tri-Services Uniformed University of the Health Sciences Nursing Research Program. The investigators would also like to recognize the contributions of research nurses, Mary Kay Burnette, M.S., R.N., and Ken Farr, B.S., R.N., to this project.

than did those who received sham TT. Lymphocyte subset analyses on blood from eleven subjects showed a decreasing total CD8 +lymphocyte concentration for the TT group. There was no statistically significant difference between groups on medication usage.

INTRODUCTION

Each year, approximately 100,000 burns occur in the United States that require inpatient management. The pain from burn injuries requiring hospitalization is prolonged and severe. The discomfort associated with debridement and lengthy healing process is often accompanied by severe anxiety. Thus, the problems of pain and anxiety management are paramount in the nursing care of burn patients.

Burns may be categorized into four types by the primary mechanism of injury (thermal, radiation, electrical, or chemical) and by wound depth (first, second, or third degree) as well as by the extent of the body surface involved. Burn injuries are unique from other trauma and surgical wounds because of the extensive physiological and psychological damage occurring in severe cases (Dyer and Roberts, 1990), which gives rise to complex medical and nursing management problems. High doses of opioids are required to bring pain under control, but even then, patients may experience pain that is relatively refractory to opioid use (AHCPR, 1992). Patients are often anxious and uncomfortable as they experience the prolonged and painful recovery period. This study was conducted to determine whether TT would increase the pain relief achieved from analgesic medications, reduce anxiety, and beneficially influence immune function among, persons hospitalized for burn injury, and whether selected covariables would influence this relationship.

RELATED LITERATURE

Characterized as a wound with tissue loss, the burn wound heals by secondary intention, which produces prolonged pain and protracted anxiety. There is a wealth of literature on the care of burn patients.

Pain and the Burn Patient

Pain is difficult to define and includes numerous physiological, psychological, sociocultural, and behavioral considerations. The simplest definition is that pain is "whatever the experiencing person says it is, existing whenever the person says it does" (McCaffery and Beebe, 1989). Unresolved pain can destroy quality of life resulting in *high levels* of anxiety. It can also act to impair sleep and appetite, thereby producing fatigue and reducing the availability of nutrients essential for healing. Thus pain may impede recovery, and in weakened or elderly patients, make the difference between survival and death (Melzack, 1990).

Pain of varying severity is common to patients with severe burns (Andreasen et al., 1972; Kinsella and Booth, 1991; and Marvin et al. 1992). In a study of the characteristics of pain experienced by burn patients, Choiniere and colleagues (1989) reported that pain began either at the time of injury or in the first six hours following the injury. Subjects in the Choiniere study reported more intense pain from therapeutic procedures than from the injury itself and that even large doses of analgesia administered prior to these procedures often failed to relieve pain. Further, pain levels of these burn subjects did not decline over time in the hospital, and no correlation was found between pain scores and burn sizes or the extent of the injury (Choiniere et al., 1989).

Anxiety and the Burn Patient

Marvin et al. (1992), Miller et al. (1992), Patterson (1992), Steiner and Clark (1977), and Andreasen et al. (1972) have all reported that fear and anxiety are frequently present in patients with severe burns. Choiniere et al. (1989) found that high levels of anxiety were not necessarily related to higher pain ratings during therapeutic procedures, but that patients who were more anxious tended to report more pain when at rest. Miller and colleagues (1992) contend that pain is exacerbated by anxiety.

Limited research has been done on nonpharmacological interventions to reduce pain and anxiety in severely burned patients. Some success in achieving reduced burn pain and anxiety has been reported with biofeedback training (Knudson-Cooper, 1981), teaching burn patients to cope (Tobiasen and Hiebert, 1985), and showing a video during dressing changes (Miller et al., 1992). Decreased anxiety in burned children has been reported with the use of relaxation training (Knudson-Cooper, 1981), and Tidwell (1996) reported reduced pain in hospitalized burn patients with the use of a deep breathing relaxation technique, music, and additional room warming during wound care.

Immune Function and the Burn Patient

Thermal injury shatters the mechanical barrier provided by the skin and interrupts both nonspecific and specific defenses. Alterations in neutrophil function include a change in adherence to blood vessel endothelium, clumping of cells, slowed chemotaxis (Griswold, 1993), and a decrease in all of the metabolic activities associated with intracellular killing of microorganisms (Warden, 1987). Profound alterations in specific cellular immunity include a decrease in total T-cell count but an increase in suppressor to helper T-cell ratio (Griswold, 1993). A decrease in the cytotoxic activity of macrophages and natural killer cells is also seen (Blazar et al., 1986; Belcher, 1996). The major humoral immunity deficit is a subnormal concentration of IgG, which may occur by twenty-four hours after the burn and may last several weeks (Griswold, 1993). Immunosuppression from these and other immune system alterations is believed to be the major contributor to infection in burn patients (Belcher, 1996), which slows healing and contributes to protracted pain.

Therapeutic Touch

The practice of TT consists of learned skills in which the practitioner consciously directs or sensitively modulates human energies (Krieger, 1993). The name Therapeutic Touch is really a misnomer because actual touch or physical contact with the patient's skin is not necessary. The technique can be implemented by holding the hands two to five inches from the patient's body since the therapy is based on the assumption of a human energy field which extends beyond the skin. Not having to touch the burn patient is an advantage because it avoids the discomfort sometimes associated with direct touch.

TT has been studied as an intervention for relief of pain and anxiety in a variety of settings and with sometimes conflicting results. Clark (1992) conducted a qualitative study of perceptions of patients who had received TT for stress management, and reported that five out of nine patients claimed they received relief of chronic low back pain or joint pain as an additional and unexpected benefit. Meehan (1993) measured postoperative pain in 108 patients in a single-blind clinical trial, comparing the effect of a single TT treatment with that of a placebo control or the standard use of narcotic analgesia. The hypothesis that TT would significantly decrease postoperative pain compared to the placebo control was not supported, but secondary analysis revealed that TT may have reduced patients' need for analgesic medication.

In an experimental pretest/posttest study of ninety hospitalized cardiovascular patients, Heidt (1981) assessed the effect of TT on anxiety as compared to that of casual touch or no touch. Patients who received TT reported a statistically significant decrease in anxiety when compared to the other groups. Quinn (1984) reported that TT reduced anxiety in hospitalized adults, and Kramer (1990) reported that TT lessened stress among hospitalized children. However, in separate experimental studies designed to test the effect of TT on anxiety of hospitalized adults, Parkes (1985) and Hale (1986) reported no significant results. When Keller and Bzdek (1986) used TT to treat tension headaches, they found a highly significant decrease in pain reported by TT subjects as compared to those in the placebo control group.

Two studies have been done that suggest TT may alter immune function. Quinn and Strelkauskas (1993) reported that bereaved patients treated with TT experienced a decrease in suppressor T-lymphocytes. Garrard (1995), working with ten matched pairs of HIV infected men, reported significantly higher CD4+ T-lymphocyte counts for the subjects who received TT than for those in each pair who received a sham treatment.

Summary

In summary, although TT is a highly controversial nursing intervention for which mechanisms and modes of action are currently unknown, the data discussed above indicate that TT may ameliorate pain perception, reduce anxiety, and enhance immune function. In light of this evidence, it is incumbent upon nurse scientists to investigate this technique and subject it to scientific rigor.

CONCEPTUAL APPROACH

Reduction of pain and anxiety are two of the leading nursing management problems in burn patients, and TT is an intervention available to nurses that may potentially address both of these problems. During a TT treatment, the practitioner assumes the existence of a human energy field (Rogers, 1970, 1990), and intervenes to enhance and balance that field. The idea behind TT is that the human energy field is abundant and flows in balanced patterns in health, but is depleted, blocked, and/or unbalanced in injury or illness. During TT, the practitioner replenishes depleted energy and clears and rebalances the energy flow in the injured person through conscious intent and hand movements which repattern the energy flow. This repatterning of energy flow is thought to result in manifestations of physical and psychological healing in the injured or ill person. It was hypothesized that in the burn injured person, TT reduces anxiety, and that TT relieves pain either directly and/or indirectly through the reduction of anxiety. TT has been shown to alter T-lymphocyte concentrations (Quinn and Strelkauskas, 1993; Garrard, 1995), and if this occurs in the burn patient, investigators speculate that these changes may enhance immune function.

METHODOLOGY

Subjects and Setting

Subjects for this study were patients on the Burn Unit at a university medical center in the southeast United States. Selection criteria dictated that subjects must be between fifteen and seventy years of age, hospitalized for treatment of burn injuries, and able to speak English and communicate verbally. Subjects were disqualified if they had greater than 75 percent total body surface area burned, had an active psychiatric disorder or mental retardation, were expected to stay less than nine days in the hospital, were unable to see or hear, or were participating in a conflicting clinical trial.

Of the 115 patients on whom data collection was begun, 99 remained in the study at least 3 days, met all study criteria, and were entered into the study sample. Subjects were invited to participate voluntarily in this research study designed to determine the usefulness of TT on pain, anxiety, and infection among burn patients. They were given a brief explanation of TT as a nursing intervention in which the therapist moves his or her hands over the patient's body without touching in order to help the patient. Subjects were informed that they would be randomly assigned to a group of patients who received TT or to a group of who received a substitute treatment, and that they would not be informed about which group they were in. Outcome measurements to be used were also described. Written informed consent was obtained by one of the investigators, and then subjects were randomized by coin toss to a TT group (n = 62) or a sham TT group (n = 37).

Subjects ranged in age from fifteen to sixty-eight, and the majority were white and male. Only two subjects in the TT group (3 percent) and one subject in the sham group (3 percent) had diabetes. Because each pain comparison included a baseline value, which would adjust for any underlying alteration in pain sensation due to diabetic neuropathy, subjects with diabetes were included in the study sample. Approximately 30 percent of either study group were noted to have other medical conditions which were unlikely to affect pain sensation or anxiety. Demographic and study characteristics of the two study groups are shown in table 1.

Because the burn patients sometimes had one or more days of treatment at another facility before arrival an the Burn Unit, or required one or more days for physiological stabilization, the mean number of days between injury and administration of baseline instruments (on study day one) was ¯6. If a subject requested not to participate in the study on

Table 1: Characteristics of subjects in the TT and sham groups

Characteristic	TT group (n=62)	Sham group (n=37)	P
Age			
Mean (SD)	36.3 (12.7)	39.2 (11.4)	0.256
Range	15-68	20-64	
Race			
%Black	26	24	0.869
%White	74	76	
Sex			
%Male	76	78	0.769
Other conditions			
%with diabetes	3	3	1.000
%with other conditions	34	30	0.669
Burn characteristics			
%of total body surface burned			
Mean (SD)	19.2 (18.1)*	15.6 (12.0)	0.244
Range	1-75*	1-60	
Proportion of burn area which is second degree burn			
Mean (SD)	0.68 (0.26)†	0.78 (0.26)‡	0.107
Range	0-1†	0-1‡	
Days from injury to study day 1			
Mean (SD)	5.7 (4.3)	6.3 (12.1)	0.696
Range	1-22	1-76	
Days in study			
Mean (SD)	6.2 (1.7)	6.4 (1.2)	0.538
Range	3-12	3-9	
Refused treatment or assessment on one or more days			
N (% of total patients in group)	7 (11.5%)§	6 (16.2%)	0.548

The P values for differences in mean were determined by t-test; P values for differences in n were determined by χ^2 test or Fischer's exact test. *n=60, †n=59, ‡n=36, §n=61

---

a given day or was not able to participate due to surgery, the day in question was not counted in the timing of interventions or outcome measures. Therefore, each subject who completed the study had a total of five days of TT or sham treatment, followed by the "day six" outcome measures, no matter how many consecutive days this required. The mean number of days required was approximately 6.3, with a maximum of 12 days. There was no significant difference between the TT and sham groups in the total number of days in the study, and there was also no significant difference between groups for any of the demographic or study participation characteristics (see table 1).

Of the ninety-nine subjects in the sample, 81 percent completed all assessments in the study and the remainder were discharged from the unit before day six assessments were done. However, their day three assessments were still available for analysis.

Instruments

A patient data sheet was developed by the researchers for recording of demographic and clinical data from the subject's medical record, and the following six instruments were utilized in this study for data collection.

McGill Pain Questionnaire

This instrument, designed by Melzack (1975), contains seventy-eight words that pertain to sensory, affective, evaluative, and miscellaneous aspects of pain. The words are divided into twenty groups of three to six words each, and subjects are asked to choose one word (or no word) from each group to describe their pain. In each of the twenty groups, the words are ranked from least to most intense and are given a corresponding score from one to six, depending upon the number of words in the group. A Pain Rating Index (PRI) (originally designated as PRI [R]), can be calculated by summing the rank scores of the words chosen. The PRI was found to correlate highly with a second score, the Number of Words Chosen (NWC), $r = 0.89$ (Melzack, 1975). In a separate section of the instrument, the subject is asked to chose one of the following five words to express overall intensity of pain: mild, discomforting, distressing, horrible, or excruciating. From this response, a present pain intensity (PPI) is calculated by assigning values of one to five to the respective descriptors. In data from 248 subjects, PPI scores were found to correlate significantly with both PRI and NWC scores, but the r-values were 0.42 and 0.32, respectively (Melzack, 1975). Melzack (1975) attributed this finding to the fact that the PRI and NWC scores give a more extensive description of the pain and are less sensitive to momentary fluctuations in psychological parameters.

Visual Analogue Scale for Pain (VASP)

This instrument consists of a 20 cm vertical line with the descriptors "no pain" at the bottom and "worst possible pain" at the top. When using the VASP, the subject was asked to mark a point (or to indicate a point) which reflected the amount of sensation experienced at the time. The intensity of sensation was scored by measuring the distance in millimeters from the low end of the scale to the subject's mark. The vertical scale was chosen because it has been shown to be easier for subjects to use than a horizontal scale, and it has also been shown to be more sensitive (Gift, 1989).

The major strength of the VASP is that its use avoids the pitfalls of reliance on language for assessment (Sriwantanakul et al., 1983). It has also been shown that subjects who have been medicated for pain are sufficiently dexterous to use a visual analogue scale (Revill et al., 1976). To avoid recall bias, subjects were asked to rate the pain which they were currently experiencing. The VASP possesses both concurrent validity and discriminant validity (Gift, 1989) and has been validated for rating the pain of burn patients (Choiniere et al., 1989). Reliability of the VASP has also been demonstrated using a test-retest method (Revill et al., 1976).

Visual Analogue Scale for Anxiety (VASA)

The VASA, an adaptation of the VASP, consists of a 20 cm vertical line with the descriptors "no anxiety" at the bottom and "worst possible anxiety" at the top. Subjects were asked to indicate how anxious they were feeling "right now" by marking or pointing to the appropriate place on the line.

Credibility of Therapy Form (CTF)

At the beginning of the study each subject completed the CTF (adapted from Borkovec and Nau, 1972) to assess whether subject expectations were related to outcome of the therapy. The five questions on the form pertain to (1) how logical TT seems to be, how confident the subject is that TT will be successful in (2) relieving pain, (3) reducing stress, and (4) preventing infection, and (5) whether or not the subject would be willing to pay for TT as an optional treatment. Responses are "Not logical" (earns one point), "Somewhat logical" (earns two points), and "Very logical" (earns three points) for the first four questions, and "No," "Maybe," and "Yes" (one to three points, respectively) for the fifth question. The summed score for the five questions was used as a covariable in data analysis. A Cronbach's alpha was calculated on subject responses to ascertain reliability of the instrument, yielding an alpha of 0.74.

Visual Analogue Scale for Satisfaction with Therapy (VASS)

This instrument, another adaptation of the VASP, consists of a 20 cm vertical line with the descriptors "not at all satisfied" at the bottom and "very satisfied" at the top. At the end of the study period, subjects were asked to indicate how satisfied they were with their TT treatment by pointing to the appropriate place on the line. This instrument and the one subsequently described were added to data collection procedures several months after the initiation of the study in an effort to document quantitatively numerous comments being made by subjects about their satisfaction with study treatments.

Effectiveness with Therapy Form (ETF)

At the end of the study period each subject was asked to complete the ETF, which is an investigator-adapted variation of the Borkovec and Nau (1972) CTF. The ETF was included to determine how satisfied subjects were with the outcome of the therapy as it relates to pain and stress, and whether they would be willing to pay for the therapy as an optional part of their hospital treatment, a further indication of the effectiveness of their treatment. Scoring was identical to the scoring of the CTF, except that scores for separate items were analyzed separately rather than summed. As was done for the CTF, subjects indicated their responses, each of which had a preassigned value.

Physiological Measurement

The original protocol of the study dictated that blood samples would be obtained on day one and day six of the study from consenting patients who had a vascular access line or who were willing to have a needlestick. However, most burn patients either had their intravenous lines removed by forty-eight hours after admission or were unwilling to have a needlestick for the sole purpose of research. For consenting patients, approximately 10 mL of blood was obtained by the subject's nurse, making sure that the blood was drawn prior to the TT treatment on day one, and also prior to or at least two hours after the subject's painful daily dressing change. In addition, to assure that the samples for any given patient were drawn at approximately the same time of day, the blood sample for day six was drawn within seventy-five minutes of the time of day at which the day one sample had been drawn.

Due to all of these constraints, usable blood samples were obtained from a convenience sample of eleven subjects. Samples were delivered to the medical center's immunocytology laboratory, where concentrations of CD4+ and CD8+ T-lymphocytes were determined using fluoresceintagged monoclonal antibodies and flow cytometry. As an AIDS Clinical Trial Group certified laboratory, the immunocytology laboratory meets predetermined standards for the reliability of its tests. A portion of each blood sample was also delivered to the hospital clinical laboratory where total white blood cell and differential white blood cell counts were made by standard laboratory techniques.

Procedure

Subjects in both the TT group and the sham group received five TT or sham treatments, given on five separate days at the convenience of the subject. Treatments were usually administered in the afternoon since dressings changes were scheduled at various times during the morning. TT treatments were provided by one of three experienced TT practitioners, trained in the Krieger-Kunz method. Sham treatments were administered by research assistants (RAs) who had no previous knowledge of TT. RAs were trained to make the same hand movements as the TT practitioners, and were not allowed to perform the sham treatment until uninformed observers could not tell whether TT or sham was being performed in a staged demonstration. Training and monitoring of the TT and sham treatments was done by one of the investigators, using a written protocol to assure integrity of the intervention.

Persons who administered TT and sham asked visitors to leave the room and made the subjects as comfortable as possible, either lying in bed or sitting in a chair before beginning the session. The subjects were encouraged to relax and close their eyes. Room lighting was dimmed and soft relaxing instrumental music was played during both the TT and sham procedures. Thus, subjects in both groups experienced the "presence" (Hines, 1992) of another and heard instrumental music while the TT and sham procedures were being performed.

Therapeutic Touch Intervention

The TT practitioner began by centring or becoming relaxed and calm and focusing on assisting the subject. Using hands held with palms facing the subject and approximately two to five inches from the subject's body, the TT practitioner assessed the energy field and implemented techniques such as clearing, directing, or balancing the energy flow, based on the assessment. Treatment length varied from five to twenty minutes depending on the practitioner's subjective judgement of the state of the subject's energy field. Upon completion of the session, the subject was allowed to rest for five to ten minutes.

Sham

The RAs who administered the sham did not center and did not assess or attempt to therapeutically manipulate the subject's energy field, but counted backwards from 100 by serial sevens as they made random mimic TT movements for a random length of time, not to exceed 20 minutes. Even though this time was allowed to vary, as was the TT treatment time, all sham group patients were given the illusion that they were receiving a therapeutic treatment. Neither the patients nor the staff on the Burn Unit knew which of the interventions were TT and which were sham.

Protocol

All patients on the Burn Unit who met study criteria were contacted as early as possible after admission to the unit, and informed consent to participate was obtained. On the next day (day one), the following baseline instruments were administered: the VASP, VASA, McGill Pain Questionnaire, and CTF. For consenting subjects, blood samples were obtained by the patient's nurse and delivered to the laboratories for lymphocyte subset and white blood cell analyses. Following administration of the instruments, the first TT or sham treatment was given, and treatments were repeated for a total of five days. On day three, the VASP was administered before and after the TT or sham treatment. On day six, the day after the final treatment, the following instruments were administered: VASP, VASA, McGill Pain Questionnaire, VASS, and ETF. Day six blood samples were also collected. For all subjects, the person administering the study instruments was different from the person administering the TT or sham treatment. Demographic and clinical information, including a record of the use of pain and other medications that affect the nervous system were obtained from the subject's medical record.

Statistical Analysis

Descriptive methods, t-tests, chi-square, and Fisher's exact tests were used to characterize the sample and test the study hypotheses. Scores for outcome variables from days three or six were analyzed with multiple regression using treatment group assignment (TT or sham) as the independent variable, with the respective baseline scores as a covariable, if appropriate. Other covariables (listed below) were allowed to enter the regression equation in stepwise manner. The P for the t-test for treatment group assignment (TT or sham TT) in the final equation was used to determine whether there was a significant difference between the mean scores of the two treatment groups, and an alpha level of 0.05 was set. This use of regression analysis yields the same results as analysis of covariance (ancova) and allows the stepwise entry of covariables. One-tailed P-values were used because the intent of the research was to test whether TT is more effective than sham TT in producing desirable outcomes.

RESULTS

Pain and Anxiety

To determine the effect of TT on subjects' pain and anxiety, outcome measurement scores recorded on days three or six were analyzed, using treatment group (TT or sham) as the independent variable, with respective baseline scores as covariables. Other covariables, which were allowed to enter the equation stepwise, included age, sex, race, days from injury to study day one, score on the CTF, whether or not pain medication had been administered within four hours before the respective baseline or outcome measurements were made, and whether or not medication for anxiety, depression, sleep, or psychosis had been administered within four hours before the measurements were made. Results are shown in table 2.

Mean scores for the outcome variables, adjusted for the effect of significant covariables, are shown for each treatment group. Higher scores indicate more pain or anxiety.

The McGill Pain Questionnaire

This was administered to subjects on days one (baseline) and six, and provided an assessment of the long-term effect of TT treatment. Ther-

Table 2: Effects of TT versus sham TT on pain and anxiety

Outcome variable		Covariables	n	Adjusted mean score		P (1-tailed)
				TT group	Sham group	
Pain measures						
McGill PRI	Day 6	Day 1, pm1	65	27.9	36.3	0.004**
McGill NWC	Day 6	Day 1, pm1	65	13.3	16.3	0.005**
McGill PPI	Day 6	Day 1, om1	61	2.11	2.50	0.064
VASP	Day 6	Day 1	65	77.3	88.4	0.197
VASP	Day 3 or 6†	Day 1	83	81.2	95.0	0.117
VASP	Day 3	Day 3 (pre Rx)	81	66.9	77.7	0.147 (post Rx)
Anxiety measure						
VASA	Day 6	Day 1	65	59.5	81.4	0.031*

Outcome variable scores were regressed on treatment group (sham or real TT) and on baseline score. The following covariables were allowed to enter the regression stepwise if P<0.10: age, sex, race, days from injury to study day 1, Credibility of Therapy Form score, administration of pain medication within 4 hours before measurements were made, administration of other medication (for anxiety, depression, sleep, or psychosis) within 4 hours before measurements were made. Covariables = covariables, in addition to treatment group, which entered the regression equation: Day 1=day 1 (baseline) score, pm1=pain medication administered within 4 hours before measurements were made on day 1, om1=other nervous system medication administered within 4 hours before measurements were made on day 1. Adjusted mean score=mean score for each treatment group, adjusted for the covariables which entered the regression equation. Post Rx=measurement done subsequent to TT/sham treatment on the day indicated. Pre Rx=measurement done before TT/sham treatment on the day indicated.

†Day 3 or 6 = day 6 score, if available; otherwise day 3 (pre Rx) score.
**P<0.01; *p<0.05.

apeutic Touch produced a significantly lower pain score than the sham treatment for two of the three indicators in the questionnaire. A significant reduction in pain was reported by TT subjects for the PRI, t (61) = 2.76, P = 0.004, and for the NWC, t (61) = 2.75, P = 0.005. For PRI, the

TT group adjusted mean score was 8.4 units lower than that of the control group (compared to a mean baseline score of 38.4 units), and for NWC, the TT group score was 3.0 units lower than that of the control group (with a mean baseline score of 15.6 units). Thus the TT group exhibited 21.9 percent and 19.2 percent more desirable scores, respectively, for the two pain measurements. Results for the McGill PPI scores on day six also indicated less pain for the TT group. However, the difference between treatment group scores approached but did not achieve statistical significance (P = 0.064).

When the VASP was used to assess the long-term effect of TT by comparing pain scores for day six, using the day one scores as covariables, no statistically significant difference was found between the TT and sham groups (see table 2). In order to use data from a maximum number of subjects, a "day three or six" variable was created, consisting of the day six score, if available. If the subject did not remain in the study through day six, the day three (before TT/sham treatment) score was used. Therefore, this variable represents the final VASP score available for each subject. When scores for "day three or six" were compared, using the day one score and other previously mentioned covariables, a difference of 13.8 units was found between the mean scores of the TT and sham groups, compared to a mean baseline score of 86.1, with t (80) = 1.20, P = 0.117 (see table 2). This represents a 16.0 percent more favorable score for the TT group, but was not statistically significant.

The immediate effect of TT on pain was examined on study day three by administration of the VASP before, and again after, the TT/sham treatment. The group which received TT reported ‾10.7 percent less pain after treatment than did the control group (a pain score of 10.8 units lower than the control group, compared to a pretreatment mean of 101 units), but this difference was not statistically significant, t (78) = 1.06, P = 0.147.

The Effect of TT on Anxiety

This effect was examined with the VASA, administered to subjects on study days one and six. The difference in adjusted mean scores for the two treatment groups was significant, t (62) = 1.90, P = 0.031, with the TT group indicating 21.9 units less anxiety than the sham group (see table 2). Since the mean baseline (day one) score for the VASA was 95 units, a difference of 21.9 units represents a 23.1 percent more favorable score for the TT group.

Measures of Satisfaction with Therapy

Two instruments were administered on study day six, to assess subjects' level of satisfaction with their TT/sham treatment: the Effectiveness of Therapy Form and the Visual Analog Scale for Satisfaction with therapy. Use of these instruments was begun at approximately one-fourth of the way through the data collection period; therefore n = 44 – 52. Results are shown in table 3. A higher score indicates greater subject satisfaction with the outcome of the treatment. When subscale scores of the ETF were compared, differences in perceived relief of pain and willingness to pay for, treatment approached statistical significance, with t (43) = -1.50, P= 0.070 for pain relief and t (44) = -1.39, P = 0.087 for willingness to pay. In both cases, scores for subjects who received TT reflected more satisfaction with the treatment than did scores for subjects who received sham. Measurement for relief of stress revealed no difference between groups, and no difference was seen when satisfaction was measured by VASS.

Medication Usage

Medication usage recorded by the hospital pharmacy in the patient chart was noted for each subject who remained in the study through day six. For opiate pain medication, mean morphine equivalents per day for days one to five were calculated (DuBé and Koo, 1988) and were 25.6 and 25.0, respectively, for the TT and sham groups, t (72) = 0.15, P = 0.882, 2-tailed. For sleep, anxiety, and antidepressant medications, mean doses per day for days one to five were recorded. The mean doses per day of medication for sleep and depression were 0.12 or less for subjects in both treatment groups, which was too low for meaningful comparison. The mean doses per day of antianxiety medication were 0.75 and 0.89, respectively, for the TT and sham groups, t (75) = -0.93, P = 0.356, 2-tailed t-test. Thus no significant differences in medication use were noted between the two treatment groups.

Physiological Measurements

Useable blood samples for both days one and six were obtained for a convenience sample of eleven subjects, six who received TT and five who received sham TT. Mean day one and day six values for percentage CD4 + cells, percentage CD8 + cells, total CD4 + cells, total CD8 + cells, CD4 + /CD8 + cell ratio, total lymphocytes, and total white blood cells were calculated. Due to the small sample size, statistical comparison

Table 3: Satisfaction with therapy following TT or sham TT

Outcome variable	n	Covariables	Adjusted mean score TT group	Sham group	P (1-tailed)
Effectiveness of Therapy Form					
Pain	45	—	2.39	2.07	0.070
Stress	44	—	2.61	2.46	0.204
Willingness to pay for treatment	47	CTF	2.37	2.05	0.087
VASS	52	CTF	159.1	166.4	0.326

Outcome variable scores were regressed on treatment group (sham or real TT) and the following covariables: age, sex, race, Credibility of Therapy Form (CTF) score, and days from injury to study day 1. Covariables were allowed to enter the regression stepwise if P<0.10. Covariables = covariables which entered the regression equation. Adjusted mean score = mean score for each treatment group, adjusted for the covariables which entered the regression equation.

between values for the TT and sham TT groups was not done. However, when the change in mean values from day one to day six was calculated for the TT and sham groups, the greatest difference between the groups was noted for the total CD8+ cell concentrations.

Total CD8+ cells/cu mm decreased by 13.0 percent from day one (mean value 462/cu mm, SE 142) to day six for patients who received TT, but increased by 46.5 percent (mean day 1-value = 312, SE 67.7) over the same period for patients who received sham TT. Total CD4+cell concentration increased by 15.2 percent from day one (mean value = 782, SE 141) to day six for the TT group, but increased 48.3 percent for the sham group (mean day 1-value = 642, SE 150). Total lymphocyte count increased 1.1 percent from day one (mean day 1-value = 1959/cu mm, SE 518) to day six for the TT group, but increased by 38.6 percent for the sham group (mean day 1-value = 1437, SE 350). Differences between the TT and sham group results for the other blood cell measurements were much smaller.

DISCUSSION

Subjects who received TT reported a significantly greater reduction in pain on the McGill PRI and NWC after receiving five days of therapy than did those who received the sham treatment. Because there was no statistically significant difference in the amount of analgesic medication taken per twenty-four hours between TT and sham group subjects, the greater pain relief reported by the TT subjects suggests that the combination of TT and analgesic medication was able to produce a more complete pain relief than analgesic medication alone.

The finding of significantly greater pain relief reported by TT subjects as compared to sham subjects is consistent with results reported by Keller and Bzdek (1986), who studied the effects of TT on tension headache pain, and Meehan (1985), who studied the effects of TT on acute postoperative pain. In another study, Meehan (1993) found that TT alone was not sufficient to relieve postoperative pain, but that it did reduce the amount of pain medication requested by patients. These results, along with the results of this study, suggest that in acute pain, TT is most effectively used as an adjunct, as opposed to a substitute, for analgesic medication.

The study design did not include a "treatment as usual" control group due to the limited number of potential subjects at the research site. Therefore it is not possible to determine whether a portion of the pain relief experienced by either TT or sham subjects was due to the Hawthorne effect. However, because subjects were not aware of whether they were receiving actual TT or the sham the statistically significant difference in pain relief reported by TT, subjects as compared to the sham subjects can be attributed to treatment effects.

Another factor that may have influenced reported pain relief is that both groups experienced presence and music while TT or sham TT was being administered. Presence is recognized as a nursing intervention capable of producing positive outcomes (Hines 1992). Although the soft music was used primarily to mask the background noise on a busy acute care hospital unit, it may also have had a beneficial effect. Even though subjects who received TT as compared to those in the sham group reported significantly greater pain relief, further study is needed to determine the relative contribution made to pain relief by presence and music.

Subjects who received TT, as compared to the sham treatment, also reported significantly less anxiety after five days of therapy. This finding is consistent with several previous studies (Heidt, 1981; Quinn, 1984; Kramer, 1990). As part of the conceptual approach, we hypothesized that anxiety reduction might contribute to pain relief, but the degree to which it contributes is unknown and needs to be investigated. Also, factors contributing to anxiety, such as cause of burn injury or area of body burned, were not examined in this study and should be considered in future studies.

Although the number of subjects from whom blood samples were obtained was too small to allow any conclusions to be drawn, the finding of a decrease in CD8+ cell concentration among TT subjects as compared to an increase in sham subjects was noted. This result is consistent with results reported by Quinn and Strelkauskas (1993), in which TT decreased the OKT8 (now called CD8+) cell counts of both bereaved persons and their TT practitioners. These investigators reported decreases in CD8+ cells ranging from 10 to 23 percent, whereas a 13 percent decrease in total CD8+ cell concentration was found in response to TT in this study. Although the impact that this change may have upon immunity is not known, the finding is of interest and should receive further exploration.

Also of interest are TT group subjects' perceptions (as reported on the ETF) of greater perceived pain relief and a greater willingness to pay for treatment, as compared to those in the sham group. Although these differences were not statistically significant at the 0.05 level, they did approach significance and do warrant further exploration. The degree of willingness to pay for treatment may provide clues as to the receptivity of patients in acute care settings to complementary therapies such as TT.

The positive findings of this study add support to the growing body of evidence on the effectiveness of TT in ameliorating pain perception and reducing anxiety. A major effort in future TT research should be directed toward elucidating underlying mechanisms and modes of action. This knowledge would provide valuable information regarding the conditions under which TT is most likely to be effective. Additional information is also needed regarding the best specific protocol for administering TT to patients hospitalized with severe burns. Replication of this study should include a treatment as usual control group and should exclude the background music during treatment in order to obtain a more precise measure of the effect of TT. Study of the long-term effects of TT administered during the acute period following a severe burn injury on subsequent physical and psychological recovery would also be useful.

CONCLUSION

Therapeutic Touch appeared to be effective in increasing pain relief as an adjunct to analgesic medication and in reducing anxiety for the burn patients in this study. Additional research is needed to explore the mechanisms for these effects and the relationships among outcomes. Therapies that reduce pain and anxiety can be particularly significant for hospitalized burn patients. If the findings of the current study are supported by subsequent research, TT may become an important part of nursing care for hospitalized burn patients, as well as for other patients for whom pain and anxiety are major problems.

REFERENCES:

Agency for Health Care Policy and Research (AHCPR). 1992. "Acute Pain Management: Operative or Medical Procedures and Trauma, Part 2." *Clinical Pharmacy* 11: 391–414.

Andreasen, N. J., R. Noyes, and C. E. Hartford. 1972. "Management of Emotional Reactions in Severely Burned Adults." *New England Journal of Medicine* 286: 65-69.

Belcher, H. J. C. R. 1996. *Immunological Responses: Principles and Practice of Burns Management.* Edited by J. A. D. Settle. New York: Churchill Livingstone, pp. 163–75.

Blazar, B. A., M. L. Rodrick, J. B. O'Mahony et al. 1986. "Suppression of Natural Killer-Cell Function in Humans Following Thermal and Traumatic Injury." *Journal of Clinical Immunology* 6 (1): 26–36.

Borkovec, T. D., and S. D. Nau. 1972. "Credibility of Analogue Therapy Rationales." *Journal of Behavioral Therapy and Experimental Psychology* 3: 257–63.

Choiniere, M., R. Melzack, J. Rondeau et al. 1989. "The Pain of Burns: Characteristics and Correlates." *The Journal of Trauma* 29 (11): 1531–39.

Clark, A. J. 1992 "Client Perceptions of Therapeutic Touch." Abstract. *Proceedings of the West Alabama Annual Nursing Research Conference*. Tuscaloosa, Alabama, p. 16.

DuBé, J. E., and P. J. Koo. 1988. "Pain." In *Applied Therapeutics*. Edited by L. Y. Young and M. A. Koda-Kimble. Vancouver, pp. 49–70.

Dyer, C., and D. Roberts. 1990. "Thermal Trauma." *Trauma* 25(1): 85–117.

Garrard, C. 1995. "The Effect of Therapeutic Touch on Stress Reduction and Immune Function in Persons with AIDS." Ph.D. diss., University of Alabama at Birmingham, Birmingham, Alabama.

Gift, A. G. 1989. "Visual Analogue Scales: Measures of Subjective Phenomena." *Nursing Research* 38(5): 286–87.

Griswold, J. A. 1993. "White Blood Cell Response to Burn Injury." *Seminars in Nephrology* 13(4): 409–15.

Hale, E. 1986. "A Study of the Relationship Between Therapeutic Touch and the

Anxiety Levels of Hospitalized Adults." *Dissertation Abstracts International* 47 1928B. University Microfilms no. 8618897.

Heidt, P. 1981. "Effect of Therapeutic Touch on Anxiety Levels of Hospitalized Patients." *Nursing Research* 30(2): 32–37.

Hines, D. R. 1992. "Presence: Discovering the Artistry in Relating." *Journal of Holistic Nursing* 10(4): 294–305.

Keller, E., and V. Bzdek. 1986. "Effects of Therapeutic Touch on Tension Headache Pain." *Nursing Research* 35: 101–105.

Kinsella, J., and M. G. Booth. 1991. "Pain Relief in Burns: James Laing Memorial Essay." *Burns* 17(5): 391–95.

Knudson-Cooper, M. S. 1981. "Relaxation and Biofeedback Training in the Treatment of Severely Burned Children." *Journal of Burn Care and Rehabilitation* 2 (2): 102–10.

Kramer, N. 1990. "Comparison of Therapeutic Touch and Casual Touch in Stress Reduction in Hospitalized Children." *Pediatric Nursing* 16 (5): 483–85.

Krieger, D. 1993. *Accepting Your Power to Heal: The Personal Practice of Therapeutic Touch*. Santa Fe, N.Mex.: Bear & Company.

Marvin, J. A., G. Carrougher, E. Bayler et al. 1992. "Burn Nursing Delphi Study: Pain Management." *Journal of Burn Care and Rehabilitation* 13 (6): 685–94.

McCaffery, M., and A. Beebe. 1989. *Pain: Clinical Manual for Nursing Practice*. St. Louis: C.V. Mosby.

Meehan, T. C. 1985. "The Effect of Therapeutic Touch on the Experience of Acute Pain in Postoperative Patients." *Dissertation Abstracts, Intl.* (46): 795B. University Microfilms no. 8510765.

———. 1993. "Therapeutic Touch and Postoperative Pain: A Rogerian Research Study." *Nursing Science Quarterly* 6(12): 69–78.

Melzack, R. 1975. "The McGill Pain Questionnaire: Major Properties and Scoring Methods." *Pain* 1: 277–99.

———. 1990. "The Tragedy of Needless Pain." *Scientific American* 262 (2): 27–33.

Miller, A. C., L. C. Hickman, and G. K. Lemasters. 1992. "A Distraction Technique for Control of Burn Pain." *Journal of Burn Care and Rehabilitation* 13 (5): 576–80.

Parkes, B. 1985. "Therapeutic Touch as an Intervention to Reduce Anxiety in Elderly, Hospitalized Patients." *Dissertation Abstracts International* (47): 473B. University Microfilms no. 8609563.

Patterson, D. R. 1992. "Practical Applications of Psychological Techniques in Controlling Burn Pain." *Journal of Burn Care and Rehabilitation* 13 (1): 13–18.

Quinn, J. 1984. "Therapeutic Touch as Energy Exchange: Testing the Theory." *Advances in Nursing Science* 6 (2): 42–49.

Quinn, J., and A. J. Strelkauskas. 1993 "Psychoimmunologic Effects of Therapeutic Touch on Practitioners and Recently Bereaved Recipients: A Pilot Study." *Advances in Nursing Science* 15 (4): 13–26.

Revill, S. I., J. O. Robinson, M. Rosen et al. 1976. "The Reliability of a Linear Analogue for Evaluating Pain." *Anesthesia* 31: 1191–98.

Rogers, M. 1970. *An Introduction to the Theoretical Basis of Nursing.* Philadelphia: F.A. Davis.

———. 1990. "Nursing: Science of Unitary, Irreducible, Human Beings: Update 1990." In *Visions of Rogers' Science-Based Nursing.* Edited by E. A. M. Barrett. New York: National League for Nursing, pp. 5–22.

Sriwantanakul, K., W. Kelvie, L. Lasagna et al. 1983. "Studies on Different Types of Visual Analogue Scales for the Measurement of Pain." *Clinical Pharmacology and Therapeutics* 34 (2): 234–39.

Steiner, H., and W. R. Clark. 1977. "Psychiatric Complications of Burned Adults: A Classification." *Journal of Trauma* 17: 134–43.

Tidwell, B. B. 1996. *Effects of an Intervention Plan on Burn Wound Care.* Dissertation, the University of Alabama at Birmingham, Birmingham, Alabama.

Tobiasen, J. M., and J. M. Hiebert. 1985. "Burns and Adjustment to Injury: Do Psychological Coping Strategies Help?" *Journal of Trauma* 25 (12): 1151–55.

Warden, G. D. 1987. "Immunologic Response to Burn Injury." In *The Art and Science of Burn Care.* Edited by J. A. Boswick. Rockville, Md.: Aspen, pp. 113–20.

14.

The Effects of Therapeutic Touch on Patients with Osteoarthritis of the Knee

Andrea Gordon, Joel H. Merenstein, Frank D'Amico, and David Hudgens

Background. The purpose of this study was to determine if Therapeutic Touch, an alternative medicine modality, is effective in the treatment of osteoarthritis of the knee.

Methods. A single-blinded randomized control trial was conducted in a family practice center of a community hospital family practice residency program in Pennsylvania. The patients were between the ages of forty and eighty, had been given a diagnosis of osteoarthritis of at least one knee, had not had knee replacement, and had no other connective tissue disease. The patients were randomized to Therapeutic Touch, mock Therapeutic Touch, or standard care. The main outcome measures were pain and its impact, general well-being, and health status measured by standardized, validated instruments, as well as the qualitative measurement of a Depth interview.

Results. Twenty-five patients completed the study. The treatment group had significantly decreased pain and improved function as compared with the placebo and control groups. The qualitative Depth interview confirmed this result.

Conclusion. Despite the small numbers, significant differences were found in improvement in function and pain for patients receiving Therapeutic Touch. A larger study is needed to confirm these results. Alternative therapies can neither be accepted nor rejected without being subjected to the scientific method.

Originally published in the *Journal of Family Practice* 47, no. 4 (October 1998): 271–77. Copyright © 1998 Appleton & Lange. Reproduced by permission from the *Journal of Family Practice*.

Osteoarthritis is the most common joint disease and the leading cause of chronic disability in developed countries (Wilson et al., 1991), yet our treatment options for this disorder are limited. Osteoarthritis patients may be among those who are looking to alternative medicine for additional possibilities for relief from their symptoms. In 1991, the National Institutes of Health (NIH) acknowledged the range of alternative options now available and created the Office of Alternative Medicine to begin evaluating these therapies.

Therapeutic Touch, a form of complementary medicine that the NIH categorizes as a "manual healing method," is an intervention that could benefit patients with osteoarthritis. Developed by Krieger and Kunz in the 1970s (Krieger, 1990), TT has since been taught in more than eighty universities and is a part of the nursing protocol in an increasing number of hospitals (Williams, 1992). The theory states that everyone has an energy system that may become imbalanced with illness. Like acupuncture or other schools of healing that postulate such a theory, TT attempts to bring the body system back into balance.

TT has been the subject of several studies that support its effects on anxiety (Heidt, 1981) and pain (Keller, Bzdek, 1986), and it is being used in diverse medical settings. Because there is some doubt, however, about its biologic plausibility (Rosa et al., 1998), the most rigorous methods are necessary to test its value.

The purpose of this study was to investigate the effects of TT on pain, level of functioning, and general well-being in patients with osteoarthritis of the knee. Qualitative measures were used in addition to quantitative measures to assess clinical significance and patient experience.

METHODS

Data Collection

Our study was a randomized controlled trial comparing TT, sham treatment (mock TT), and no treatment. Data collection ran from August 1995 to November 1995 at the Lawrenceville Family Health Center, one of two residency offices affiliated with the University of Pittsburgh Medical Center, St. Margaret Memorial Hospital, Family Practice Residency Program. Approximately 14,000 low- to middle-income patients are seen there each year.

Patients recruited for this study were between the ages of forty and eighty, had been given a diagnosis of osteoarthritis of at least one knee, and were able to read and speak English. Those patients with a diagnosis of connective tissue disorder, bilateral total knee replacement, or total knee replacement of their only affected knee were excluded from the study. Patients were identified by a chart review of those with relevant diagnoses over the past year, and were then recruited by telephone. Thirty-one patients met the inclusion criteria and agreed to participate. Informed consent was obtained. These patients were assigned a rating of mild, moderate, or severe osteoarthritis, according to their responses on the Osteoarthritis of the Knee form (Health Outcomes Institute, 1991) and a rheumatologist's reading of their bilateral knee radiograph. The questionnaire and radiograph readings were equally weighted in describing the severity of the arthritis. Subsequently, the patients within each rating were assigned to one of the three study groups, using a proportionate randomization. This insured that there were equal numbers of patients with each severity rating in each group.

Baseline data were gathered on all patients, using the Stanford Health Assessment Questionnaire (HAQ) (Ramey, Raynauld, Fries, 1992), the West Haven-Yale Multidimensional Pain Inventory, version 2.1 (MPI) (Kearns, Turk, Rudy, 1985), and two visual analog scales to measure pain and general well-being. The HAQ is a general questionnaire regarding the patients' health status, functional status, medications, and use of medical services. The MPI addresses the patient's pain and the perception of its impact, and his or her functioning and social interactions. The visual analog scales are horizontal lines with the extreme responses printed at either end that allow patients to identify their level of pain or well-being on a scale from one to ten. These scales were completed before and after each treatment or placebo treatment as interim measures in both groups. The visual analog scales were not administered to the control group because we wanted to minimize any inadvertent placebo effect resulting from this contact.

All groups continued to receive their usual care throughout the study period. In addition, the treatment group received a TT treatment once a week for six weeks, and the placebo group received a mock treatment at the same rate, for identical amounts of time.

Since much of TT deals with the practitioner's perceptions, it appears as though he or she is simply moving her hands a few inches away from the patient's body. Previous studies have taken advantage of this fact by designing a series of movements to be done as a mock treatment, while the performer focuses on a cognitive task rather than on the patient (Keller, Bzdek, 1986; Meehan, 1991). We used this method with the placebo group. The actual TT practitioner did not give the mock treatments because it is theorized that some of the therapeutic process becomes automatic, and it is difficult for trained practitioners to go through the motions and not do TT (Quinn, 1989; Horrigan, Quinn, 1996). The mock Therapeutic Touch (MTT) practitioner was chosen to resemble the TT practitioner in several ways; both were women of approximately the same age with experience in health care.

Before the study, both actual and mock TT treatments were videotaped and reviewed to insure that objective observers could not tell the difference.

Outcome measures were pain and its impact, general well-being, and health status. These measures were obtained using visual analog scales before and after each treatment, the HAQ, the MPI, and the qualitative technique of the Depth interview (Crabtree, Miller, 1991). The Depth interviews were designed to further investigate the patients' experiences and ascertain whether they noted any changes that were not adequately addressed by our instruments. These interviews were piloted prior to the study. They were administered by an anthropology doctorate student who was previously unacquainted with the patients. In addition, an auditor was used to review the interviews once the analysis had been completed. This was done to insure that there was no evidence in the transcribed interviews that contradicted our conclusions.

All groups completed the HAQ, MPI, and the two visual analog scales in the first week. In addition, the treatment and placebo groups had a TT or MTT treatment and then completed both visual analog scales again afterward. During weeks two through five, only the treatment and, placebo groups were seen. The subjects completed the two visual analog scales before and after each weekly treatment. At the sixth week, they also participated in a Depth interview. At week seven, all subjects (treatment, placebo, and control groups) again completed the HAQ, MPI, and the two visual analog scales. There was then no contact by the investigators with any of the groups until week thirteen, when all subjects completed the HAQ, MPI, and both visual analog scales for the final time. The treatment and placebo groups also had their second Depth interviews at this time.

Stastical Analysis

Initially, one-way analysis of variance was used to compare treatment, placebo, and control groups at baseline for continuous-level measured variables obtained from the HAQ, MPI, and visual analog scales. Chi-square tests of homogeneity of proportions were used to compare categorical variables. Assumptions of these procedures were examined using residual diagnostics.

The HAQ and the MPI were examined between groups over time by using a 2-factor repeated-measures analysis of variance. Post hoc individual tests (such as comparing the treatment group at week one with itself at week thirteen) were performed using Fisher's least significant difference method.

The visual analog scales, given before and after each treatment session, were studied within groups using the paired *t*-test. The differences between the before and after scores were tested between groups over time using analysis of variance.

All statistical tests used SAS software (SAS Institute, 1989). Levels of significance were considered at P < 0.05. The Depth interviews were analyzed by the method described by Crabtree and Miller (Crabtree, Miller, 1991).

RESULTS

Thirty-one patients were enrolled and randomized. All were white and English-speaking. No significant differences were found in the ages or the severity scores of the groups (see table 1). Of these thirty-one, two were unable to participate because of schedule conflicts. One patient was found to be unqualified for this study, and one left without explanation after looking at the questionnaire. Of the remaining twenty-seven patients, twenty-five completed the entire study. The other two patients, one from the treatment and one from the placebo group, completed treatments and the first two sets of data collection only. They were unable to be reached to schedule the final interview and set of questionnaires.

Pain and function were evaluated by analysis of the MPI, HAQ Functional Disability Index, and Depth interviews. The MPI consists of thirteen scales that evaluate different aspects of pain, coping with pain, and function (Kearns, Turk, Rudy, 1985). The sections of the HAQ that

TABLE 1			
Subject Characteristics (N=27), by Randomized Group			
Characteristic	**Treatment Group (n=8)**	**Placebo Group (n=11)**	**Control Group (n=8)**
Age			
Average, in years	64.38	64.45	68.75
Sex			
Female, no. (%)	5 (62.5)	8 (72.7)	5 (62.5)
Severity score*			
Average (SD)	2.7 (.6542)	2.84 (.8774)	2.82 (.8534)

SD denotes standard deviation.
*Average severity scores were assigned on a scale of 1 to 5, where 5 is the most severe.

deal with pain, function, and general health status make up the HAQ Functional Disability Index, which has been previously used in studies to report on arthritis patients (Pincus et al., 1983; Thompson, Pegley, 1991; Fries, Spitz, Young, 1982).

The treatment group had significantly decreased pain and improved function as compared with both the placebo and control groups. This was demonstrated by repeated-measures analysis on ten of thirteen scales on the MPI (see table 2). Several of the scales showed some improvement in the placebo group and additional improvement in the group that received the actual treatment (see figures 1 and 2). The treatment groups began to relapse after the treatment had stopped, but remained generally improved above baseline. An analysis of these results that included the two patients who did not complete the study did not change the results.

There were no significant differences noted on the HAQ Functional Disability Index (see table 3). There were, however, significant improvements seen on the HAQ, general health status questions. The treatment group did statistically better than the placebo group on two measures of current health status (continuous and ordinal, P = 0.05 and P = 0.001, respectively), dealing with the frustrations of arthritis at week seven (P = 0.05), and number of tender joints (P = 0.02). They improved significantly more than the control group on measures of energy level (P = 0.02), coping with the frustrations of arthritis at week 13 (P = 0.02), mood (P = 0.04), and general health status. The placebo group did not

---

TABLE 2

MPI Repeated Measures Results

Scales in which increasing score indicates clinical improvement:

	Groups			P values	
	Treatment	Placebo	Control		
Scale	Average (SD)	Average (SD)	Average (SD)	T vs P	T vs C
Life control	4.95 (.191)	4.35 (.168)	4.08 (.178)	.0259	.0085
Support	3.65 (.304)	3.15 (.268)	2.98 (.284)	.2255	.2656
Solicitous responses	2.94 (.245)	2.65 (.183)	3.04 (.224)	.3497	.7727
Distracting responses	2.42 (.230)	1.92 (.171)	2.75 (.209)	.0975	.3036
Household chores	4.77 (.244)	4.65 (.182)	3.67 (.223)	.6988	.0043
Outdoor work	2.57 (.225)	1.39 (.167)	1.78 (.205)	.0005	.0178
Activities away from home	3.72 (.237)	2.41 (.177)	2.18 (.217)	.0003	.0003
Social activities	3.05 (.202)	2.51 (.150)	2.36 (.184)	.0443	.0510
General activity level	3.53 (.161)	2.74 (.120)	2.50 (.147)	.001	.0005

Scales in which decreasing score indicates clinical improvement:

	Groups			P values	
	Treatment	Placebo	Control		
Scale	Average (SD)	Average (SD)	Average (SD)	T vs P	T vs C
Pain severity	2.14 (.196)	3.27 (.173)	3.06 (.183)	.0002	.002
Interference	1.50 (.214)	2.36 (.189)	2.65 (.201)	.0056	.0016
Affective distress	1.32 (.255)	2.67 (.225)	2.32 (.239)	.0005	.0081
Punishing response	0.67 (.345)	1.84 (257)	1.72 (315)	.0137	.0365

Note: Averages represent the average score across all three time points.

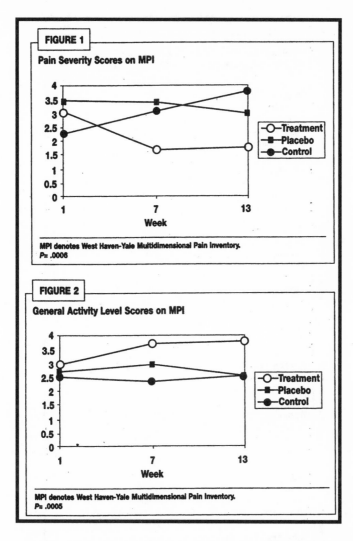

FIGURE 1

Pain Severity Scores on MPI

MPI denotes West Haven-Yale Multidimensional Pain Inventory.
P= .0006

FIGURE 2

General Activity Level Scores on MPI

MPI denotes West Haven-Yale Multidimensional Pain Inventory.
P= .0005

improve significantly more than the control group on any of these measures. There was no difference between the groups in the change in pain scores on visual analog scores before and after TT or MTT, except once when the placebo group improved more than the treatment group. The average scores on each visual analog scales question did demonstrate greater improvement over time in the TT treatment group than in either the placebo or the control groups (see figures 3 and 4).

The qualitative data supported the improvement in the treatment group that was noted on the MPI. One patient in the treatment group

TABLE 3

Results of the Stanford Health Assessment Questionnaire Functional Disability Index

	Week 1	Week 7	Week 13
Dressing and grooming			
Treatment group	0.25	0	0.07
Placebo group	0.35	0.18	0.3
Control group	0.13	0.07	0.56
Arising			
Treatment group	0.75	0.38	0.29
Placebo group	0.9	0.65	0.65
Control group	0.69	0.07	0.94
Eating			
Treatment group	0	0	0
Placebo group	0.23	0.18	0.18
Control group	0.04	0	0.21
Walking			
Treatment group	0.88	0.44	0.21*
Placebo group	0.95	0.8	0.5
Control group	0.71	0.86	1.21*
Hygiene			
Treatment group	0.33	0.04	0.09
Placebo group	0.53	0.36	0.46
Control group	0.37	0.52	0.46
Reach			
Treatment group	0.25	0.13*	0.14
Placebo group	0.65	0.73*	0.65
Control group	0.44	0.36	0.56
Grip			
Treatment group	0	0*	0
Placebo group	0.27	0.45*	0.23
Control group	0	0.09	0.17
Activities			
Treatment group	0.33	0.08	0.05
Placebo group	0.89	0.63	0.75
Control group	0.75	0.48	0.71

* Significant difference between groups; $P < .05$.

who had only rare pain at baseline noted little change. All the other patients in the treatment group reported decreased pain and arthritis symptoms with a concomitant increase in activity. Patients' comments included: "But for all the time I was coming here the pain was very small," and "Everything [has changed]. I can walk. I have no pain. I have no swelling." Many described an increased activity level or increased ease of participation in their activities. When one subject was asked if she was able to be more or less active since the treatment, she replied, "Oh, more, definitely. . . . I don't mind my job so much."

Several patients in the treatment group also noted that they were

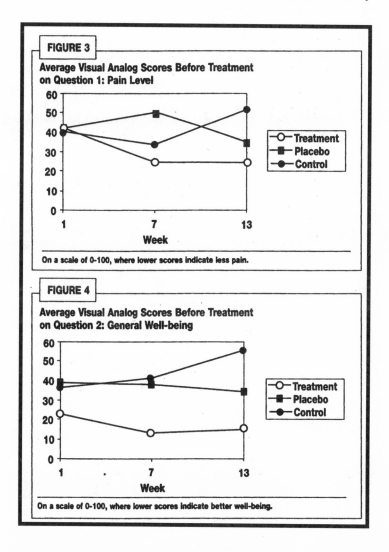

FIGURE 3

Average Visual Analog Scores Before Treatment on Question 1: Pain Level

On a scale of 0-100, where lower scores indicate less pain.

FIGURE 4

Average Visual Analog Scores Before Treatment on Question 2: General Well-being

On a scale of 0-100, where lower scores indicate better well-being.

able to delay or decrease other measures that were usually needed to control their symptoms. One patient said during her first interview, "I was at one point taking four doses a day of Extra Strength Tylenol. Each time since having the therapy I only take two tablets in the morning and don't have to take any the rest of the day." Weeks later this patient felt that having had TT may have "changed the fact that I might have to get a knee replacement as quickly." Other patients in the treatment group also noted that TT had allowed them to delay steroid injections or medications or walk farther without subsequent pain and swelling. During their second interview (seven weeks after the treatments had stopped), most patients in the treatment group felt that their symptoms had begun to worsen but that they were still improved compared with their pretreatment status. All the patients in the treatment group found TT a pleasant experience, and many commented that they wished it would continue.

The placebo group described a more heterogeneous response. Five of eleven patients had some decreased pain, but three of these were guarded in their descriptions: "It has let up a little bit, but not that much," and "I think I feel better." Four other patients noted that they felt better, but described the effect as one of "relaxation," "at peace," or "it is like something has been lifted." The remaining patient in the placebo group did not note any changes. Two patients did note a decreased "tightness in the joints." One patient stated that she felt it helped her and that she "would pay to do this." Most of these patients enjoyed the treatments and wished they could continue, but described a variety of reasons for this, such as "I miss coming out [to the office]," and "They were calming . . . even if they didn't take the pain away, something about them felt good."

During their second interviews, patients in the placebo group who had previously improved were more likely to describe symptoms as long-standing than were those in the treatment group, who described their experience in terms of what had happened during the treatments and since the treatments ended, commenting on the differences between these periods. Patients in both groups who spontaneously commented on their practitioner expressed positive feelings about her.

DISCUSSION

This study was designed as a randomized controlled trial in an attempt to clarify the effects of TT, with the knowledge that the placebo effect may account for the improvements seen with many pain treatments (Turner et al., 1994). The mock treatment was designed to be as similar to TT as possible from the patients' perspective, to elicit the same placebo effect. Patients' expectations of the treatment may also have contributed to their response. By the random assignment of patients to one of the three groups, the bias due to self-selection was eliminated. It was possible to make this only a single-blinded study, since the TT practitioner cannot be blinded to the treatment she is giving. The study duration was chosen because six weeks was felt by practitioners to be a sufficient period to show any short-term change due to TT.

Our results showed that TT decreased arthritis pain, and improved function and general health status in these patients. This improvement was significantly greater than that seen in the placebo group. The treatment group also demonstrated a slower return to baseline than did patients who improved with the MTT. These results were demonstrated with both quantitative and qualitative measures. The qualitative findings reinforced the quantitative findings and assured the clinical impact of this magnitude of improvement.

The fact that there was no difference in the amount of change between groups on the interim visual analog scales implies that there was no greater effect with either MTT or TT immediately following a treatment. If any of the effects were due to a greater placebo effect or rapport with the practitioner, one would expect to see greater improvement in that group immediately after treatment.

The HAQ Functional Disability Index, however, did not demonstrate improvement in any of the groups, which was not consistent with the rest of our findings. This may be because each scale consists of only two or three questions, most of which are extremely task-specific (e.g., "Are you able to bend down to pick up clothing from the floor?"). Each MPI scale contains between three and eleven questions, making this a more powerful instrument. Measures of general health status on the HAQ did show significant changes that were all consistent with the findings of the MPI and interviews in the direction of improvement of the treatment group.

The difference in outcomes between treatment and placebo groups allows us to distinguish the effect of TT from that of the relationship with the practitioner. The treatment group clearly improved, and more so than the placebo or control group. If additional improvement was not due to TT, then some other factor would have had to affect the treatment group differently. The practitioner was a variable that was different between groups, but this was controlled for in several ways that have been described previously. Two visual analog scales measuring the patients' perception of their practitioner as either warm or concerned showed no difference between groups. The interviews supported this, as patients in both groups spontaneously expressed positive feelings about their practitioner.

Changes in use of medications over time were analyzed to insure that this had not influenced one group more than another. There was no significant difference between groups in the change of number of medications.

Other studies have investigated the effects of TT on pain (Keller, Bzdek, 1986; Meehan, 1991), stress or anxiety (Vaughan, 1995; Quinn, 1984; Kramer, 1990; Heidt, 1981), and wound healing (Wirth, 1990, 1995; Quinn, 1988, 1989; Brandt, 1993). Criticisms of these studies have included the lack of control for placebo effect, time limitations on practitioners, inappropriate measurement tools, and the lack of both subjective and objective data (Clark, Clark, 1984; Fries, Spitz, Young, 1982; Turner et al., 1994; Vaughan, 1995). This study was designed so that there would be both a baseline control and a placebo group. The time limitations on the TT were removed, but the placebo treatments matched. Previously validated instruments were used, and a qualitative component was employed to confirm the clinical impact of quantitative findings.

Our study did have the limitation of a small sample size. Despite this, many of our measures achieved statistical significance. Some of the absolute changes on the ordinal scales are only one to two points (on six- or ten-point scales), but the interviews have assured us that changes of this magnitude are clinically significant and, indeed often seemed dramatic to the patients.

Our positive findings have several implications. Although large studies are needed to confirm the effect, TT may offer a means of symptom control for osteoarthritis patients without the side effects caused by current modalities such as NSAIDs and corticosteroid injections (Brandt, 1993). Complementary therapies are often rejected because of a lack of belief in their theory, even when well-designed randomized controlled trials show evidence of their efficacy. The authors of a 1991 meta-analysis of controlled trials of homeopathy stated, "Based on this evidence, we would be ready to accept that homeopathy can be efficacious, if only the mechanism of action were more plausible" (Kleijnen, Knipschild, Riet, 1991). If we are confident that the methodology of a randomized controlled trial is our best tool for discerning objective evidence, then we must be prepared to reconsider our theoretical framework if we find that it conflicts with the evidence.

Future research could study larger groups and answer subsequent questions on the efficacy of TT in several ways. TT is thought to help with healing, but osteoarthritis is a condition in which there are chronic structural changes, so the gradual return of symptoms after the cessation of treatment is not surprising. Future studies could use other conditions with more defined end points, such as following the healing rate of similar operative incisions. Other issues that will need to be addressed include the amount of training required to perform TT effectively and its effects on other commonly seen patient complaints.

It may well be that TT works in a different way than by manipulating energy fields. If other, larger studies confirm our findings of the effectiveness of this treatment, it will be important to design studies into the mechanism of action. In the meantime, it would be imprudent to reject a safe and effective therapy because we do not understand or do not accept its mode of action.

REFERENCES

Brandt, K. D. 1993. "NSAIDS in the Treatment of Osteoarthritis, Friends or Foes?" *Bulletin on the Rheumatic Diseases* 42: 14.

Clark, P. E., and M. J. Clark. 1984. "Therapeutic Touch: Is There a Scientific Basis for the Practice?" *Nursing Research* 33: 3741.

Crabtree, B., and W. Miller. 1991. "A Qualitative Approach to Primary Care Research: The Long Interview." *Family Medicine* 23: 145–51.

Fries, J. F., P. W. Spitz, and D. Y. Young. 1982. "The Dimension of Health Outcomes: The Health Assessment Questionnaire, Disability, and Pain Scales." *Journal of Rheumatology* 9: 789–93.

Health Outcomes Institute. 1991. "Osteoarthritis of the Knee." *Form*.

Heidt, P. R. 1981. "The Effect of Therapeutic Touch on the Anxiety Level of Hospitalized Patients." *Nursing Research* 30: 32–37.

Horrigon, B., and J. F. Quinn. 1996. "Therapeutic Touch and a Healing Way." *Alternative Therapies* 2: 70.

Kearns, R. D., D. C. Turk, and T. E. Rudy. 1985. "The West Haven-Yale Multidimensional Pain Inventory." *Pain* 23: 345–56.

Keller, E., and V. M. Bzdek. 1986. "Effects of Therapeutic Touch on Tension Headache Pain." *Nursing Research* 35: 101–106.

Kleijnen, J., P. Knipschild, and G. Riet. 1991. "Clinical Trials of Homoeopathy." *British Medical Journal* 302: 321.

Kramer, N. A. 1990. "Comparison of Therapeutic Touch and Casual Touch in Stress Reduction of Hospitalized Children." *Pediatric Nursing* 16: 483–85.

Krieger, D. 1990. "Therapeutic Touch: Two Decades of Research, Teaching, and Clinical Practice." *NSNA/Imprint* (September–October): 83–88.

Meehan, T. C. 1991. "Therapeutic Touch and Postoperative Pain: A Rogerian Research Study." *Nursing Science Quarterly* 6: 69–78.

Pincus, T., J. A. Summer, S. H. Sorac Jr., K. A. Wallston et al. 1983. "Assessment of Patient Satisfaction in Activities of Daily Living Using a Modified Stanford Health Assessment Questionnaire." *Arthritis and Rheumatism* 26: 1346–53.

Quinn, J. 1984. "Therapeutic Touch as Energy Exchange: Testing the Theory." *Advances in Nursing Science* (January): 42–49.

———. 1988. "Building a Body of Knowledge: Research on Therapeutic Touch." *Journal of Holistic Nursing* 6: 3745.

————. 1989. "Future Directions for Therapeutic Touch Research." *Journal of Holistic Nursing* 7: 19–25.

Ramey, D., J. P. Raynauld, and J. Fries. 1992. "The Health Assessment Questionaire 1992, Status and Review." *Arthritis Care Res*, 5: 119–29.

Rosa, L., E. Rosa, L. Sarner et al. 1998. "A Close Look at Therapeutic Touch." *JAMA* 279: 1005–10.

SAS Institute, Inc. 1989. *SAS/STAT User's Guide*. Version 6, 4th ed. Volume 1. Cary, N.C.: SAS Institute, Inc.

Thompson, P. W., and F. S. Pegley. 1991. "A Comparison of Disability Measured by the Stanford Health Assessment Questionnaire Disability Scales in Male and Female Rheumatoid Outpatients." *British Journal of Rheumatology* 30: 398–400.

Turner, J. A., R. A. Demayo, J. D. Loeser et al. 1994. "The Importance of Placebo Effects in Pain Treatment and Research." *JAMA* 271: 1609–14.

Vaughan, S. 1995. "The Gentle Touch." *Journal of Clinical Nursing* 4: 359–68.

Williams, G. 1992. "The Lowest-Tech Medicine Ever." *Longevity* (January): 61.

Wilson, J. D., E. Braunwald, K. J. Isselbacher et al. 1991. *Harrison's Principles of Internal Medicine*. 13th ed. New York: McGraw-Hill, Inc, p. 1692.

Wirth, D. P. 1990. "The Effect of Non-Contact Therapeutic Touch on the Healing Rate of Full Thickness Dermal Wounds." *Subtle Energies* 1: 1–20.

————. 1995. "Complementary Healing Interventions and Dermal Wound Reepithelialization: An Overview." *International Journal of Psychosomatics* 42: 14.

15.

Perception of Conventional Sensory Cues as an Alternative to the Postulated "Human Energy Field" of Therapeutic Touch

Rebecca Long, Paul Bernhardt, and William Evans

Abstract Background. Therapeutic Touch proponents claim that humans emit a metaphysical "human energy field" that TT practitioners can sense and manipulate via their hands even without direct physical contact between practitioner and patient. As evidence, proponents note that TT practitioners commonly report various tactile sensations as they sweep their hands just above their patients' bodies. An experiment was conducted to determine if, and under what conditions, human subjects could detect via their hands the presence of a nearby human body that they could not see or touch.

Methods. Twenty-six subjects were tested to determine whether or not they could detect the presence of an investigator's unseen hand that was steadied just above one of the subject's hands. Subjects were tested at various distances between hands of subject and investigator and in trials in which various sensory cues were systematically added and removed.

Results. Subjects performed well at three inches between hands, offering correct guesses regarding the location of the investigator's unseen hand more than 70 percent of the time. Subjects' abilities remained strong at four inches between hands but diminished at six inches between hands. Subjects performed no better than chance

Originally published in *Scientific Review of Alternative Medicine* 3, no. 2 (fall/winter 1999). Copyright © 1999 Prometheus Books. Reprinted with permission from authors and publisher. The authors thank Jon Cadle, Dale Heatherington, Beth Holley, J. Sandefur, Rebecca Steinbach, and Harry Taylor for their assistance in conducting the experiment. They send special thanks to Béla Scheiber and other prominent skeptics for their consultation and support.

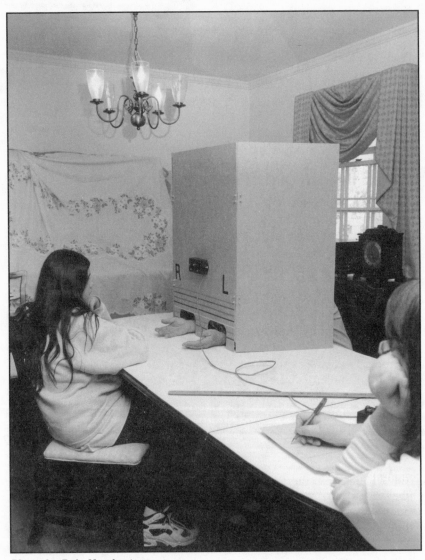

Photo by Dale Heatherington

would predict when body heat was shielded. Subjects who were purposefully miscued by investigators performed significantly worse than subjects who were not miscued.

Conclusions—Participants in Therapeutic Touch sessions may be mistaking conventional sensory cues such as radiated body heat for evidence of a metaphysical phenomenon.

Practitioners of the alternative nursing practice known as Therapeutic Touch claim that they use their hands to sense and manipulate a metaphysical "human energy field" that emanates from their patients. TT practitioners claim that manipulation of the HEF can facilitate physical and psychological healing. Moreover, TT practitioners contend that they can sense and manipulate the HEF without touching their patients. Indeed, TT is typically conducted with the practitioner's hand a few inches from the patient's body.

Despite this lack of direct physical contact between TT practitioners and patients, both practitioners and patients often report feeling sensations of warmth and tingling during TT sessions. TT proponents claim that these sensations stem from perception of a special type of energy that cannot be accounted for by conventional science. These sensations are often adduced by TT proponents as evidence of the efficacy of TT and the validity of its metaphysical constructs. For their part, some skeptics suggest that TT practitioners and patients may be merely imagining the sensations of warmth and tingling that are so often reported in TT testimonials. In this view, TT participants are victims of the power of suggestion and their desire to find corroborating evidence for their metaphysical worldview.

This article reports the results of an experiment designed to address these issues. More specifically, our experiment assessed (1) whether or not human subjects can detect, without using sight or touch, the presence of a human hand when the hand is placed just above the subjects' hands, and (2) the role that conventional sensory cues such as radiated body heat may play in subjects' abilities to detect the presence of a human hand that they cannot see or touch. If subjects are unable to detect the presence of a nearby human hand when all significant sources of conventional sensory cuing have been eliminated, this would constitute evidence against the claim that humans can sense (or manipulate) a metaphysical HEF.

BACKGROUND

TT is today among the most commonly utilized alternative health therapies. TT has enjoyed particular success in the nursing community, where it has been embraced by several mainstream nursing organizations and utilized by nurses in many hospitals in North America and around the world (Meehan, 1998; Rosa et al., 1998). TT enjoys frequent and largely favorable coverage in nursing journals and periodicals (Meehan,1998).

The success of TT in terms of the number and prestige of its practitioners has drawn the attention of researchers who have attempted to empirically assess the effectiveness of TT, especially in treating stress, pain, and a variety of mood disturbances. Rosa et al. report that eighty-three research studies that focus at least in part on TT had been published through 1997 (Rosa et al., 1998). As Meehan notes, this research has been inconclusive (Meehan,1998). The relatively few studies to report positive results for TT have been beset with methodological problems. These problems include the lack of control groups, failure to use blind protocols, the use of only a small number of subjects, and an overreliance on subjects' self-reports regarding the effectiveness of TT interventions. Meehan suggests that much of the TT research conducted to date has done too little to control for possible placebo effects (Meehan,1998). In a recent meta-analysis, Peters reports that the many methodological limitations of the existing TT research make it difficult or even impossible to say anything conclusively about the effectiveness of TT (Peters,1999). Earlier literature reviews, such as a report commissioned by the University of Colorado Health Sciences Center (Claman et al., 1994), have also noted similar methodological problems and limitations.

Perhaps in frustration with the great methodological difficulties (and high financial costs) associated with TT research that examines health outcomes, some researchers have moved from attempts to assess TT's therapeutic effectiveness to investigations of the TT practitioner's avowed ability to sense and manipulate the HEF.

Within the theoretical constructs of TT the HEF is a metaphysical manifestation of the flow of vitalistic life energy through the body. Persons who are ill are said to have deficits, blockages, or imbalances in their vital energy flow. TT practitioners claim they can use their hands to detect disturbances in the HEF, correct blockages by "unruffling" the field, and correct imbalances by channeling healing energy (Krieger, 1992). Again, the HEF is said to be sensed and manipulated without physical contact between practitioner and patient. Practitioners typically move their hands over the patient's body at a distance of two to four inches (Rosa et al., 1998), although slightly greater distances are cited by some proponents.

Dolores Krieger, one of the cofounders of TT, notes that TT practitioners almost always describe their perceptions of disturbances in the HEF in one of the following six ways: "heat," "cold," "tingling," "pressure," "electric shocks," or "pulsations." The phrase most often used is "temperature differential" (Krieger, 1992). TT proponents do not believe that these sensations are responses to ordinary sensory stimuli. Instead, they maintain that TT participants perceive an energy force that scientific instruments cannot detect and that conventional scientific theories cannot explain. For example, Krieger writes that the terms used by TT practitioners to describe the sensations "indicate a common experience for which we do not as yet have an adequately expressive language" (Krieger, 1992). According to Krieger, the sensation of heat "is not the sense of heat one feels when a hot stove is touched or a finger is passed through a flame." Rather, Krieger explains, "Therapeutic Touch deals with a very different aspect or conception of temperature differential than the one we currently understand in biophysics" (Krieger, 1993).

To determine whether or not TT practitioners can sense an HEF, Rosa et al. (1998) designed an experiment in which TT practitioners were asked to detect the presence of an unseen human hand that hovered above one of the practitioner's hands. Subjects and investigator were seated at a table divided by an opaque partition. Subjects placed their hands through holes in the partition. Twenty-one TT practitioners were tested. In 280 trials, these TT practitioners could correctly identify the hand over which an investigator's unseen hand hovered only 44 percent of the time, a rate that is no better than that which would be expected by chance. Ball and Alexander (1998) conducted an experiment in which a single blindfolded TT practitioner was asked to detect the presence or absence of a human body that, when present, was positioned (on a massage table) four inches from the practitioner's hands. This practitioner was successful in seven out of ten trials, a success rate that Ball and Alexander deemed insufficient to warrant concluding that the TT practitioner was able to detect HEFs.

The results reported by Rosa et al. (1998) and Ball and Alexander (1998) make sense in terms of science. Given what we know about electromagnetic fields and human physiology, it does indeed seem unlikely that HEFs exist and function in the manner that TT proponents believe them to. But science would also suggest that several sensory cues might be readily available to help humans determine when an unseen human body is in very close proximity. For example, radiant body heat might provide a salient sensory cue. Similarly, rustling of clothing or movements of air caused by even the slightest body movements might provide cues that a body is nearby. In this context, it might seem strange to expect that subjects would fail to perform at better-than-chance rates when asked to discern the presence or absence of an unseen but very close human body.

In order to adequately blind a test of whether or not human hands can detect the HEF of a nearby human body, it is necessary to eliminate any conventional sensory stimuli that could either (1) cue the subjects as to the presence of the body, or (2) miscue the subjects. The experimental apparatuses and procedures themselves may introduce confounding sensory cues. Investigator speech and behavior during experimental protocols may introduce them. Cuing often creeps into experimental protocols in the most surprising and sometimes seemingly inexplicable ways (Rosenthal, 1976). The seeming inevitability of subtle but nonetheless confounding cues such as rustling shirt sleeves and investigator tone of voice have led experimenters in sciences such as medicine, psychology, and sociology to adopt double-blind conditions whenever possible.

We discovered during pilot testing that subjects could seemingly be cued (and miscued) by investigators' body movements. For example, subtle sounds associated with the rustling of clothing or paperwork by the investigator were sufficient to cue some test subjects. In addition, some subjects could detect a very slight flow of air onto their hand if the investigator's hand was placed over it too rapidly or with a downward movement. Curiously, this slight breeze cued some subjects and miscued others who interpreted the sensation as coolness and therefore selected the wrong (i.e., warmer) hand. Similar subtle but significant cuing and miscuing effects were observed with some test subjects when an air conditioning system was running and the placement of the investigator's hand over the subject's hand blocked the flow of air.

Subjects were seemingly cued (and miscued) when the investigator rested an elbow on the experimental table, which turned out to be a common investigator tendency, especially when testing time was lengthy. Subjects displayed an ability to sense the vibrations or slight change in table alignment caused by this practice, and tended to preferentially guess the hand in front of the investigator's elbow. This resulted in both cuing and miscuing because the investigator's elbow was not always in front of the subject's hand over which the investigator's hand was placed.

Subjects were also seemingly cued and miscued when investigators gave a verbal signal (e.g., "okay," "ready") to indicate that their hand was in position. Investigators tended to look at the hand they were holding in place and subjects could seemingly detect the direction from which the audible signal was issued. We found evidence to suggest that investigators could miscue subjects by issuing an audible signal while looking at the wrong hand, as investigators did on occasion.

Rosa et al. (1998) asked subjects to place their palms in an upward position, a procedure we adopted (even if the palms-upward position is not typically used in TT practice). However, we discovered that subjects who were asked to keep their palms turned upward often complained of discomfort and reported "tingling," "pulsating," and "electrical" sensations in their hands. Subjects understandably expressed concerns that these sensations might interfere with their ability to detect sensations relevant to the experiment.

In short, there is a danger that experimental designs of this type may introduce sensory cues that threaten the validity of the study. Investigators may intentionally or (more likely) unintentionally introduce confounding sensory cues, and subjects may consciously or unconsciously make use of these cues. Because it is impractical to double-blind such an experiment, it is especially important to rigorously blind the subjects with respect to the investigator. In designing our experiment, we tried to minimize these threats to validity. We also designed our experiment in part to assess the potential role of investigator cuing and miscuing in experimental assessments of TT practitioners.

METHODS

Twenty-six subjects were tested under blinded conditions to determine if they could detect the presence of an investigator's hand that they could neither see nor touch. Subjects were recruited from among acquaintances of Rebecca Long (the first author of this report). There were thirteen male and thirteen female subjects, ranging in age from ten to eighty-one years. (A twenty-seventh subject was tested but his data were excluded from our analysis because he did not follow the protocol as instructed.) None of the subjects were TT practitioners, and none had ever been treated by a TT practitioner. None had more than a superficial familiarity with TT practices and claims.

The experiment utilized an apparatus very similar to that used by Rosa et al. (1998). Subjects were seated at a table and placed their hands through holes in a large opaque screen. Subjects rested their hands on the table, palms upward. The position of the screen and the placement of holes in the screen were informed by the pilot testing discussed above and designed to minimize physical sensations caused by the awkward hand position. To further minimize potentially confounding hand sensations, care was taken to minimize testing time. Subject comfort was verified before and after each set of experimental trials.

A towel was placed over subjects' forearms to prevent them from seeing through the holes in the screen. All reflective surfaces visible to subjects while they were in place for testing were covered to preclude the possibility that subjects would receive visual cues via reflected light. No air conditioning or heating system was run while testing was in progress. Room temperature was 64°F during all trials on one of the two days on which subjects were tested; it was 74°F during the second day of trials.

Two investigators participated in the experiment. Investigator 1 was Rebecca Steinbach, an eleven-year-old female. Investigator 2 was Rebecca Long, a female adult. Another person stood nearby to monitor subject and investigator adherence to experimental protocols and to verify the accuracy of the recorded data. Data were recorded by an individual other than the investigator. This individual was shielded from view of the subjects and operated the LED device utilized in the experiment (described below).

Investigators 1 and 2 each tested a different group of thirteen subjects, one week apart. Each subject underwent ten trials in each of the experimental conditions under which he or she was tested. In each trial, an investigator steadied her hand in place over one of the subjects' hands. Whether the investigator placed her hand over the subjects' left or right hand was determined in advance using a random number table (odd-numbered integers were associated with the subject's right hand and even-numbered integers with the subject's left hand). To avoid creating air movement, the investigator's hand was moved into position over the subject's hand slowly and with a horizontal movement, parallel to the table. Investigators wore clothing that did not rustle. Investigators were not permitted to lean on the table.

To eliminate the possibility of verbal cuing, a red "ready" light was used to signal the subject that the investigator's hand was in place. An LED device was also used to signal the investigator regarding whether to place her hand over the subject's left or right hand. The lights used to signal investigators were enclosed in a box that prevented light leakage that might have cued subjects. Pilot testing confirmed that the LEDs generated no light or heat that was detectable by subjects.

Trials were conducted at each of three different distances between the hands of subjects and investigators: three, four, and six inches. Hand distances were measured from the center of the subject's palm to the palm of the investigator's hand. A series of colored lines were placed on the investigator's side of the partition to help investigators judge where to place their hands.

In addition to varying the distance between hands, we used two additional experimental manipulations to assess the possible role of conventional sensory cues in subjects' guesses. In one set of trials, the possible role of body heat as a sensory cue was evaluated by interposing a thin piece of glass (from a picture frame) between the hands of subject and investigator. The glass was placed three inches above the palm of the subject. The investigator's hand was placed on the surface of the glass.

In a separate set of trials, conducted at a distance of six inches between hands, deliberate investigator miscuing was introduced. Instead of using the "ready" light to signal subjects, the investigator spoke the word "okay" while looking in the direction of the *incorrect* hand. At the same time, the investigator gently rested her elbow on the table in front of the incorrect hand.

Although subjects were given no time limits, all made their guesses rather rapidly, and in all cases the sets of ten trials were completed in less than one minute per set. After testing, each subject was invited to comment about the trials. These comments were recorded, as were all unsolicited comments made by the subjects during the trials.

RESULTS

Subjects were assessed in six different experimental conditions. Subjects could be expected to make correct guesses 50 percent of the time based on chance alone. Results are reported in table 1, where reported significance levels are based on two-tailed t-tests against the null hypothesis of chance accuracy (five out of ten correct guesses).

Subjects performed significantly better than chance would predict at distances of three and four inches between hands. At three inches, subjects tested by Investigator 1 made correct guesses an average of 7.62 times out of 10, with a standard deviation of 1.76 ($t = 5.36$; $df = 12$; $p = 0.0002$). Subjects tested by Investigator 2 offered correct guesses an average of 7.69 times out of 10, with a standard deviation of 1.32 ($t = 7.38$; $df = 12$; $p < 0.0001$). Fifteen of the twenty-six subjects offered at least eight out of ten correct guesses. Three subjects scored a perfect ten out of ten. No subject guessed incorrectly more than five times out of ten. One subject who scored ten out of ten was retested and proved able to offer correct guesses thirty out of thirty times (these retesting data are not included in our statistical analyses).

At four inches between hands, subjects made correct guesses an average of 6.54 times out of 10, with a standard deviation of 1.90 ($t = 6.54$; $df = 12$; $p = 0.0128$). At this distance, five of thirteen subjects

Table 1: Mean correct subject guesses, by experimental condition

Experimental Condition [a]	Mean Correct Guesses Out of 10	Standard Deviation	t(df)	Significance [b]
3 inches [c]	7.62	1.76	5.36(12)	$p = .0002$
3 inches [d]	7.69	1.32	7.38(12)	$p < .0001$
4 inches [c]	6.54	1.90	2.92(12)	$p = .0128$
6 inches [c]	5.77	1.42	1.95(12)	$p = .0751$
3 inches, with glass barrier [e]	5.20	1.21	0.64(14)	$p = .5314$
6 inches, with negative cuing [f]	3.90	1.66	−2.09(9)	$p = .0660$

[a] Inches refers to distance between hands of subjects and investigator
[b] Based on two-tailed t-test against the null hypothesis of chance accuracy
[c] Investigator 1; 13 subjects
[d] Investigator 2; 13 subjects
[e] Investigators 1 and 2; 15 subjects
[f] Investigator 1; 10 subjects

achieved scores of at least eight out of ten, and one subject scored ten out of ten.

At six inches between hands, subjects did not perform better than chance would predict, although the results could be interpreted as marginally significant. At this distance, subjects made correct guesses an average of 5.77 times out of 10, with a standard deviation of 1.42 (t = 5.77; df = 12; p = 0.0751). One subject who scored eight out of ten correct guesses at this distance was retested and achieved a total score of twenty-seven out of thirty correct guesses (this was the same subject who scored thirty out of thirty at three inches between hands).

When a glass barrier was interposed between the hands of subjects and investigator, subjects performed neither better nor worse than chance would predict, making correct guesses an average of 5.20 times out of 10, with a standard deviation of 1.21 (t = 0.64; df = 14; p = .5314). Fifteen subjects were tested at three inches between hands both with and without the glass barrier. A repeated-measures analysis of variance reveals that these subjects were significantly more likely to offer correct guesses when the glass barrier was not in place (F = 26.62; df = 1,14; p < 0.0001).

When deliberate miscuing was introduced subjects performed neither better nor worse than chance would predict, although the results could be interpreted as marginally significant. Subjects made correct guesses only 3.90 times out of ten, with a standard deviation of 1.66 (t = -2.09; df = 9; p = 0.0660). Again, this condition involved a distance of six inches between hands. A repeated-measures analysis of variance indicates that there was a significant difference in subjects' abilities to offer correct guesses at six inches between the uncued and miscued conditions (F = 9.875; df = 1,9; p = 0.012). That is, subjects made significantly more successful guesses when deliberate miscuing was absent.

To assess whether or not subjects manifested significantly different results for either one of our two investigators, a between-subjects t-test was conducted on the results obtained at three inches between hands (the only distance at which both Investigators 1 and 2 tested subjects). No significant differences were found between results obtained by the two investigators (t = 0.126; df = 24; p < 0.0001).

To determine if the accuracy of subjects' guesses declined as a function of distance between the hands of subjects and investigators, a regression of accuracy on distance was computed, albeit only for Investigator 1 (who was the only investigator to assess subjects at three, four, and six inches) and only for her uncued subjects. The resulting equation was:

Accuracy = 9.16 – 0.58(Distance)

The adjusted R-square coefficient for this equation was 0.14. This coefficient was statistically significant (t = -2.68; df = 37; p = 0.01). Accuracy does indeed seem to decrease significantly as distance between the hands of subjects and investigators increases.

We next attempted to determine if this negative relationship between distance and accuracy could be modeled using the inverse-square relationship between distance and intensity manifested in many natural phenomena such as gravity, magnetic flux, and radiant heat transfer. Accordingly, an inverse-square of distance was regressed onto accuracy. The resulting equation was:

Accuracy = 5.15 + 22.15($1/\text{Distance}^2$)

The adjusted R-square coefficient for this equation was 0.15. This coefficient was statistically significant (t = 2.83; df = 37; p = 0.008). This equation would predict that perfect accuracy would be obtained at a distance of 2.14 inches between hands and that near-chance accuracy would result at large distances between hands.

In describing the sensations they felt during the trials, most subjects referred to sensations of heat. In fact, "body heat" was the phrase most commonly used by subjects—both during and after the trials—to refer to their perceptions. Many subjects reported that they made their guesses on the basis of a heat differential they perceived between their hands when the "ready" light signaled them. Two subjects reported "tingling" feelings in their palms, but most subjects identified the sensations as heat.

DISCUSSION

The simplest explanation for our findings is that subjects were using radiant body heat to discern the presence of the investigator's unseen hand. The experimental protocol was designed to eliminate all salient sources of sensory cuing other than body heat. Subjects' abilities to discern the investigator's hand where high when the distance between the hands of subject and investigator was small. Subjects' abilities diminished as the distance was increased. Regression analysis confirmed that subjects' abilities were indeed a function of distance between hands, as would be expected if real energy such as radiant body heat was involved. Subjects performed no better than chance would predict when a piece of glass was interposed between the hands of subject and investigator, a finding that also suggests that body heat was the most salient cue. Finally, in their self-reported accounts of their sensations subjects routinely used the term "body heat" and spoke of discerning heat differentials between their hands when an investigator's hand was in place over one of the subject's hands. Both the trial data and subjects' self-reports are consistent with the explanation that body heat provided a highly salient and effective cue.

Our subjects manifested substantial variation in individual ability to detect the investigator's unseen and untouched hand. Moreover, subjects' scores in the test trials were consistent with their self-reported ability to detect body heat. A number of subjects volunteered that they felt body heat at three inches but not at four inches. Others stated that they felt body heat at three and four inches but did not feel body heat at six inches. Some reported that they could distinctly feel body heat at six inches. No subjects reported that they could feel body heat at six inches but not at four inches. And in all cases, subjects guessed more accurately in trials in which they professed to feel body heat than in trials in which they offered no such professions.

Our findings regarding investigator cuing suggest that such cuing can influence and even potentially contaminate experimental results.

We tested the effects of only two sources of cuing: voice signaling and leaning on the table. Future research would be needed to evaluate the effects of other potential sources of investigator cuing or miscuing.

The results reported here would seem consistent with Ball and Alexander's (1998) report in which a single blindfolded subject made correct guesses regarding the presence or absence of human body in seven out of ten attempts. In attempts where a body was present, Ball and Alexander maintained a distance of four inches between the body and the subject's hands. The subjects in our experiment made successful guesses an average of 6.54 times out of 10 at a distance of four inches between the hands of subject and investigator.

The results reported here are inconsistent with results reported by Rosa et al. (1998), who report that the TT practitioners they tested could not perform at better-than-chance rates when asked to discern the presence of an investigator's hand placed eight to ten centimeters (approximately three to four inches) above one of the subject's hands. Additional research would seem to be required to address these discrepancies and to provide conclusive evidence regarding the abilities of humans to detect nearby but unseen and untouched human bodies.

CONCLUSION

The results of our experiment provide evidence against the claim that humans can perceive (or manipulate) a metaphysical HEF which emanates from the human body. When salient sources of conventional sensory cuing were eliminated, our experimental subjects could not discern the presence of an unseen human hand.

Our experiment has demonstrated that individuals who are untrained in TT can readily discern the presence of an unseen human hand at the distances at which TT is typically practiced (i.e., three to four inches) when body heat is not shielded. Although TT practitioners may detect an "energy field" of sorts, the most parsimonious explanation is that the "heat-like" sensations perceived by TT practitioners are due to radiant body heat. In addition, our pilot testing suggested conventional explanations for the "tingling," "pulsating," and "electrical " sensations sometimes reported in the TT literature. We found that such sensations may be caused by the hand position used in TT (palms and fingers flattened and stretched), and by the continual back-and-forth movements of the hands. Certainly, our findings suggest that one can readily explain the sensations reported by TT practitioners without recourse to metaphysical theories that invoke unconventional energy fields.

TT proponents may dispute our conclusions because our experimental subjects were not trained TT practitioners. TT proponents may also object that we have not conclusively ruled out the possibility that our subjects were sensing the HEF rather than body heat. Indeed, we do not claim to have definitively falsified the claim that TT practitioners can sense an HEF. However, within the theoretical system of TT, the universal vital energy force of which the HEF is a manifestation is said to transcend matter and to be everywhere. Although glass effectively shields the transmission of radiant body heat, a universal vital energy such as is postulated in TT would presumably penetrate glass just as it penetrates other matter. If the HEF exists and functions as TT proponents claim, then trained TT practitioners should be able to sense the HEF when conventional sensory cues such as body heat have been eliminated. The burden of proof now rests with the practitioners of TT, who must demonstrate an ability to detect the HEF that is distinct from an ability to detect radiant body heat.

Our findings suggest that skeptics should no longer discount the sensory experiences reported in TT testimonials as being entirely the products of wishful thinking or autosuggestion. Rather, the implications of these perceived sensations should be accounted for in future TT research. During TT sessions, participants who have embraced TT may fully expect to sense the HEF and its manipulation. The conventional sensory cues that our research suggests are readily available might then provide TT participants with sensations they interpret as "proof" of the efficacy of TT. This process could likely facilitate a placebo effect among TT patients.

Our findings regarding variation in subjects' abilities to sense cues such as body heat also have implications for future research on TT. Perhaps this individual variation accounts for the fact that proponents of TT differ in the hand distances they recommend or utilize for the practice of TT, a fact that has seldom been noted (let alone addressed) in previous research. Researchers should test TT practitioners under conditions (e.g., hand distance) that the TT practitioner feels are optimum. Differences in subjects' abilities to detect sensory cues, and the relationship of this ability to distance, should also be accounted for in designing clinical studies that involve comparisons of treatment and control groups.

Finally, the findings reported here regarding investigator cuing and miscuing clearly indicate that TT researchers must be vigilant in identifying and controlling for potential sources of sensory cuing which could confound test results. This caution would apply not only in tests of subjects' abilities to detect an unseen human body, but also in clinical studies that utilize "sham" TT as a placebo. Confounding sensory cues may be subtle, and they may or may not be consciously generated or interpreted by participants in experimental protocols. Because of the inherent difficulties in double-blinding TT experiments, it is critical to effectively blind the subjects from cuing by the investigators. Future research on TT must control and account for the many, varied, and often subtle sources of cuing.

We applaud the move toward testing the specific claims of alternative medical practitioners. But as with all new research trajectories, researchers (including the authors of this paper) may have only begun to uncover some of the unanticipated difficulties inherent in research designs and protocols such as ours. Still, this difficult work must continue if we hope to obtain solid evidence regarding the efficacy and validity of alternative medical therapies.

REFERENCES

Ball, T. S., and D. K. Alexander. 1998. "Catching up with Eighteenth Century Science in the Evaluation of Therapeutic Touch." *Skeptical Inquirer* 22 (4): 31–34.

Claman, H. N., R. Freeman, D. Quissel et al. 1994. *Report of the Chancellor's Committee on Therapeutic Touch*. Denver: University of Colorado Health Sciences Center.

Krieger, D. 1992. *The Therapeutic Touch: How to Use Your Hands to Help or Heal*. New York: Prentice Hall.

———. 1993. *Accepting Your Power to Heal: The Personal Practice of Therapeutic Touch*. Santa Fe, N.Mex.: Bear.

Meehan, T. C. 1998. "Therapeutic Touch as a Nursing Intervention." *Journal of Advanced Nursing* 28: 117–25.

Peters, R. M. 1999. "The Effectiveness of Therapeutic Touch: A Meta-Analytic Review." *Nursing Science Quarterly* 2: 52–61.

Rosa, L., E. Rosa, L. Sarner et al. 1998. "A Close Look at Therapeutic Touch." *JAMA* 279: 1005–10.

Rosenthal, R. 1976. *Experimenter Effects in Behavioral Research*. New York: Irvington.

16

Therapeutic Touch: Investigation of a Practitioner

Robert Glickman and Ed J. Gracely

INTRODUCTION

For a century or more, nursing, along with its sister health professions, has combined personal caring and technology. Nursing demands a high level of expertise whether it is routine bedside medical-surgical nursing or more advanced work in dialysis, oncology, cardiology, and critical care. In recent years, however, nurses have been increasingly involved with unproven therapeutic systems that do not meet the usual standards of scientific medicine. Nursing publications print papers on foot reflexology (Lynn, 1996), Reiki (Van Sell, 1996), homeopathy (Skinner, 1996), and "Therapeutic Touch" (Mackey, 1995).

Proponents of TT claim that an "energy field" surrounds the human body. Depending on the practitioner, the "energy field" is said to extend two to eight inches from the surface of the skin, and some claim to be able to feel it from farther distances. Although no one has demonstrated or measured this field, TT practitioners claim to be able to assess the field and "heal" people by "balancing" it. They state that TT has five phases. They are: (1) centering (the therapist focusing one's own consciousness); (2) assessment/scanning (using the hands to assess the patient's dynamic energy field); (3) unruffling/clearing (vigorously "stirring" the area immediately surrounding the person in order to "improve" the field); (4) treatment/balancing; (5) evaluation.

PhACT, the Philadelphia Association for Critical Thinking, and its committee, Philadelphia Area Nurses and Skeptics Alliance (PANSA), a

Originally published in *Scientific Review of Alternative Medicine* 2, no. 1 (spring/ summer 1998). Copyright © 1998 Prometheus Books. Reprinted with permission from authors and publisher.

group of nurses, other healthcare workers, and skeptics, concluded that if nurses are to be involved with TT, the first question asked should be: Can a nurse detect a human energy field? At the time of a recent review by Scheiber, TT research was minimal, and most writings were commentary and speculation (Scheiber, 1997). Research was either flawed in design, such as having inadequate sample sizes or blinding, or was not supportive. There was no convincing evidence that claims of healing by TT was anything other than a placebo effect.

More important, TT research has focused on alleged healing by TT when no one has yet established that a practitioner could actually detect an HEF. We therefore investigated the claim that practitioners can detect an HEF.

On January 25,1995, an "in-service" (an educational demonstration) held at Frankford Hospital in Philadelphia featured TT specialist Linda Degnan, R.N., BSN, of the Mind/Body Connection in King of Prussia, Pennsylvania. In two hours of lecture and demonstration, Degnan made several unusual and testable claims, including her ability to feel the difference between a migraine headache and a tension headache simply by feeling the person's HEF.

On the basis of Degnan's claims, we proposed several tests to determine the presence of these special skills. Degnan refused testing that could prove whether or not she could feel an energy field. This refusal became the basis for an editorial in *RN* magazine and the first time in sixteen years that an article critical of TT appeared in a major large-circulation nursing journal (Glickman and Burns, 1996).

Since further attempts to find practitioners willing to be tested were fruitless, PhACT contacted James Randi, a professional magician who has investigated paranormal and pseudoscientific claims including homeopathy, faith-healing, and psychics. Randi had previously offered a reward to anyone able to demonstrate a paranormal event under mutually agreed upon test conditions. Randi had extended this reward of $742,000 to any TT practitioner who could prove detection of an HEF under test conditions. As a result of Randi's efforts, we were able to recruit one TT practitioner who was willing to be tested. (Randi subsequently acted as a moderator for the test.)

METHODS

A simple two-sleeved mold was constructed of cardboard and fiberglass (the same type of fiberglass used for orthopedic casts that TT practitioners claim to be able to feel through). The mold was placed on a table with the participant to be seated at the table, hidden by a cloth sheet through which protruded the mold. After a coin-flip, the right or left sleeve would be occupied by the participant's corresponding arm. Without the use of visual cues, the practitioner would approach the table and assess the HEF flowing from the construct.

A test was scheduled on November 8,1996, in the Short Procedure Unit of the Frankford Campus of the Frankford Hospital in Philadelphia. Over sixty individuals and organizations that use and promote TT were sent announcements of the reward, both written and by e-mail. Recipients included the National League of Nurses (NLN), American Nurses Association (ANA), the Office for Alternative Healthcare at Columbia-Presbyterian Medical Center, New York, and the New York Theosophical Society, which included Dr. Dolores Krieger as a member. The reward was also listed on the Martha Rogers e-mail service. After several inquiries and discussions, N. W., a massage therapist and TT practitioner from California, volunteered to fly to Philadelphia at her own expense to be tested. The protocol and purpose were explained to N. W. in advance. After her arrival in Philadelphia and further discussion, all agreed that the focus would be limited to energy-field detection.

The protocol was modified to accommodate some of N. W.'s methods. N. W. claims that a normal limb does not have a palpable field, but an injured or painful limb creates a hot, cold, or "pulling" sensation. First, an "open test" was conducted with the identity of the participant known. N. W. stated that she could tell the difference between the fields of a woman with a painful wrist and that of a man with no symptoms. A coin-flip determined which participant subject would place an arm in the apparatus. In this open test, N. W. was able to correctly distinguish between the two participants ten out of ten times (see table 1).

We proceeded to a preliminary closed test. In the closed test, we implemented the same procedure, except for the curtain that barred N. W. from visually identifying the participant.

RESULTS

In the closed test, N. W. was able to identify the "correct field" only eleven times out of twenty attempts (see table 2). This result was consistent with chance. N. W. did not qualify for the final definitive test.

TABLE 1: OPEN TEST

Trial	Participant	Subject's Comments
1	PM	Feels coolness on (participant's) left (L); nothing on right (R)
2	BS	Doesn't feel a whole lot ("Not a whole lot"); less than PM
3	PM	"She's changed . . . warm on L . . . less on R . . . totally different"
4	BS	She is drawn to his L elbow and not much else
5	BS	Seems to take longer . . . feels L elbow and nothing else
6	BS	Similar to before—L elbow
7	PM	Feels cold on top L . . . thinks PM is more tense
8	BS	L elbow . . . nothing else . . . gets more subtle with each one
9	BS	He's cold (referring to elbow) . . . nothing else
10	BS	Felt cool on left toward wrist area and nothing on right

BS and PM indicate the two participants in this study.

DISCUSSION

The single test reported here was negative. It does not rule out the possibility that energy fields exist, or that some other TT practitioners can detect them, or that some other mechanism explains perceived benefits of TT. However, the likelihood of HEF existence and the ability to detect HEFs remains extraordinarily low.

TT was seemingly created as a nursing procedure and is now supported by major nursing organizations such as the ANA and the NLN. "Energy-field" disturbance is now listed as a nursing diagnosis by the North American Nursing Diagnostic Association and appears in nursing textbooks. The movement boasts over 40,000 practicing nurses in North America alone. The use of TT ranges from quiet performance behind closed doors in hospitals to open performance in office settings with a $75 fee.

Nursing journals contain articles praising and encouraging TT. The nursing journal *Today's O.R. Nurse* featured an article favoring TT being incorporated into the routine of operating room nurses (Jonasen, 1994). The journal also published an accompanying test on TT sponsored by the University of Maryland School of Nursing for Continuing Education Units (CEUs) (CE quiz, 1994).

TABLE 2: CLOSED TEST

Trial	Actual	Response	Subject's Comments
1	PM	BS	Feels heat on L . . . cold on R . . . "He's different"
2	PM	PM+	Feels warm then "it got hot" on L
3	PM	BS	"My first thought is . . . nobody is here"
4	PM	PM+	Feels cold
5	PM	PM+	"It's a girl" . . . feels cold
6	BS	BS+	"Very subtle change here . . . I'm toying . . . having to struggle . . . difficult to guess . . . I'm going to say a guy"
7	PM	PM+	"It's a girl" . . . feeling cold at top L
8	PM	BS	"It's a guy . . . nothing . . . he is less whacked"
9	BS	PM	"It's her" . . . feels cold on lower L
10	PM	BS	"Not much of anything . . . more of a turkey shoot now because they've changed so much"
11	PM	PM+	Focuses on L . . . "It's a girl" but feels torn . . . feels something on upper L
12	BS	PM	"It's a girl" . . . she senses something on lower L but can't go up because of curtain
13	PM	PM+	Again female . . . doesn't feel drawn to L side
14	BS	BS+	Her hand wants to go up into the curtain (to elbow)
15	PM	PM+	Cold on lower L . . . not drawn to elbow . . . "this is interesting"
16	BS	PM	No desire to "go up" . . . cold on lower L
17	BS	BS+	Doesn't feel cold . . . drawn to elbow
18	PM	BS	Touches elbow . . . "Cold up here"
19	PM	BS	"I'm not drawn to the L elbow but I think it's the guy . . . don't feel much"
20	BS	BS+	"I think it's the guy . . . didn't notice a whole lot"

TT's creators are Dolores Krieger R.N., Ph.D., and Dora Kunz, a "fifth-generation sensitive" (a psychic-type "medium") who claims to have been clairvoyant since birth. Dora Kunz came to the United States from Java in the 1960s. She was president of the American Theosophical Society and held that position for many years. Kunz met Krieger sometime in the mid to late 1960s, and through Kunz's influence, Krieger became a Theosophist.

Theosophy is a theology created in 1875 by Madame Helena Blavatsky. Theosophists see themselves as transcending both religion and science. Blavatsky was heavily influenced by the spiritualist movement of the time. She claimed to be visited by spirits and astral beings who imparted special knowledge on how to form theosophy (Ellwood, 1996). Theosophy borrows heavily from Hindu and Tibetan philosophies and religions; from the Kabala, or Jewish mysticism; and from astrology (Randi, 1995). Theories of psychic powers and the concept of prana, the Hindu name for life energy or the "vital force," are important ideas in theosophy. Prana is said to be responsible for all bodily functions from the cellular to basic locomotion. Pranic "healing" occurs by the "healer" transmitting the prana to the patient. Yoga, a part of Hinduism, includes several exercises, meditations, religious practices, and beliefs that are designed to keep prana flowing well through the chakras and the five sheaths of existence (Barrett, Jarvis, Kroger et al., 1997).

Krieger and Kunz collaborated to test the healing powers of a Hungarian healer named Oskar Estabany. In 1973, Krieger presented a paper based on this work at an ANA conference. She explained in the paper that prana was the source of the healing in the technique that would later be called "Therapeutic Touch" (Krieger, 1973). In her latest book *Therapeutic Touch Inner Workbook*, Krieger (1997) continues to expound on the importance of prana to the TT concept. She devotes an entire chapter to "The Reality of Chakras" (pp. 49–71) where human physiology, TT, and Hindu and Theosophical religious concepts are melded into a single system. Another chapter introduces prana and its various subsystems and explains how TT uses these systems (pp. 73–94).

TT is pseudoscience. Pseudoscience is a system of false or unsubstantiated claims that uses the jargon of science to sound convincing. Using quantum mechanics to explain extrasensory perception is one example (Chopra, 1989; Stenger, 1997). Other types of pseudo- and pathological science use inadequate research designs, misinterpretation and selection of data, and inadequate quality control. Proponents often are unwilling to perform definitive studies, fail to recognize and respond positively to challenges, or do not recognize negligence and contrary evidence (Barrett, 1993; Krieg, 1997).

Krieger's first published scientific research was a study of the effect of healer Estabany's laying on of hands on hemoglobin levels (Krieger, 1972). The study had statistical and methodological weaknesses including the fact that it was nonrandomized and that the control group also experienced a rise in hemoglobin, an outcome that was not adequately addressed (Clark and Clark, 1984). Further studies by Krieger still did not address these shortcomings (Krieger, 1973). In spite of these problems, this study is still quoted as "proof" of TT effectiveness.

Most TT writings do not report on whether TT works but on which illnesses it can be used for. Negative results in TT research (Meehan, 1993) are rarely referred to. These are two more characteristics of pseudoscience. In 1994, a Chancellor's Committee was formed to determine the appropriateness of teaching TT at the University of Colorado School of Nursing. The Committee (Claman, 1994) [see appendix 3] found that, "To date, there is not a sufficient body of data, both in quality and quantity, to establish TT as a unique and efficacious healing modality" (p. 6). As quoted in 1995 in the *Washington Post*, TT promoter Janet Quinn, R.N., Ph.D., admitted, "There's no Western scientific evidence at this point for the existence of an energy field" (Glazer, 1995).

TT researcher Therese Meehan, R.N., Ph.D., stated, "What current research tells us, according to Popper's principles of refutation and verification, is that there is no convincing evidence that TT promotes relaxation and decreases anxiety beyond a placebo response, that the effects of TT on pain are unclear, and replication studies are needed before any conclusions can be drawn. Other claims about outcomes are, in fact, speculation" (Meehan, 1995).

Martha Rogers's Science of Unitary Human Beings is another philosophically based approach to nursing. It introduced to nursing such concepts as the unitary man, "Homo Spacialis" (the next evolutionary plateau for humankind, humans in outer space), transcendence, pandimensionality, and other speculative abstractions. "From the science of unitary human beings, Rogers has derived a theory of paranormal phenomena. This theory posits that in a pandimensional, unitary world, there is no linear time and no separation of human and environmental fields. It provides an explanation for phenomena such as clairvoyance and telepathy and for interventions such as TT that need not involve physical contact. According to this theory, action-at-a-distance phenomena are normal rather than paranormal" (Meehan, 1993).

TT's association with Rogers's ideas came after Krieger received criticism for her third hemoglobin study and the prana explanation for TT (Krieger, 1973). Krieger dropped the prana explanation and embraced the HEF concept then being developed by Rogers (Rosa, 1994). To recruit TT practitioners for testing, we contacted the Nurse Rogers e-mail service, which discusses nursing from a "Rogerian" perspective. This led to a series of written exchanges. We found that the Rogerians feel that not all TT is alike and that Rogerian TT can be different from the TT others are using. This only served to cloud the issue further and will discussed at a later point.

Martha H. Bramlett, R.N., Ph.D., stated, "The energy field he

[Glickman] is trying to measure is not the one we're saying we feel." Also part of this discourse was Francis C. Biley, R.N., Ph.D., of University of Wales College of Medicine, a contributing author of *The Theory and Practice of Therapeutic Touch* (Churchill Livingstone, 1995) and Coordinator of the International Region of the Society of Rogerian Scholars. She stated, "I think a Rogerian would say that they 'perceive' a field manifestation, rather than feel a field, i.e., we chose to call what ever [sic] is going on a perception of an energy field rather than say that it is an energy field or is energy."

So there is a blurred area where TT science and Rogerian science "overlap." Yet proponents have not clarified the differences in the TT HEF that can be "felt" and the Rogerian HEF that can be "perceived."

Claims of TT proponents represent a dramatic deviation from usual scientific and ethical standards. One scientific standard is that a single piece of evidence cannot prove or disprove a proposition, but serves instead to change the odds in one way or the other by a factor proportional to the quality of its evidence. For example, a "good" piece of evidence in support of a proposition might change the odds in its favor by twenty-fold (say, from 2-1 in favor up to 40-1 in favor). A weak piece of evidence might only increase the odds by a factor of 2.

For ordinary medical claims, many of which have a fifty-fifty or better likelihood of being true before the study is conducted, even modestly good evidence shifts the balance enough that one may regard the claim as probable. On the other hand, for a therapy whose validity would require inventing a new branch of physics, the claim may start with a 10,000-to-1 odds against it. Even strong evidence of the ordinary sort does not suffice to move such a proposition to the plausible range. Repeated and consistent evidence from well-designed research by different researchers can turn an implausible claim into a believable one. In the case of TT repeatedly positive studies would bolster the likelihood of TT validity, but more negative studies would further decrease the likelihood of the claims.

In order to bolster the validity of TT claims or to falsify them, more trials were planned. An invitation to be tested during the week of December 8–11, 1996, was sent by certified letter to Dolores Krieger's home address. It invited Krieger and an associate to be tested in Fort Lauderdale, Florida, with expenses paid by the James Randi Educational Foundation (JREF). It was received on November 19,1996. She did not respond or acknowledge the request. E-mail to the New York Theosophical Society was not helpful.

A second large-scale test of any willing TT practitioner was scheduled for June 2, 3, and 4, 1997. An award of $1,100,000 was offered by the JREF for any practitioner demonstrating the ability to detect an HEF

The testing was to be supervised and videotaped by "Scientific American Frontiers" (SAF) for a program to be broadcast on PBS TV in November 1997. SAF, an objective third party unaffiliated with either skeptics groups or proponents of TT, was to be the official judge for this test. Also to have been present for the test were *Time* magazine and *Der Spiegel* magazine (Germany). Invitations were again sent out to as many groups and individuals as possible. It was mentioned on Dr. Dean Edell's nationally syndicated radio show. Three nonnurse practitioners inquired, but no one volunteered to be tested.

The SAF program of 1997, however did include a blinded test of thirty TT practitioners. The test was devised by Emily Rosa of Loveland, Colorado, and negative results were obtained. The results of this test was combined with a previous test and published (Rosa et al., 1998).

In testing a phenomenon, one adapts the test to fit the nature of the phenomenon. For example, we modified our procedure for N. W. when she said that some of the fields were changing as she worked with them. If part of the objection to testing was some detail of the procedure, we invited TT practitioners to talk to us about that.

Perhaps, for example, it is the need to get twenty out of twenty correct which is the problem. Certainly there are many legitimate perceptual skills (such as the ability to identify a bird from its song or a disease from its symptoms) for which an occasional error may be made even by an acknowledged expert. But this is a solvable problem. If a TT practitioner were confident, say, of getting 90 percent right, a variation on the procedure could be developed to provide a fair test while not requiring 100 percent accuracy.

TT proponents have spent twenty years focusing on which ailments TT can be used for, without first determining if anyone could actually detect an HEF. Practitioners have made a poor showing in the few times they have allowed themselves to be tested, and the large majority has been silent.

CONCLUSION

At this time, there is no reason to assume that TT practitioners have the ability to feel or detect alleged HEFs. A possible outcome of assuming the existence of HEFs is that TT could become part of mainstream nursing, and performing TT could become a requirement in education and for licensure.

On the other hand, some practitioners accept money for performing TT. If one cannot prove the detection of the HEF, continuing to perform TT at best could be willful ignorance or incompetence. At worst, if performed by less scrupulous individuals with knowledge of TT's ineffectiveness, and with intent to mislead the subject, it could be considered a fraud. Either way, if present standards of care were to be applied to TT, it would logically be unacceptable and below the standard of practice. Allowing oneself to be deceived as a health professional is usually regarded as a potential danger to patients.

The authors would like to thank James Randi, Béla Scheiber, DeeAnne Wymer, and Linda Rosa for their participation and contributions to this project.

REFERENCES

Barrett, S. 1993. "Homeopathy: Is it Medicine?" In *The Health Robbers*. Edited by S. Barrett and W. Jarvis. Amherst, N.Y.: Prometheus Books, pp. 191–202.

Barrett, S., W. Jarvis, M. Kroger, and W. London. 1997. *Consumer Health: A Guide to Intelligent Decisions*. Madison, Wis.: Brown & Benchmark, p. 165.

CE quiz. 1994. *Today's O.R. Nurse* 1: 50–51.

Chopra, D. 1989. *Quantum Healing: Exploring the Frontiers of Mind/Body Medicine*. New York: Bantam.

Claman, H. N. 1994. *Report of the Chancellor's Committee on Therapeutic Touch*. Denver: University of Colorado Health Sciences Center (July 6).

Clark, P., and M. Clark. 1984. "Therapeutic Touch: Is there a Scientific Basis for the Practice?" *Nursing Research* 1: 37–41.

Ellwood, R. 1996. "Theosophy." In *The Encyclopedia of the Paranormal*. Edited by O. Stein. Amherst, N.Y.: Prometheus Books, pp. 1555–72.

Glazer, S. 1995. "The Mystery of 'Therapeutic Touch.' " *Washington Post Health*, 11(51): 16–17.

Glickman, R., and J. Burns. 1996. "If Therapeutic Touch Works—Prove It!" *RN* 12: 76.

Jonasen, A. M. 1994. "Therapeutic Touch: A Holistic Approach to Perioperative Nursing." *Today's O.R. Nurse* 1: 7–12.

Krieg, E. 1997. "Examining the Amazing Free-Energy Claims of Dennis Lee." *Skeptical Inquirer* 4: 34–36.

Krieger, D. 1972. "The Response on In-Vivo Human Hemoglobin to an Active Healing Therapy by Direct Laying on of Hands." *Human Dimensions* 1: 12–15.

———. 1973. "The Relationship of Touch, with the Intent to Help or to Heal, to Subjects' In-Vivo Hemoglobin Values: A Study in Personalized Interactions." ANA, pp. 39–59. Paper presented March 21, San Antonio, Tex.

———. 1997. *Therapeutic Touch Inner Workbook*. Santa Fe, N.Mex.: Bear & Company Inc.

Lynn, J. 1996. "Using Complimentary Therapies: Reflexology." *Professional Nurse* 11 (5): 321–22.

Mackey, R. 1995. "Discover the Healing Power of Therapeutic Touch." *American Journal of Nursing* 4: 27–33.

Meehan, M. 1993. "Therapeutic Touch and Post-Operative Pain: A Rogerian Research Study." *Nursing Science Quarterly* 6 (2): 69–78.

———. 1995. "Letter." *American Journal of Nursing* 75 (7): 17.

Randi, J. 1995. *An Encyclopedia of Claims, Frauds, and Hoaxes of the Occult and Supernatural.* New York: St. Martin's Press, pp. 232–33.

Rosa, L. 1994. "Therapeutic Touch: Skeptics in Hand to Hand Combat over the Latest New Age Health Fad." *Skeptic* 3(1): 40–49.

Rosa, L., E. Rosa, L. Sarner, and S. Barrett. 1998. "A Close Look at Therapeutic Touch." *JAMA* 279: 1005–10.

Scheiber, B. 1997. "Therapeutic Touch: Evaluating the 'Growing Body of Evidence' Claim." *Scientific Review of Alternative Medicine* 1: 13–15.

Skinner, S. 1996. "How Homeopathy Works." *RN* 12: 53–56.

Stenger, V. 1997. "Quantum Quackery." *Skeptical Inquirer* 1: 37–40.

Van Sell, S. 1996. "Reiki: An Ancient Touch Therapy." *RN* 2: 57–59.

17

Replication of TT Research: A Case Study

Dale Beyerstein

Replication in science is rightly considered to be a necessary condition for acceptance of experimental results. That a result in an individual experiment is statistically significant, even highly so, is not very interesting if the research design is poor. Even if the design is excellent, there are often subtle differences between the design of an experiment and its actual implementation. People often believe that they are following the protocol when in fact they are not. They may *think* that they have controlled for other variables which may have influenced their results, or even been the sole cause of them, but in fact they have not. Carelessness, inattention, miscalculation, or any number of human frailties to which humans are occasionally prone can cause even the greatest of theoreticians or experimental designers to err.

Or there is just plain bad luck. To say that the results of an experiment are statistically significant at the 0.0001 level is just to say that there is one chance in 10,000 that these results are due to "chance," which, if we are determinists, is just a nice way of describing those frailties described in the previous paragraph that we have not been able to identify. If we are believers in some type of indeterminism, then the practical point is still the same: that is, there is no way of getting around the fact that the results in question could be that one that statistics predicted out of 10,000 would in fact be from chance alone.

This chapter discusses a series of five experiments offered in support of the hypothesis that Therapeutic Touch aids wound healing which were carried out by Daniel Wirth, M.S., J.D., of Healing Sciences Research International of Orinda, California, and members of his group. Four replications of this research were attempted subsequently by this group. Because of my difficulty in communicating with Wirth [see chapter 9 in this volume], these remarks are confined to the publications of this group that describe these experiments. Before discussing these publications, some remarks about replication and the different roles it plays in science *versus* pseudoscience are in order.

There are two types of replication: hard and soft. The former involves replicating as many of the features of the original experiment as is possible by using the same controls to exclude confounding variables; that is, variables that would provide evidence for some other causal factor than the one being tested for. The same types of subject and the same condition (i.e., the healing of a similar wound in the same part of the body) must also be present. In a soft replication, the hypothesis is tested under different circumstances to see whether it can be extended to cover a new sort of case; that is, to see whether a treatment that was found to work for one condition will also work for another. A different protocol or method of measurement may be introduced to provide independent evidence for the effect.

These two cases are best thought of as extreme ends of a common scale rather than two mutually exclusive and jointly exhaustive categories. Not many studies are purely hard replications or purely soft. At the hard end of the scale there may be slight modifications in the protocol of the second study because the second group has a slightly different hypothesis in mind. There may be practical reasons making it impossible for the second study to have exactly the same conditions as the first. For instance, it may not be possible for the second group to have access to the same type of subject as the first or the second group may not have the financial resources, expertise or equipment to duplicate the protocol of the first. Or the first group may have made some error which the second group will routinely correct. In some hard replications, the subject pool may be much larger because the first may have produced an effect which is statistically significant but the number of subjects may have been too small to reliably indicate the magnitude of the effect. Thus, the second experiment may use more subjects in order to get a more reliable measure of the effect. Many experiments intended as soft replications will share many of the protocols with the first experiment.

The distinction between hard and soft replication is very important for the following reason: When a group announces a novel result, especially one that was not anticipated by most scientists in the field, it is important that another group do a hard replication. There is always the possibility of some innocent error which was not detected by the first group producing an artifact (something that was not noticed or expected to be present) which accounts for the result, rather than the hypothesized cause. A second hard replication is not likely to have the same artifact present.

Hard replication is especially important when examining evidence for TT where its proponents admit that neither the bioenergetic field with which the TT practitioner interacts nor the force she or he exerts on that field can be measured by any known instrument. It is also very important to have this hard replication carried out by an independent group. If the first group allowed an artifact into their protocol without noticing it, there is a fairly strong probability that they will make the same mistake again.

It is also important to keep the design of the original experiment as simple as possible. Where one is unsure of the mechanism of TT, it will be difficult to distinguish an artifact from an essential component of TT. Therefore, one must eliminate variables that are not, according to TT theory, thought to be essential to its practice. Obviously such variables would include other treatments offered along with TT, whether part of standard medical procedure or rival alternative therapies, such as *laying-on of hands, Reiki,* or *creative visualization.* But, as we shall see, Wirth's group did all three things in his replications of his original experiment.

It is interesting to contrast the role that replication plays in mainstream scientific research with pseudoscience. In the former, even results considered unlikely by the majority in the field are taken seriously enough to replicate if they come from reputable scientists. For example, in 1962, a chemist from Kostroma in the USSR, Nikolai Fedyakin, announced that he had discovered a new type of water with properties (such as viscosity) differing from pure H_2O. A leading Russian chemist, Boris Deryagin, took Fedyakin's work seriously and replicated it. He announced his replication in England in 1966 and by 1968 interest spread to the United States. Despite the a priori implausibility of a new kind of water (except for Kurt Vonnegut Jr. in *Cat's Cradle* [Vonnegut, 1963]), hundreds of experiments attempting to replicate Fedyakin's findings, published in such journals as *Nature* and *Science,* were conducted. Many did succeeded in replicating these findings but some did not. The controversy raged until 1972, when the number of failed replications indicated that an alternative hypothesis was more plausible.

Fedyakin maintained that polywater formed only in the tiniest of capillary tubes which are extremely difficult to keep clean. In addition, when measuring the properties of minuscule samples of water, it was very difficult to separate minuscule amounts of glass leached from the tubes from the pure water. The consensus became that the anomalous properties of Fedyakin's water were the result of these impurities (Franks, 1982).

A more relevant example comes from psychology (Singer, 1981). By 1962 the consensus among neuroscientists specializing in memories was, as it still is, that memories of specific events or skills are encoded in the organization of the neurons of the brain. That year, James

McConnell announced the results of an experiment which favored the hypothesis that chemicals stored in the brain encoded memories. Planaria (flatworms) can be conditioned to scrunch up when a light is flashed on them. McConnell claimed that he trained one group of flatworms to perform this trick. He then took advantage of the fact that they are cannibalistic. He fed already-trained flatworms to an untrained group of flatworms and reported that the second group displayed the scrunching behavior despite never having been taught. This, of course, suggested that they had picked up the memories, chemically encoded, from the previous group.

Neuroscientists at Berkeley, Singer among them, bent over backward to give McConnell the benefit of the doubt. They invited a colleague of McConnell's to supervise their replication on the chance that there was some subtle detail that accounted for McConnell's success but which he failed to note in his paper. The Berkeley group could not replicate the findings. The likely explanation for McConnell's "success" in the first instance was mislabeling of the jars containing the worms. One group of flatworms is quite difficult to tell from another, and perhaps McConnell fed neophyte flatworms to experienced ones and, as one would expect, some of the previously schooled flatworms simply remembered their skill.

These examples illustrate four points about the role replication plays in bringing controversies in mainstream science to closure. First, scientists are willing to attempt to replicate experimental results even when they seem to lend support to hypotheses which are implausible given the state of current knowledge. Second, and more important, large numbers of scientists are willing to put aside other research commitments to design attempted replications independently. Third, and more important yet, these attempted replications zero in on the most essential claims of the hypotheses under consideration. For example, in polywater, the viscosity of the substance was the main issue, while in the chemical hypothesis of memory, the issue was whether or not the flatworms could really learn the scrunching behavior without having been conditioned to it. Time is not spent examining auxiliary hypotheses or designing complicated experimental protocols involving mechanisms which could interfere with the results predicted by the hypothesis at issue.

Another important feature of mainstream science is that, if a replication fails because of some mistake made in the original experiment, there are no data to explain the hypothesis that is inconsistent with mainstream theory. The controversy is at an end.

Pseudoscience or parascience, on the other hand, can be identified by its failure as a collective enterprise on all four of these criteria. How well does TT as a collective research program fare on these criteria? The answer is that although TT does not so much fare poorly, it fails to have a research community at all. The Rosa et al. (1998) experiment published in the *Journal of the American Medical Association* (*JAMA*) and the wound healing experiments of Daniel Wirth illustrate this point. We shall discuss the Rosa et al. paper first, and then those of Wirth because the TT response, or more properly, nonresponse, to Rosa et al. is part of the problem with the inconclusive results presented by Wirth.

The Rosa et al. paper is a parallel to the examples discussed above in that in all of these cases research data are presented that, if they stand the test of replication, threaten an entire discipline because they are inconsistent with the fundamental hypotheses on which that discipline rests. In the case of TT, the notion that there is a bioenergetic field which can be detected and manipulated by the TT practitioner is central to TT, as the idea that memories are structurally encoded in patterns of neurons is to modern theories of memory. The experimental results of Rosa et al. are inconsistent with this hypothesis. One would expect, therefore, that the TT community would devote at least some resources to finding methodological flaws in the experiment or to attempt to replicate the experiment. But no such effort on the part of the TT community has been undertaken. Contrast this avoidance of internal criticism and replication with the behavior of skeptics. When the Rosa et al. study was published, skeptics were not shy about discussing its weaknesses (Selby, 1998). In fact, Long et al. (1999) followed expected scientific behavior by attempting to recreate many aspects of the Rosa study. This is exactly how science is supposed to work. [See chapter 15 in this volume.]

The next case study of TT replication concerns five experiments conducted by Dr. Wirth. The first two in the series provided statistically significant results in favor of the claim that TT aids in healing of wounds but three further experiments did not. Two studies showed no statistically significant differences between the rate of wound healing in the experimental group receiving TT and the control groups receiving other modes of treatment or no treatment at all. The last four in the series are soft replications of the original study in that the measurements of wound healing differed from the original and other experimental conditions differed in important ways. None of these experiments have been replicated, to our knowledge, by independent groups.

The experiment described in Wirth (1990) [see chapter 9 in this volume] was double blind. Forty-four subjects appeared at the lab every day for sixteen days and placed their arms through a gasket-like device in a door. There was a practitioner on the other side administering TT for the twenty-three subjects in the experimental group and for the twenty-one subjects in the control group there was not. Since TT doesn't involve actually touching the subject this is a perfect way to blind the subjects. But Wirth went beyond this to guarantee that his subjects would be ignorant of what was happening. He told them that there was some sort of Kirlian measuring device on the other side of the curtain measuring bioelectric energy emanating from the hole in their arms (they were led to believe that this was why the wound was put there!).

Forty-four subjects is a very small sample on which to base a conclusion about the efficacy of TT for any type of healing, unless the difference between the two groups is very great. Where the difference is great, this would certainly suggest that TT has some effect and this result, in turn, would call for a hard replication of the experiment with a much larger sample. Such a replication, as we shall see, has never been reported, but Wirth (1990) certainly qualifies as an adequate sample size for a preliminary experiment to determine whether a larger-scale experiment is worth contemplating; it also serves to iron out unforeseen practical problems that may arise.

The subjects were examined on the eighth and sixteenth days by an M.D. who was not only unaware of which subjects had TT and which did not, he was also unaware of the purpose of the experiment. He was given the same story about measuring bioelectric fields and thought that the point of his measurements of wound sizes was to have them correlated with the measurements of the amount of energy escaping through them. One might object that playing with the doctor's gullibility is unnecessary, since all that is required is that he not know which subjects received TT and which were controls. It is not a criticism of the experiment to say that Wirth was overly cautious. He alone kept the code which revealed which subjects had the TT and which did not. There was a third investigator, referred to enigmatically as EI (for experimental investigator), who led the subjects to the door that they put their arm through. Again, this person was kept unaware of whether there was a TT practitioner behind the door. She came and went by a separate entrance. The TT practitioner, the fourth member of this group, was also unaware of which subject was attached to the arm she saw.

Wirth reports that by the eighth day not only were the wounds of those given TT significantly smaller—3.90mm^2 *vs.* 19.34mm^2 ($p < 0.001$) for the control group, the standard deviation of the wound sizes of the TT subjects was much less—2.95 mm^2 *vs.* 4.46mm^2 for the control group ($p < 0.05$). By the sixteenth day, not only were more than half of the experimental group fully healed versus none of the control group ($p < 0.001$), the average wound size decrease in the experimental group was

99.3 percent but 90.9 percent in the experimental group. These results are highly significant statistically but again the size of the sample permits the results of just a few subjects to affect the aggregate results significantly. Randomization of subjects into control or experimental group is obviously crucially important and evidence of the fairly small size of the standard deviations within each group suggests that the subjects were relatively homogeneous.

The main methodological flaw in this design is one that was an obvious concession to practicality. The subjects were run in two blocks, one of twelve treatment subjects and ten controls, and a second consisting of eleven in each group; the data were pooled. The first block went through the sixteen days of treatment, then the second were incised and treated. Nothing wrong with that. But here is the dicey part: the subjects were divided into a morning and an afternoon session and to reduce the time the TT practitioner had to be present, all the TT subjects were run together in one of these sessions. Presumably, then, on the eighth and sixteenth days when the wounds were measured, the TT subjects came to the doctor *en bloc*, followed or preceded by the control subjects. Now, Wirth assures us that the doctor was kept blind about which were the TT subjects. Wirth's protocol was designed to minimize the contact between the experimenters, thus minimizing the chances of a slip that would unwittingly give away crucial information. Nevertheless, if Wirth had any contact with the doctor at all during the month of the experiment, it would be possible for the doctor to receive subtle, unintentional cues. For example, the morning subjects were expected to have similar wound sizes or that those in the afternoon might resemble each other more closely on average than they resemble the morning ones.

It is also important to know who was in charge of the code that kept the experimenters blind to which were experimental subjects and which were controls. Someone who was involved neither in the handling of subjects nor the measurement of their wounds nor with the TT practitioner would nevertheless have to keep the data on these three correlated so that they could be matched up at the completion of the experiment. For example, if someone wanted to skew the results in favor of TT, at the conclusion of the experiment they would rank the subjects in order of wound healing and call the first twenty-three therapeutically touched and the next twenty-one controls. Or, if they saw positive results for TT and wanted to skew them against TT, they would shuffle the results again and then there would appear to be no difference between the two groups. In order not to be accused of doing either of these things, our group that was considering replicating Wirth's experiment [see chapter 9 in this volume] resolved to put the original list of code numbers of those subjects who were receiving TT and those who were controls into a safety deposit box before the experiment started and have someone witness my removal of it when the two groups were to be compared. Our group wanted to ask Wirth what procedure he used to rule out this type of data fudging, but as I indicated elsewhere in this book, we did not receive his cooperation in discussing his experiment, so we have not replicated his experiment.

It is crucial to be clear on how Wirth matched his controls with his experimental subjects. He reports that he received 175 responses from university students, suggesting that he solicited them through the traditional ways—notices on bulletin boards, ads in the university newspaper, and so on, at his alma mater, John F. Kennedy University. From these he chose forty-four, all male. Of course he did not go into details in the paper about how these subjects were chosen (perhaps these were the only ones to volunteer once the degree of commitment became clear to them). He does not describe any subject matching that may have been done to insure that controls and experimental subjects were correlated with some relevant characteristics in common.

Another consideration is Wirth's choice of a method to measure wound sizes. The doctor who examined the patient's wound—identified only as "Dr. M"—traced the wound parameters on a clear acetate sheet with a pen by holding the sheet over the wound and drawing on it. These wound tracings were then sent to an independent laboratory, not named in the article, to be scanned by a computer which produced a measurement of the surface area of each wound. These data were then sent to an independent statistician, again not named.

The crucial stage of this three-step procedure is, of course, the original tracings of the wounds. How thick was the pen? Did the doctor consistently trace on the outside of the wounds, on the insides, or on the border? Was the acetate sheet always kept flat or was it pressed onto the wound, thus changing the shape of the sheet while the tracing was done?

These details matter when we remember that the average difference in surface area of the experimental group wounds versus the control ones on the sixteenth day was only $1.56mm^2$ ($2.95 mm^2$ for the experimental group versus $4.46mm^2$ for the control group). This is a highly statistically significant difference but only meaningful if we can be assured that the doctor's tracings of these very tiny areas were extremely accurate. To be fair, the average difference in surface area between control and experimental groups was much greater on the eighty day—$15.44mm^2$—but here we are talking about a difference the size of an average match head.

Unfortunately, although Wirth is very precise about stages two and three, he tells us no more than I have described about how the tracings were done. The only detail he provides about the tracings applies to those done after the original wound was made. He says, "Tracing was performed by Dr. M. after the incision was made by using a transparent acetate plastic sheet. The acetate sheet was laid over the wound and the edge traced with a pen" (Wirth, 1990, p. 4). Compare this to the detail he provides about the analysis of the tracings:

> After all the sessions had been run, Dr. M sent the wound tracings to an independent laboratory technician who was skilled in calculating surface areas of tracings using a Planix 5000 Digitizing Line-Area Meter. The surface area of each tracing was measured three, and the resultant mean figures were forwarded to a independent statistician who was asked to analyze the data. (p. 10)

It is much more important to know how accurate the wound tracings were than the exact compute hardware that did the digitizing of the tracings.

The more common alternative method to determine wound sizes is to take a photo of the wound with a ruler as a scale. It is interesting to note that this was the method used in Wirth's replication (Wirth et al., 1993). The advantage of this method is that the photos are available for reexamination if there are any questions about the measurements. The patients' wounds, of course, disappear, but the photos of them remain. Provided that the photos are taken in a standard way, the areas of the wounds can be remeasured by independent investigators.

The advantage of the digitized results is that they are subject to quantitative measurement—that is, we get a precise measurement of how much more or less one wound has healed than another. Even better, after pooling the measurements of the two groups, we can have a quantitative measure of how much better or worse the experimental group healed *versus* the control group. The tracing method also could be done from the photos just as well as from the original wounds and these results digitized by Wirth's method. Note that if the wounds are traced but not photographed, it is impossible for independent investigators to retrace wounds which have long since healed. Thus, the ideal procedure would have been to combine the two methods and provide both the photographs of the wound next to a ruler and the digitized results. Neither of Wirth's papers (1990, 1993) used this combined strategy.

Wirth et al. (1993) reports a replication of Wirth (1990). The replication used twenty-four healthy subjects, ranging in age from thirty-five to sixty-three, with a mean age of forty-seven, as opposed to forty-four subjects in the original study. Perhaps there were practical difficulties in obtaining subjects, but given this even smaller sample, we could not determine the effect size of TT in this experiment. Subjects came from a group which met twice a week to practice progressive relaxation and meditation, so were dedicated to "new age" healing techniques. Wirth et al. (1993) states that the subjects were blind to the purpose of the study. They were initially told that they would be measured with "a noncontact diagnostic device which measured biopotentials associated with the body," and were informed of the true nature of the experiment only upon its completion. The TT practitioner is again not identified but is described as "an R.N. trained in the use of TT with over five years experience." No mention is made as to whether the TT practitioner was the same as the one involved in Wirth (1990).

The subjects were given a wound in the shoulder with a skin biopsy instrument as in the first experiment, again by a doctor who was blind to the protocol. The wound was dressed at that time by the doctor. This experiment lasted ten days, as opposed to sixteen in Wirth (1990). Patients in the experimental group were subjected to a five minute session of TT each day while the control group received no treatment. This time the patients sat with their wounds exposed against a door with a two-by-three-foot one-way mirror. The TT practitioner could see the patient but not vice versa. The experimenter running the program was also unaware whether the TT practitioner was behind the door. This differs from the earlier procedure in that in this case there was a barrier (the mirror) between patient and practitioner.

Patients' wounds were assessed on days five and ten (as opposed to eight and sixteen in Wirth [1990]) by the doctor who originally made and dressed the wound, as well as by three other physicians, all blind to the purposes of the experiment. Instead of measuring the actual size of the wounds and then aggregating the results, an entirely different procedure was used. Six criteria for assessment were followed: (1) presence or absence of infection, (2) estimate of reepithelialization (regeneration of the layer above the membrane that separates the skin from connective tissue), (3) percentage of wound closure, (4) normal scar formation versus irregular, (5) pigmentation of scar, and (6) cosmetic appearance.

This would seem to be an inferior method of measurement for determining wound healing to the one reported in Wirth (1990), because these measurements are based on the clinician's subjective judgment rather than a quantitative measure. For the third measure, that of wound closure, the clinician who measured the amount of closure (the same one who administered the biopsy in the first place but was blinded to which groups the subjects belonged) simply scored it on a five-step scale, consisting of "0–25 percent," "26–50 percent," "51–75 percent," "76–99 percent" and "100 percent." There were three other physicians, again blind as to whether the patients they examined belonged to the experimental or control group, who independently rated the wound closure. Their ratings appear to be fairly close to those of the first physician. However, table 1 in Wirth et al. (1993) makes it difficult to determine this, since the figures for the first physician are conflated into three groupings, "0–50 percent," "51–99 percent" and "100 percent." The figures for the other three physicians are further conflated into two groupings, "100 percent" and "unhealed." Thus the *p*-values published in this paper are impossible to verify and the precise inter-rater reliability of the four physicians is impossible to determine. Nevertheless, Wirth et al. (1993) reports the results as being statistically significant.

This seems like an impressive number of variables to consider but they are not independent of each other and two variables were not, in fact, measured independently in this study. These were two of the most significant criteria, (2) reepithelialization and (3) percentage of wound closure. As Wirth et al. (1993) put it:

> The categories of wound reepithelialization and wound closure were combined into one category due to the fact that clinical estimates of both reepithelialization and wound closure were identical on both day five and day ten. . . .

and

> Determining whether or not a wound is healed as evidenced by complete reepithelialization is demonstrated by full wound closure. (pp. 129, 131).

Pigmentation of scar (variable 5) is not clearly defined in Wirth et al. (1993). The four categories with which the clinicians were to judge were "unhealed," "normal," "hyperpigmented" (which presumably means that the wound area appeared darker than the surrounding skin), and "hypopigmented" (lighter).

Cosmetic appearance (variable 6) seems to be an otiose variable to include in this study. Wirth et al. (1993) state:

> The overall cosmetic appearance of cutaneous wounds was included in this study in order to provide valuable biological information on the wound healing process.

But they do not state what this valuable biological information is that is independent of the more precise measurements given by three other variables—scar formation, wound closure, and reepithelialization (as estimated by wound closure). The categories given to the doctors to assess this variable were "unhealed," "poor," "fair," "good" and "excellent." The first has an operational meaning, if it is defined in terms of the three variables mentioned above, but the other four seem lacking in operational meaning.

There was no statistically significant difference in the two groups with respect to infection. One case in the control group was reported to have a minor wound infection on day ten, while no infections were reported in the TT group. Wirth et al. (1993) do not state what counted as a "minor" infection. In any case, the patients were not in a common environment for the duration of the study, and therefore the likelihood of different environmental sources of infection could not be controlled. Of course, this infection would influence the rate of wound healing for that patient and thus this uncontrolled factor could very well be the reason why there was one less healed wound—out of only twelve—in the control group. But Wirth et al. (1993) report this statistically insignificant difference in a way that minimizes its importance: "Upon analysis of the results, the category of wound infection was eliminated from the study due to insufficient data."

The data do not appear to be insufficient at all; they appear to show *no statistically significant difference*. To eliminate the infected wounds from the study is to ignore an alternative explanation for the differences found in the category on which they place the weight of their findings—reepithelialization. We have no information about whether just this one patient, or perhaps more than one of them, was in an environment which subjected him, her, or them to more sources of infection than the experimental group and whether fighting off infection slowed their rate of wound healing. This is, of course, the bane of all studies with small samples (the largest subject pool in any of Wirth's studies was forty-four).

The single category of interest in this study is the combined one of percentage of wound healing combined with the clinical estimate of reepithelialization (the former estimated from the latter). Wirth reports the difference between the control and experimental groups as significant but we would have to have access to his raw data to see how he computed this. As a replication of Wirth (1990) this study has so many differences in methodology and measurement that it cannot count as strong confirmation of the original results. It fares better as independent evidence for the claim that TT is of some use in wound healing, and as an extension of their research program which provides some evidence as to whether clinicians can detect a difference in wound healing in the course of normal patient examination outside of a laboratory setting. No independent group has announced a replication of either Wirth (1990) or Wirth et al. (1993) to date.

Wirth's group, however, has conducted three further experiments, measuring the same independent variable, the reepithelialization of a wound induced with the same 4 mm punch biopsy device. The third and fourth experiments in the series have more complex protocols. The third study, Wirth et al. (1994), consisted of only twenty-five subjects, all of whom received biofeedback, visualization and relaxation exercises during the course of the wound healing. The purpose of this study was to determine whether TT's healing effects vary with distance between healer and subject and whether or not the subject has direct visual contact with the healer.

The subjects received TT under each of four different conditions but in different orders: (1) through a one-way mirror, as in Wirth et al. (1993); (2) through a one-way mirror covered by a plastic sheet; (3) via a video monitor image with the healer and subject in adjacent rooms; and (4) via video monitor where the healer is in a room one floor below the subject. Given that the point of this experiment is to test TT under different conditions, the flaw in its design is that all subjects were given the biofeedback, visualization, and relaxation exercises. If one is a skeptical about these treatments, then their inclusion is simply one further complication in the design which could introduce artifacts. On the other hand, if one believes that they have some efficacy in wound healing, one would expect that they would minimize the differences in wound healing under the other four conditions, since all subjects would heal faster than if the wounds were untreated by anything. Thus, it is no surprise that there were no statistically significant differences between the four phases of treatment. Wirth, however, considers another explanation which he also applies to his group's next study.

The fourth study, Wirth and Barrett (1994) suffers from the same defects as the third, in addition to some other ones. First, the subject pool was only fifteen. Second, in this study the subjects were not blinded as to whether they were receiving treatment as was the case in the other four experiments. The subjects were treated under four different conditions. Under two, they were treated by a TT practitioner who formulated the intention to heal before treating the subjects; under two conditions they were treated by a practitioner who went through the same motions as the first, but who did not form this intention to heal. This served as the control. Subjects were also treated with LeShan healing, intercessionary prayer, and Reiki in various combinations under the four conditions, and under one condition, both healers received Reiki before doing their treatments. There was a statistically significant rate of healing for subjects when treated under "sham" TT as opposed to "real" TT; but they healed *better* while being treated with sham TT.

In a literature review discussing these five studies, Wirth (1995) suggests that placebo effects and experimenter effects may explain the negative results for TT in this study. But this presupposes that Wirth's group was sending signals to the subjects that suggested to those in the control group that they expected them to heal better, and to the experimental group that they expected them to heal worse. How plausible is this? But Wirth himself is a TT practitioner, a fact which he does not disclose in these studies. However, he does disclose this fact in another study, Wirth and Cram (1993). In discussing the protocols used in this study, he writes:

> For eight of the subjects, the NCTT [NonContact Therapeutic Touch] and mimic segments were performed from behind by an independent TT practitioner without contact and without the subject's knowledge. For the remaining four subjects, the NCTT and mimic segments were performed from behind by the first author (D. W.) without contact and without the subject's knowledge. Both individuals were experienced practitioners formally trained in the traditional TT method with over thirteen years of combined experience.

In addition, the fact that he and his group have invested so much time and energy in exploring TT (as well as the other complementary therapies examined in the third and fourth studies) would indicate that his group finds these methods promising. As well, Wirth's unpublished M.S. thesis (in the now defunct Consciousness Studies program at John F. Kennedy University outside of San Francisco) is very uncritical of complementary healing in general. So at least Wirth, if not the rest of his research group, appear committed to TT, a fact which discounts any conclusions. If anything, they would indicate that the experimenters expectations should influence the subjects in favor of TT. And finally, if these factors influenced the results against TT in the fourth study, there is no reason why they could have not have influenced the positive results for TT in the first and second studies.

A second explanation, which Wirth (1995) offers for the third experiment as well, is that:

> The use of multiple healers working simultaneously might have served to reduce or cancel the effectiveness of the treatment intervention. . . . Although the healers utilized in the two studies appeared to be compatible, there was a degree of ego investment involved as to which healing system was superior.

But Wirth offers no way of independently predicting when healers will be incompatible (if he had such a test, presumably he would not have used these healers); the only test is whether they fail.

Yet another set of explanations which Wirth (1995) cites for the failure of both experiments are ones that result from multiple healing interventions being given to subjects over the short duration of these experiments. These factors are: inhibitory, cancellation, carryover and learning effects. These would be equally likely if the effects were positive for TT which calls into question Wirth's group's experimental design as much as they help explain the negative results.

The fifth experiment, Wirth et al. (1996), was a hard replication of Wirth et al. (1993). There were thirty-two subjects in this study as opposed to twenty-four in the earlier one and for this reason was the better of the two studies. In fact, the results were statistically significant for the control group receiving no TT and were not for the group receiving TT. By way of explanation for this setback for the TT hypothesis, Wirth (1995) postulates:

> The reverse significance demonstrated by the control group could have been due to the ill health of the healer which might have inhibited the wound healing process for the treatment group.... This theoretical premise appears to be supported by the fact that the treatment group subjects reported experiencing the same physiological symptoms during the study as the NCTT healer and also concomitantly demonstrated no fully healed wounds. In contrast, the control group subjects exhibited four fully healed wounds with no accompanying ill effects.

The symptoms reported by the healer were so vague that she reported that she had lost the ability to concentrate on the healing; unfortunately they weren't serious enough to cancel the trial. It was not reported that either the practitioner or the complaining subjects received any medical attention for these symptoms. The complaints would appear to be of the sort that, had there been no need to explain the unfavorable results for TT, there would have been no need to take notice of them.

What conclusion should we draw from this set of five studies? Wirth's own conclusion about the three studies which failed to support TT is:

> The inhibitory, cancellation, carryover, learning, experimenter and placebo effect explanations introduced above are, at best, theoretical postulates for the reverse significant and nonsignificant effects demonstrated in [experiments three, four and five]. An equally valid

explanation, however, is that the healing interventions utilized might have been ineffective with the results simply indicating the range of possible outcomes inherent within the research design.

The first four conditions on the list hold only for the third and fourth experiments, not the fifth which provided negative results for TT. And the last two, experimenter and placebo effects, apply equally to the first and second experiments which gave positive results, as they do to the fifth, which produced negative ones.

In other words, his group has not provided much at all by way of evidence in favor of TT. It is interesting that this is not the way that Wirth's group's research is thought of among those who defend TT. Wirth's first paper (1990), which presents the strongest evidence for TT, continues to be cited by proponents of TT, while the others are very rarely cited. All six papers are published in obscure journals which are not carried by the majority of university libraries, and therefore they are not readily accessible even to those in the medical, nursing, and scientific community. Therefore the information they have on Wirth's group's research is subject to selective reporting from secondary sources.

The more serious problem is that the wider research community has let Wirth's group down in two ways: First, they have not independently replicated any of these studies. Of course, Wirth's group cannot be blamed for this failure on the part of others—except for the lack of cooperation with this author reported by me elsewhere in this book. The net effect is that his group has carried on with other soft replications of his original study as part of a research program to determine the extent to which TT might affect wound healing without any of his data being confirmed. Second, the problem still remains with the central claim of TT addressed by Rosa et al. (1998) and Glickman et al. (1998). That *someone* in the TT community ought to replicate Rosa's findings is clear but it is by no means clear that Wirth's group ought to do it.

In the research communities of chemistry and psychology of memory discussed above, there were many research groups who carried on with their research programs while others tackled the anomalous results. Their research programs would have been put to an end if those anomalous results had stood the test of replication, especially those that were reporting data that were not self-consistent; the anomalous results were, in fact, laid to rest. So, their decision to carry on while others turned their attention to the anomalous results proved to be a sound division of labor because progress on their own projects continued during this interval. Similarly, if someone manages to demonstrate that TT practitioners can detect the bioenergetic field they postulate, then Wirth's group, or others who enter his area, have some chance of explaining the inconsistent results produced by Wirth's group in terms consistent with TT. Until this is done, the best explanation of Wirth's group's inconsistent results from their set of studies would seem to be that whatever is responsible for the differing rates of wound healing they reported, it is not Therapeutic Touch.

REFERENCES

Franks, F. 1982. *Polywater*. Cambridge, Mass.: MIT Press.

Glickman, R., and E. J. Gracely. 1998. "Therapeutic Touch: Investigation of a Practitioner." *Scientific Review of Alternative Medicine* 2: 43–47.

Long, R., P. Bernhardt, and W. Evans. 1999. "Perception of Conventional Sensory Cues as an Alternative to the Postulated 'Human Energy Field' of Therapeutic Touch." *Scientific Review of Alternative Medicine* 3 (2).

Rosa, L., E. Rosa, L. Sarner, and S. Barrett. 1998. "A Close Look at Therapeutic Touch." *Journal of the American Medical Association* 279: 1005–10.

Selby, C. 1998. "The JAMA TT Article Critiqued." *Rocky Mountain Skeptic* 15 (6): 1, 10–12. Website at: http://bcn.boulder.co.us/community/rms. Also available from the Rocky Mountain Skeptic, PO Box 7277, Boulder, CO 80306.

Singer, B. 1981. "On Double Standards." In *Science and the Paranormal*. Edited by George Abell and Barry Singer. New York: Charles Scribner's Sons, pp. 142–48.

Vonnegut, K. 1963. *Cat's Cradle*. New York: Dell Publishing Co., Inc.

Wirth, D. P. 1990. "The Effect of Noncontact Therapeutic Touch on the Healing Rate of Full Thickness Dermal Wounds." *Subtle Energies* 1: 1–20.

———. 1995. "Complementary Healing Intervention and Dermal Wound Reepithelialation: An Overview." *International Journal of Psychosomatics* 42 (1–4): 48–53.

Wirth, D. P., and M. J. Barrett. 1996. "Complementary Healing Therapies." *International Journal of Psychsomatics* 41: 61–67.

Wirth, D. P., M. J. Barrett, and W. S. Eidelman. 1994. *Complementary Therapies in Medicine II*, pp. 187–92.

Wirth, D. P., and J. R. Crum. 1993. "Multi-Site Electromyographic Analysis of Noncontact Therapeutic Touch." *International Journal of Psychosomatics* 40: 47–55.

Wirth, D. P., J. T. Richardson, W. S. Eidelman, and A. C. O'Malley. 1993. "Full Thickness Dermal Wounds Treated With Noncontact Therapeutic Touch: A Replication and Extension." *Complementary Therapies in Medicine* 1: 127–32.

Wirth, D. P., J. T. Richardson, R. D. Martinez, W. S. Eidelman et al. 1996. "Noncontact Therapeutic Touch Intervention and Full Thickness Cutaneous Wounds: A Replication." *Complementary Therapies In Medicine* 4 (4): 14–20.

18

Recent Research
on Therapeutic Touch*

Mahlon W. Wagner

The concept and technique of Therapeutic Touch were introduced in the early 1970s by Dolores Krieger. At that time, many in the field of nursing were dissatisfied with the direction that their profession seemed to be taking. Many nurses sought greater influence and respect from both patients and physicians as well as from healthcare insurance agencies.

The techniques of TT could easily be taught to nurses and soon claims were being made that patient comfort, satisfaction, and recovery from various ailments were all markedly improved by the administration of TT. Simultaneously, critics were appalled by what they perceived to be New Age mystical nonsense. While the beneficial effects of actual touch to the development of infants—the enhancement of interpersonal relations and general physical and mental health—have long been recognized, this new TT is actually the application of "nontouch" where a practitioner holds her or his hand(s) several inches above the patient's skin.

Krieger and her followers do deserve credit for recognizing that modern scientific medicine demands research to support new and controversial healthcare techniques. Adherents of TT point to more than twenty years of accumulated research that, they say, provides adequate support for the efficacy of TT. Unfortunately, this research has been plagued with significant methodological flaws (Clark and Clark, 1984). The attention paid to research by TT proponents has also been coupled with such concepts as the vaguely defined "human energy field" and, in many instances, with an outright hostility or antipathy to the requirements of science.

---

*Kevin Courcey and Dónal O'Mathúna provided invaluable assistance in tracking down some documents and giving insight into many of the shortcomings of TT research.

SCIENCE, ANTISCIENCE, AND TT

As is often the case in alternative medicine, the stance of many TT proponents toward science is inconsistent if not self-contradictory. On the one hand, proponents often give the impression that they are strongly committed to research. But when design flaws are found, or the research is not supportive of their claims, they quickly proclaim that science is irrelevant or is not necessary or that the mysterious physics of quantum mechanics surely has answers that confirm the legitimacy of TT. A pronounced suspicion of the actions and motivations of scientific medicine is also evidence among many TT proponents. One frequently hears TT advocates claim that physicians are conspiring to denigrate the noble profession of nursing and that HMOs want to hire less-educated practical nurses to save money. Krieger herself complains of the "strongly reactionary forces [based upon] materialistic and reductionistic philosophies" and of "the frankly hostile lockstep reactions of the [skeptical] media" (Krieger, 1999).

A critical editorial published in *Research in Nursing and Health* (Oberst, 1995) unleashed a firestorm of letters that clearly demonstrates the antiscientific attitudes of many TT supporters. The writer of the editorial said there was neither empirical evidence for an HEF nor credible research supporting TT. She went on to suggest that TT actually wastes time and resources in patient treatment. Her main point was that too many doubters were unwilling to publicly say that "the emperor has no clothes," perhaps for fear that they (the skeptics) would be called "politically incorrect" for discouraging diversity within the nursing profession.

Also in *Research in Nursing and Health*, one letter-writer argued against the "blind acceptance of reductionist inquiry" (Wells-Federman, 1995). Another (Bright, 1995) managed to use at least three of the standard arguments of New Agers. She suggested that women have long suffered persecution because they threaten the "interests of conventional medical men." Further, she argued that the perception of "the force of subtle energy" (the HEF) has been "dulled, even forbidden through years of Western mechanism and scientific positivism," and that Krieger has rediscovered a sensitivity "long lost through the development of Western civilization." Yet another writer (Malinski, 1995) suggested that an equally valid alternative worldview exists where "personal knowledge, feelings and values are primary sources of information," and "this diversity needs to be celebrated in nursing."

Finally, one of the more prominent promoters and researchers of TT wrote a letter to *Nursing Research* (Heidt, 1995) brimming with sexist and

New Age views. This letter alleged that "because we are primarily a woman's profession we can never be content with using a reasoning mind alone in our scientific search," and "TT was not meant to be subjected to a scientific tool." According to this letter writer, Krieger courageously "*dared* to depart from Western models and look at . . . research from the *East*." She asserted that we cannot ignore the results of homeopathic and ayurvedic treatment and concluded that we must "use structures from the higher realms of the mind and beyond the mind."

It is clear that there is a pervasive antiscience, New Age viewpoint present among TT proponents. They bring up the false dichotomies of "Eastern" versus "Western" Science and of "Female Intuition" versus "Male Science" when the actual dichotomy is between pseudoscience and science. Introducing the "successes" of homeopathy or other non-science-based treatments as evidence that TT is effective is fallacious because there is no reliable evidence for the efficacy of such treatments. Homeopathy is itself based upon discredited vitalistic assumptions of "subtle energies" similar to the HEF (or *prana*) of TT.

While the majority of TT proponents may well be more sympathetic to an intuitive, nonrational approach to the subject, a few have engaged in research. Until recently, critics could easily dismiss such research because (a) double-blind procedures were not used, (b) the critical measure was actually irrelevant to the condition being studied, (c) too few subjects were tested, and (d) results could not be replicated. However, an increasing number of TT researchers are now attempting to validate the practice of TT through sophisticated clinical studies. What follows are descriptions and analyses of two of the most current and most credible of the TT research efforts to date.

RECENT TT STUDY: TURNER ET AL.

The TT study that has received the greatest publicity was a Pentagon-funded ($355,225) burn study at the University of Alabama at Birmingham (UAB) Burn Center (Turner et al., 1998; Scheiber, 1997; Selby, 1996).

In the UAB study, either "real" TT, or "sham" TT as a placebo, was administered to ninety-nine burn patients in an attempt to alleviate pain and anxiety. Sixty-two patients received five to twenty-minute sessions of TT on up to five separate days from one of three experienced TT practitioners. Research assistants (RAs) who had no previous knowledge of TT administered the sham treatments. The RAs were trained to make the same hand movements as TT practitioners, and practiced until outside observers could not tell whether TT or sham was being performed in a staged demonstration. During the twenty-minute sham treatments the RAs were instructed to mentally count backward from 100 by serial sevens to avoid any unintentional "treatment/attention." Neither the patients nor the hospital staff knew which interventions were TT and which were sham.

Prior to the beginning of the study, a Credibility of Therapy Form (CTF) was administered to assess the subjects' outcome expectations for the TT therapy. This form included ratings of how logical the patient found TT, how effective the patient expected the treatment to be, and the patient's willingness to pay for TT treatments.

Several subjective scales were administered that measured pain, anxiety, and therapy effectiveness/satisfaction during and after the study. One was the McGill Pain Questionnaire, which contained at least three pain indices: a Pain Rating Index (PRI), Number of Words Chosen (NWC), and Present Pain Intensity (PPI). Three Visual Analog Scales (VAS) were also administered to rate pain (VASP), anxiety (VASA) and satisfaction with therapy (VASS). On each of the three VAS scales, the respondent marked the magnitude of that particular experience along a twenty-centimeter line. After the study, an Effectiveness with Therapy Form (ETF) was administered to rate how satisfactory patients found their patient to be in relieving pain and stress, and whether they would be willing to pay for the TT.

Prior to treatment on day one (baseline), the McGill Pain Questionnaire, the VASP, and the VASA were administered, along with the CTF. On day three, the VASP was administered before and after the TT or sham treatment. On day six, along with the ETF, the McGill Pain Questionnaire, the VASP, and the VASA were again administered.

On days one and six, blood was drawn for white blood cell and lymphocyte analysis but only from a convenience sample of consenting patients. Blood samples were drawn either prior to, or at least two hours after, the subject's painful daily dressing change.

A variety of statistical tests were used employing one-tailed probability values. Outcomes for the TT group and the sham TT group were assessed by a stepwise regression technique. The various outcome parameters (pain, anxiety, satisfaction with treatment) were regressed against the baseline score, then other covariables (age, sex, race, administration of medication, confidence in treatment, etc.) were allowed to enter the regressions stepwise if $P < 0.10$.

Two of the three pain indices of the McGill Pain Questionnaire (the PRI and the NWC) produced significant differences favoring TT treatment. The PPI showed less pain for the TT group, which approached but did not achieve significance ($p = 0.064$). The VASP showed more favorable scores for the TT group but was not significant when comparing day one with days three or six. The immediate effect of TT on pain relief was assessed from the taken for day three, when the VASP was given just before and just after TT, with a result of 16.0 percent less pain for TT. This, however, was not statistically significant.

Anxiety was significantly reduced by day six for the TT group ($p = 0.031$) with 26.1 percent more favorable scores. Patients receiving TT reported greater willingness to pay for treatment, but the difference was not significant ($p = 0.326$). These tests, however, weren't introduced until more than 25 percent of subjects had been tested.

There were no reported differences between the TT and sham TT groups in usage of medication for pain, sleep, anxiety, and antidepressant medications during the study.

Finally, only six TT and five sham subjects submitted their blood for analysis. Of seven blood-cell analyses, three were reported as showing advantages for the TT group (13 percent lower CD8+ cells versus 46.5 percent increase for the sham group, 15 percent increase CD4+ cells versus 48.3 percent increase for the sham group, and 1.1 percent increased lymphocytes versus 38.6 percent increase for the sham group).

The researchers concluded that their results were positive, and consistent with reports of previous TT research: "The positive findings in this study add support to the growing body of evidence on the effectiveness of TT in ameliorating pain perception and reducing anxiety."

In both their review of the literature on TT and in the discussion of their results, Turner et al. refer to at least five studies supportive of TT reducing pain, stress, and anxiety. However, it is distressing to note that these studies have been shown in a number of published reviews to be either seriously flawed or nonreproducible. (Courcey, 1999). For example, the Clark (1992) study was not quantitative (five of nine subjects "claimed" lower back pain relief), not peer-reviewed, and not blind. The Heidt (1981) and Quinn (1984) reports of decreased anxiety with TT could not be replicated. In fact, the Heidt and the Quinn results seem readily attributable to simple eye contact by the practitioner instead of to TT. Another study referenced by Turner et al., which found less stress in hospitalized children after TT (Kramer, 1990), has been disowned by many TT researchers themselves as having so many flaws in design and analysis as to be obvious to introductory college students (Meehan, 1995). And the cited study of decreased blood lymphocytes (Quinn and Strelkauskas, 1993) examined a grand total of four subjects and merely reported a percentage decrease after TT, certainly not an acceptable statistical analysis. There is, therefore, no basis in the literature cited by Turner et al. to support the efficacy of TT.

A number of aspects of the Pentagon burn study protocol also deserve comment. With respect to the methods used to assess pain and anxiety, and McGill questionnaire and VAS instruments are indeed well-recognized as valid in the literature. However, the addition of two assessment forms "several months after the initiation of the study" casts some reasonable doubt on their utility.

Treatment length for the TT group ranged from five to twenty minutes, as determined by the practitioner's assessment. Treatment length for the sham group also varied, up to a maximum length of twenty minutes. Other than to specify a twenty-minute maximum treatment length per session, Turner et al. neither demonstrate that treatment times were comparable for the TT and sham TT groups, nor demonstrate that differences in treatment time do not affect the study outcome. Further, this range of treatment length violates tenets of the "Krieger-Kunz" TT method, which Turner et al. specifically state was utilized. Krieger has explicitly cautioned that burn treatment must be done for no longer than two to three minutes at a time and that longer treatments could adversely and seriously affect the patient (O'Mathúna, 1998).

Turner claims to have conducted a single blind study because "neither the patient nor the staff on the Burn Unit knew which of the interventions were TT and which were sham." The RAs were trained to mimic TT hand movements and practiced until "uninformed observers could not tell whether TT or sham was being performed in a staged demonstration." During the sham treatment the RAs counted backward from 100 by serial sevens to avoid treatment/attention. Several questions need to be answered. First, during the staged demonstration, did the RAs also count backward? Second, could the observers see the facial features of the RAs during this concentrated backward counting or did they merely attend to the hand gestures? Third, and most critically, why were sham subjects never questioned about whether *they* knew they were receiving sham treatment? Turner et al. state that test subjects had been informed they would either receive TT or sham TT, so subjects were alerted and sensitized to the possibility. Surely the facial expressions of the calm, relaxed TT practitioners were markedly different from the RAs who were anxiously preoccupied with a mathematical problem. Therefore, we are really not given conclusive evidence that this was even a single blind study.

Were the statistical analyses appropriate? The researchers used one-tailed probability values because they intended "to test whether TT is more effective than sham TT," and "an alpha level of 0.05 was set." If, indeed, previous research was supportive of the efficacy of TT, one might expect that a much smaller alpha level would be appropriate, say 0.01 or even 0.001. A 0.05 alpha level is too easily achieved and used primarily in exploratory studies. Turner, herself, is quoted in the press as saying that this study would be "the first real scientific evidence there is for Therapeutic Touch" (Butgereit, 1994).

The essential question is whether a one-tailed test is justified instead of a two-tailed test. A one-tailed test assumes that all of the difference between groups will lie in a certain direction. It is much easier to achieve significance using one-tailed probability values since a much smaller difference between groups is needed for a statistically significant difference to be reported. It is appropriate to use a one-tail test under two conditions: (a) an accepted, logically coherent, theoretical basis exists to predict a difference in a certain direction, or (b) sufficient acceptable prior research exists as a basis for predicting the direction of the difference.

Clearly, such a theoretical basis for Therapeutic Touch does not exist. At best the theory for TT is a mixture of Eastern philosophy, anecdote, and experiential claims. TT adherents talk of a subtle metaphysical energy field that becomes unbalanced. TT practitioners maintain that, through meditation, they can detect these energy imbalances and correct them. None of this constitutes any kind of coherent theoretical basis to support use of a one-tailed test. In addition, enough doubt has been cast upon all prior research to show that for this reason, also, there is insufficient justification for a one-tailed test.

One other problem with the Turner et al. study is the frequent reporting of differences which "approach significance." Either there are significant differences or there are not. It is inappropriate to report differences that are not significant. Unfortunately, this malpractice is commonly seen in many "alternative" studies in an attempt to suggest something that simply does not exist. One other "statistical malpractice" occurs when numerous tests of significance are performed and an uncorrected $p = 0.05$ level is used. It is well known, for example, that if nothing is really happening (the null hypothesis is true), but one performs twenty t-tests, then by pure chance alone, an experimenter expects to find one that is significant. The Turner et al. paper reports no correction for multiple tests.

Not only does the rationale for the statistical analysis seems insufficient, the actual numbers themselves, as reported in the study, do even less to inspire confidence in the trustworthiness of the results. Turner et al. report that ninety-nine patients initially joined the study and remained at least three days. When subjects were randomly assigned (by "coin toss") to either the TT or the sham TT groups, sixty-two were placed in the TT group and thirty-seven in the sham group. Large differences between group sizes can cause problems in statistical analyses, yet no reason for the substantial difference in the numbers assigned to the two groups was provided.

If that were not confusing enough, the experimenters state that only 81 percent of the original subjects completed the study. They provide no breakdown of how many subjects dropped out of the TT versus the sham TT groups. Table 1 of the article provides a statistical comparison of the TT and non-TT groups at the beginning of the study, showing the groups to be equivalent with respect to various characteristics, yet there is no assurance that the groups remained equivalent at the end of the study when much of the critical data was measured. In the analysis of pain reports we are told that the total *n* varied from sixty-one to eighty-three with no breakdown of the number in each group. Even table 3, which involved instruments added after several months, reports between forty-four and fifty-two subjects, again with no breakdown of how many were in each group. Finally, only "adjusted" mean scores are given and there is no mention anywhere of variance/standard deviations which is standard procedure in any research of this kind. It is clearly impossible to evaluate such data.

At the beginning of the study, the CTF was administered to assess whether subject expectations were related to outcome of the therapy. However, although CTF scores were allowed to enter some of the statistical tests as a covariable, no evaluation was presented of the relationship of subjects' prior expectations regarding the success of TT treatments to their perceived pain reduction. It is also noteworthy that the CTF asks how logical TT seems to be. This item is crucial because one must wonder about the degree of critical thinking of the patient who responds that TT is "very logical," and subject answers to this question could strongly correlate to perceived reduction in pain and anxiety.

The last information given in the report deals with blood cell counts for six patients who received TT and five who received sham TT. Despite first admitting that these data are not amenable to statistical analyses, Turner et al. proceed to provide percentage increase/decrease values that seem to favor the TT group. But, truly, the "sham" is even to present these data at all. No meaning whatsoever can be drawn from raw percentages on this few subjects.

It is noteworthy that Turner failed to mention the fact that three times more patients had infections during or after TT than in the sham group. (This was found in their "Final Progress Report" dated May 20, 1996 [see appendix 2 in this volume].) If those data had been reversed, and reduced infection rates observed in the TT group, one might suspect that these would have been reported as an important percentage favorable to TT.

If all of the foregoing criticisms are either ignored or irrelevant and the study viewed in its most favorable light, what might the TT optimist conclude? Six tests measured pain. But only two of these (and these two were least directly involved in measuring the subjective intensity of pain) were significant. In addition, these two (PRI and NWC) are not independent measures, but are both based on the same questionnaire data and are highly correlated ($r = 0.89$), suggesting that they may simply be measuring the same thing. Anxiety reduction was not significantly reduced (if the more appropriate two-tailed test is used). The optimistic supporter of TT must reluctantly conclude that the study provides no definitive evidence that TT is of any significant help to burn patients.

RECENT TT STUDY: GORDON ET AL.

In a second study, Gordon et al. examined the effects of TT on patients with osteoarthritis of the knee (Gordon, 1998). Twenty-seven patients were randomly assigned either to continue to receive only the usual care (Control Group, n = 8), to receive TT (Treatment Group, n = 8), or receive mock TT (Placebo Group, n = 11). Severity of symptoms were randomized among all three groups, with average ages between sixty-four and sixty-nine. The TT and placebo groups received treatments (of unknown duration) once a week for six weeks. A practitioner chosen to resemble the TT practitioner (both were women of approximately the same age and healthcare experience) treated the placebo group with mock Therapeutic Touch (MTT). No information is given about the degree of knowledge about TT possessed by this person. Before the study both TT and MTT treatment techniques were video taped and reviewed to insure that unbiased observers could not see any differences. During the MTT, the practitioner counted backward from 100 by serial sevens to prevent any unintentional attention to the patient or "intent to heal."

Instruments used to measure various aspects of pain and health included two questionnaires, the Stanford Health Assessment Questionnaire (HAQ) and the thirteen-scale West Haven—Yale Multidimensional Pain Inventory (MPI). In addition, two VAS assessments were used to measure subjective pain and general well-being. Both the TT and MTT groups completed VAS scales before and after each of the six treatments. It is unclear who was present when these data were gathered. In-depth interviews were conducted at week seven and again at week thirteen. Another person who was unacquainted with the patients conducted these interviews, but his relation to the investigators is uncertain.

The various assessment instruments used in this study are widely considered acceptable for the assessment of pain and disability. On ten of the thirteen MPI scales, the treatment group showed significant improvement over the placebo and control groups. However, significant differences were not found on either the HAQ Functional Disability Index or the VAS (except for one instance in the six weeks of testing when the placebo group improved more than the TT group).

Gordon et al. gave considerable weight to selected verbal reports from in-depth interviews which seem to support the efficacy of TT treatment. They conclude that, despite the small numbers, "it would be imprudent to reject a safe and effective therapy [just] because we do not understand or do not accept its mode of action." A subsequent letter in the same journal concludes that this was a "well-designed effort to evaluate the efficacy of an unconventional treatment (TT)" (Evanoff and Newton, 1999).

In contrast to the Turner et al. study, Gordon et al. related no references to favorable results of past TT studies. In fact, the authors noted various flaws previously found by critics of other studies that they attempted to correct in their study. In many ways, this appears to be a better designed study than the more widely publicized UAB burn study. However, a closer look shows that there are, again, notable problems with the Gordon et al. study.

For exactly the same reasons pointed out earlier in the Turner et al. study, this study cannot be considered single-blind. Subject blindness cannot be presumed because it was never properly evaluated or demonstrated. The placebo subjects were never queried, nor did the independent observers examine the facial expressions of the placebo practitioner. We also do not know whether the in-depth interviewer was "blind" with regard to which patients received TT or placebo treatments.

The small sizes of the groups (as admitted by the researchers) is simply unacceptable. It is difficult to conclude that we have here random samples from a population of osteoarthritic patients. This, in itself, renders any conclusions of this study as tenuous indeed. In addition, assessment of severity of condition (used to equate the groups) was based, in part, on patient reports. Quite possibly, some patients who often tend to be overly pain-sensitive or complaining could bias any equivalence of symptom severity.

On two of the three instruments which measured pain relief (HAQ and VAS) there were no differences between the TT and the placebo groups. Considering that the VAS was given pre- and posttreatment six times to each of the two groups, one might well expect to see a significant difference (as it did once, favoring the placebo group). The fact that the control group scored lower on many measures could easily be due to the lack of attention given to them. They were not seen at all during weeks two through five. It would have been very easy to avoid this flaw by bringing them in for weekly evaluation just as the subjects in the TT and MTT groups were.

The paper's emphasis on the anecdotal reports from the in-depth interviews is somewhat troubling because these could obviously have been selected to place TT in a more positive light than might actually be the case. In addition, anecdotes are not only irrelevant in reaching scientific conclusions, they are often the refuge of last resort when there is little else available to convince a lay audience of the claims of an "alternative" or unconventional treatment. As one example, "several" TT patients reported using less medication leading the authors to conclude readily that TT may allow for reduction or cessation of medication. However, no significant effect of TT on medication requirements is found elsewhere in the literature, e.g., Turner et al. (1998). The researchers inadvertently hurt their own arguments when they seem quite willing to place more emphasis upon selected anecdotes than upon statistics.

As was the case with the Turner et al. experiment, the experiment violated the established protocol for TT. The researchers seem to be unaware that many supporters of TT (including Krieger herself) caution against using TT with the elderly (O'Mathúna, 1998). They also fail to report other research that found TT to be less effective than progressive muscle relaxation for degenerative arthritis (Peck, 1997).

Finally, it is interesting that the researchers introduced a 1991 meta-analysis of homeopathy as justification for the continued use of TT, incorrectly implying that the meta-analysis authors seem to suggest that ignorance of mechanisms of action should not hinder the use of a "safe and effective therapy." But those authors have made it abundantly clear on many occasions that almost all of the homeopathy trials were poorly designed and analyzed and that the homeopathic remedies were not effective (Kleinjen et al., 1991a; Kleinjen et al., 1991b).

CONCLUSIONS

Here we have looked at two of the most recent attempts to study the efficacy of TT for pain relief. The burn study has far too many flaws to be seriously considered. The osteoarthritic study is much better designed and analyzed, yet also suffers from weaknesses in blinding and sample size.

It still seems that researchers of TT are unaware of how to conduct a "blind" study adequately. The sham techniques used in these two studies have been criticized previously but continue to be used. We know that experimental subjects respond to eye contact, to implied suggestion and to someone with a caring personality although they may not be aware of these cues. This unawareness is the basic reason for insuring that the subjects are "blind" to the experimental treatments. There is ample evidence in the annals of psychology of subjects being unaware that they are responding to very subtle cues. One has only to remember the Hawthorne Effect, the Greenspoon Effect (subtle verbal cues) (Greenspoon, 1950), and the Carpenter Effect (ideomotor action) (Vogt and Hyman, 1959). The subtle cues supplied by the practitioners of the sham or mock TT treatments may easily explain any group differences that are found.

Subjects are most often able to respond honestly to inquiries. One has to ask why, if nursing professionals are concerned with patient well-being, that, to date, no one has bothered to ask the patients whether they are aware of the differences between sham and actual TT treatment that they are receiving. By asking the patients, it might be discovered that "blindness" was not achieved at all.

One almost wonders whether the TT researchers have gone out of their way to deny these subtle influences (other than the wondrous subtlety of TT itself) so that they can ultimately conclude that TT intervention is a "proven" success.

It is clear that we must continue to wait for a well-designed, well-conducted truly blind (preferably double-blind) study of TT. The research sophistication of some TT researchers continues to grow. They must be encouraged. However, research of substandard quality must not be accepted as evidence that practices such as TT are efficacious. If the nursing profession itself is to continue to enhance its prestige in the healthcare community, it must distance itself from New-Age mysticism and antiscientific philosophies.

REFERENCES

Bright, M. A. 1995. "Letter, Re: Therapeutic Touch." *Research in Nursing and Health* 18: 285–86.

Butgereit, B. 1994. "Therapeutic Touch: UAB to Study Controversial Treatment for Pentagon." *Birmingham News*, November 17, pp. 1A, 10A.

Clark, A. J. 1992. "Client Perceptions of Therapeutic Touch." Abstract. *Proceedings: West Alabama Annual Nursing Research Conference*. Tuscaloosa, Alabama, p. 16.

Clark, P. E., and M. J. Clark. 1984. "Therapeutic Touch: Is There a Scientific Basis for the Practice?" *Nursing Research* 33: 37–41.

Courcey, K. 1999. "Further Notes on Therapeutic Touch." Website at: http://www.quackwatch.com/01QuackeryRelatedTopics/tt2.html.

Evanoff, A., and W. P. Newton. 1999. "Letter: Therapeutic Touch and Osteoarthritis of the Knee." *Journal of Family Practice* 48 (1): 11–12.

Gordon, A., J. H. Merenstein, F. D'Amico et al. 1998. "The Effects of Therapeutic

Touch on Patients with Osteoarthritis of the Knee." *Journal of Family Practice* 47 (4): 271–77.

Greenspoon, J. 1950. "The Effect of a Verbal Stimulus as a Reinforcement." *Proceedings of the Indiana Academy of Sciences* 59: 287.

Heidt, P. 1981. "Effect of Therapeutic Touch on Anxiety Levels of Hospitalized Patients." *Nursing Research* 30(2): 32–37.

———. 1995. "Letter." *Research in Nursing and Health* 18: 377–78.

Kleinjen, J., P. Knipschild, and G. Reit. 1991a. "Clinical Trials of Homeopathy." *British Medical Journal* 302: 316–23.

Kleinjen, J., P. Knipschild, and G. Reit. 1991b. "Trials of Homeopathy." *British Medical Journal* 302: 960.

Kramer, N. 1990. "Comparison of Therapeutic Touch and Casual Touch in Stress Reduction in Hospitalized Children." *Pediatric Nursing* 16 (5): 483–85.

Krieger, D. 1999. "Viewpoint: Nursing as (Un)usual." *American Journal of Nursing* 99 (4): 9.

Malinski, V. 1995. "Letter." *Research in Nursing and Health* 18: 286.

Meehan, T. C. 1995. "Letters to the Editor." *Research in Nursing and Health* (July 18): p. 481.

Oberst, M. T. 1995. "Editorial: Our Naked Emperor." *Research in Nursing and Health* 18 (1): 1–2.

O'Mathúna, D. P. 1998. "Therapeutic Touch: What Could be the Harm?" *Scientific Review of Alternative Medicine* 2 (1): 56–62.

Peck, S. D. E. 1997. "The Effectiveness of Therapeutic Touch for Decreasing Pain in Elders with Degenerative Arthritis." *Journal of Holistic Nursing* 15: 176–98.

Quinn, J. 1984. "Therapeutic Touch as Energy Exchange: Testing the Theory." *Advances in Nursing Science* 6 (2): 42–49.

Quinn, J., and A. J. Strelkauskas. 1993. "Psychoimmunologic Effects of Therapeutic Touch on Practitioners and Recently Bereaved Recipients: A Pilot Study." *Advances in Nursing Science* 15 (4): 13–26.

Scheiber, B., and C. Selby. 1997. "UAB Final Report of Therapeutic Touch—An Appraisal." *Skeptical Inquirer* 21 (3): 53–54.

Selby, C., and B. Scheiber. 1996. "Science or Pseudoscience? Pentagon Grant Funds Alternative Health Study." *Skeptical Inquirer* 20 (4): 15–17.

Turner, J. G., A. J. Clark, D. K. Gauthier et al. 1998. "The Effects of Therapeutic Touch on Pain and Anxiety in Burn Patients." *Journal of Advanced Nursing* 28 (1): 10–20.

Vogt, E. Z., and R. Hyman. 1959. *Water Witching USA*. Chicago: University of Chicago Press, p. 132.

Wells-Federman, C. L. 1995. "Letter." *Research in Nursing and Health* 18: 472–73.

19.

Science or Pseudoscience? Pentagon Grant Funds Alternative Health Study

Carla Selby and Béla Scheiber

Consider the following: A major public university's burn center requests a grant for $317,725 from the Uniformed Services University of the Health Sciences (USUHS) (a department of the Pentagon) in order to study the "laying over of hands," or "The Effect of Therapeutic Touch on Pain and Infection in Burn Patients." One might be skeptical about the topic to be investigated and therefore not surprised that the grant was rejected. Now assume that this same university resubmitted the grant proposal revised in accordance with the suggestions of USUHS and two months later was awarded a grant of $355,225.

And, in fact, that's what happened: $355,225 was awarded September 20, 1994, to the University of Alabama at Birmingham (UAB) Burn Center for a "single blinded randomized clinical trial" to "quantify the effect of therapeutic touch (TT) on pain and infection in burn patients, and to develop a research based protocol for practice. A comparison will be made between the control group which will receive placebo intervention (mimic TT) along with the standard treatment regimen, and the experimental group will receive TT in addition to usual burn center management" (Turner, 1994, p. 35).

During the experiment, a group of burn patients—suffering from first-, second-, and third-degree burns on anywhere from 5 percent to 70 percent of their bodies—will have a nurse's hands waved over them without touching (which should relieve any anxiety about exacerbation of pain on the part of burn patients) to see if the patient is helped. This group of patients will be compared with a control group of burn patients—selected by a coin toss—who are denied the benefit of a trained practitioner's TT, but who instead get a wave of the hands from a nurse who has been trained in how to fake Therapeutic Touch.

Of course, a skeptic might ask, "What's the difference between waving your hands over a patient's body hoping to help heal him or her and *pretending* to wave your hands over a patient's body hoping to help heal him or her?" Another question might be, "What if the mimic TT practitioner feels compassion for the burn patient and accidentally performs actual TT?" How would that affect the results of the study? Granted, the UAB Burn Center deals with burn victims, but if the USUHS was going to reject the first proposal and make suggestions, why didn't they suggest that the practitioners start with a group of subjects suffering from less trauma? For example, people with mild sunburn? [See appendix 1.]

The proposal "is designed to investigate the effects of a complementary therapy" (Turner, 1994, p.35).

The "specific objectives" of the project are to:

1. Recruit 150 subjects aged 15 to 65 and randomly assign them to either the treatment or control group.
2. Compare the effects of TT on the outcomes of pain perception and nosocomial infection.
3. Develop and test a TT protocol for use as an adjunct to narcotic analgesia in lowering pain levels and the incidence of infection in burn patients. (Turner, 1994, p. 35)

Apparently, no one at USUHS raised concerns about the less-than-scientific and extremely imprecise language used in the grant proposal to describe TT and support the request. Language such as:

1. Therapeutic Touch is a contemporary interpretation of several ancient healing practices.
2. The technique ... is based on the assumption of a human energy field which extends beyond the skin. The idea behind TT is that the human energy field is abundant and flows in balanced patterns in health but is depleted and/or unbalanced in illness or injury.
3. This action is believed to place the person in an optimal position for his/her own resources to be used in self-healing.
4. In this view, the therapist acts as a human energy support system until the persons own immunological system is robust enough to take over.
5. Central to the practice is the assumption of a human energy field and an environment filled with "life energy" which is also present in all living organisms.

6. Support for this view is based entirely on a field world view.
7. Quantum theory states that all of reality is made up of energy fields and that over 99 percent of the universe is simply space.
8. Our present technology does not allow the measurement of the human energy field, but to a trained sense, primarily touch, the human energy field can be perceived and assessed.

One might well ask, "Doesn't that last point actually negate the practice of Therapeutic Touch, which involves no touching? And what was that bit about quantum theory all about?" The proposal goes on: "It is postulated that TT, which therapeutically manipulates the individual's energy pattern, stimulates the release of endorphins through the triggering of supraspinal mechanisms" (Turner, 1994, p. 42).

Perhaps the people at USUHS were impressed by the diagram of the Conceptual Model of Study that accompanied the proposal. The diagram [figure 1] shows that burn injury causes "pain," "stress," and "risk of infection." TT, on the other hand, leads to "activation of endogenous opioid system," "reduced stress," and "decreased T-suppresor lymphocytes," which in turn lead to "pain relief" and "decreased risk of infection," which together lead to "enhanced healing" (Turner, 1994, p. 45). Of course, the existence of a human energy field as well as the benefits of TT are all hypothetical. Their efficacy is the purpose of the study, after all. Unfortunately, the continued assumption of the validity of the theoretical basis of TT is to be found throughout the proposal without any comment about this logical fallacy on the part of the proposal's reviewers.

Among other criteria for selecting the subjects are the necessity of speaking English and the ability to communicate verbally. The subjects must also be able to see and hear. One might wonder if the patients need to be able to see and hear so that they will be aware when either TT or mimic TT is being administered. However, this requirement is

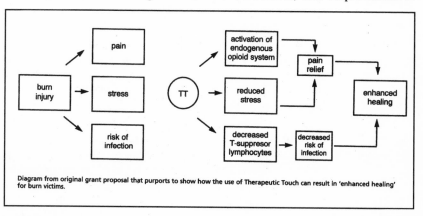

Diagram from original grant proposal that purports to show how the use of Therapeutic Touch can result in 'enhanced healing' for burn victims.

putatively added in order to determine if the TT was effective and if the mimic TT was not effective. Why? Because the results are measured by *asking* the patients if they feel better!

The proposal says the following "instruments" will be used in this study to collect data relative to outcome variables:

1. McGill Pain Questionnaire (which consists primarily of three major classes of word descriptors: sensory, affective and evaluative, and is used to specify the subjective pain experience);
2. Visual Analogue Pain Estimation Scale (which is used by having the patient mark or indicate a point on a straight line that reflects the amount of sensation the patient is experiencing at the time);
3. Visual Analogue Anxiety Estimation Scale (which is used by having the patient mark or indicate a point on a similar straight line that reflects the amount of anxiety the patient is experiencing);
4. Credibility of Therapy Form (which is used after an explanation of TT to record the patient's opinion as to how logical TT seems, how confident the patient is that TT will be successful, and if the patient would be willing to pay for TT as an optional part of hospital treatment). (Turner, 1994, p. 47)

The names of patients who answer "yes" to that last question ought to be valuable information to somebody!

The grant proposal isn't afraid to reveal the secrets of TT by describing how it works: "The TT practitioner will begin by centering" which "consists of a quieting and focusing of consciousness with the intent to help. Next, an assessment of the subject's energy field will be done to search out all areas of imbalance, blocked energy flow, congestion, or deficit in energy flow. Then TT treatment will begin, starting at the subject's crown and moving downward to the feet . . . through stimulation and augmentation, clearing of congestion or blocks in flow, or quieting the energy flow to achieve a balanced, abundant, symmetrical energy flow. The TT practitioner's hands, held about four inches above the subject, will move in a rhythmical way directing energy from central areas of the subject's energy field to peripheral ones or touching the subject lightly for short periods where additional energy is needed" (Turner, 1994, p. 49). Contrast this precision methodology with TT's exceedingly imprecise origin in Martha Rogers's "nursing theory . . . based entirely on a field world view" (Turner, 1994, p. 40) which has far more in common with revealed wisdom than with a scientific hypothesis.

An ongoing assessment by the practitioner will indicate when the treatment is completed. At the conclusion of this process, the subject will be allowed to rest quietly for about ten minutes. It is implied therefore that the subject needs this time of quiet rest at the end of TT treatment in order to recover from all the agitation caused by the practitioner's waving hands.

On the other hand, the placebo intervention of the mimic TT administered to the control group will be completely different:

> Mimic treatments will be provided to all control group subjects by the nonnurse research assistant, who does not know what Therapeutic Touch is. This research assistant will be trained to perform the same movements that will be used by the Therapeutic Touch practitioners. However, instead of centering and holding the intent to help the subject as the Therapeutic Touch practitioners will do, the research assistant will simply begin the treatment and will count back from 100 by serial sevens during the mimic treatment.
>
> To assure that the sessions are all comparable, three uninvolved lay persons will be asked to observe the research assistants and the Therapeutic Touch practitioners and identify which treatments are real. The research will not be started until observers cannot tell the real from the mimic treatments.
>
> Mimic treatments will be given in the patients' rooms approximately one hour before the daily dressing change: As in the Therapeutic Touch treatment, the patients will lie on their backs on the hospital beds. Lighting will be dim, and soft, relaxing instrumental music will be playing. Prior to the first treatment, the subject will be instructed to relax as fully as possible and a brief explanation of what will be done during the treatment will be given. The research assistant may randomly spend between five and twenty minutes doing the mimic treatment. At the end of the mimic treatment, the subject will be allowed to rest quietly for about ten minutes. Thus, with this single, blind placebo intervention, all subjects and unit personnel will perceive that subjects are receiving the same intervention. The identity of the mimic TT vs. TT intervention subjects will be known only to the researchers. (Turner, 1994, p. 52)

The proposal attempts to address some "limitations" of its study: "A frequent criticism when TT administration is used as an intervention relates to the 'placebo effect.' However, administration of a mimic intervention to control subjects helps control for placebo effect" (Turner, 1994, p. 52). In other words, a placebo treatment for a possible placebo treatment will take care of that problem!

In considering the success that the UAB Burn Center had in acquiring $355,225 to study TT, we ask whether public money is best spent on such highly speculative "alternative therapies." What is the difference, after all, in TT and "remote healing" where practitioners will patients to get better from across the room, or perhaps, over the phone. (What about e-mail?)

Further, should questions not be asked about the ethics of trying a completely speculative technique on burn patients whose pain is most severe and intractable and whose infection rate is very high? First and most important, practitioners of TT must demonstrate some basis in reality for their theory. Then, and only then, can they move to the next step—proving its efficacy.

REFERENCE

Turner, J. G. 1994. "The Effect of Therapeutic Touch on Pain and Infection in Burn Patients (N94-020A1)." *Grant Agreement* (Grant No. MDA 905-94-Z-0080), Uniformed Services University of the Health Sciences, approved 9/20/94, accepted 11/9/94. (Due to the unwillingness of UAB to provide us a copy of this grant proposal, we obtained it through a Freedom of Information Act request.)

20.

UAB Final Report of Therapeutic Touch: An Appraisal

Béla Scheiber and Carla Selby

Therapeutic Touch is a modern variant of the ancient "laying-on of hands." Ironically, this new version involves only incidental touching while the practitioner passes her or his hands over the patient's body at some distance from it in an attempt to "unruffle" the person's energy field. While the existence of a human energy field has never been scientifically demonstrated, practitioners talk and behave as if it is a fact. Founder and chief promoter of TT Dolores Krieger, has said, "My only concern when doing Therapeutic Touch is the person's energy field" (Calvert, 1994).

Infrequent attempts have been made to subject the claims of TT practitioners to some scientific rigor. None have been as ambitious as those undertaken recently at the University of Alabama at Birmingham (UAB) Burn Center (Selby and Scheiber, 1996a; Turner et al., 1998). Principal Investigator Joan Turner, D.S.N., R.N., C.I.C., undertook the challenge by proposing to study the effect of TT on pain and infection in burn patients. After an eighteen month investigation at a cost of $355,225 to taxpayers, UAB has delivered its "Tri-Service Nursing Research Grant Final Report" to the Uniform Services University of the Health Sciences, a division of the Pentagon [see appendix 2]. The Rocky Mountain Skeptics submitted an FOIA (Freedom of Information Act) request for this document after trying unsuccessfully to obtain it

---

Originally published in *Skeptical Inquirer* 21, no. 3 (May–June). Copyright © 1997 Committee for the Scientific Investigation of Claims of the Paranormal. Reprinted with permission from the authors and publisher. To obtain documents of the proposal and its final report refer to the following Websites: http://www.parascope.com/articles/1196/touch1.htm, http://bcn.boulder.co.us/community/rms. See appendix 2 for the complete May 20, 1996, "Final Progress Report" from the *Tri-Service Nursing Research Grant Final Report*.

from the principal investigator. She had refused to provide us with a copy of the report and also informed us that she would ask the Pentagon not to give it to us since she was writing an article for publication. Fortunately, the Pentagon has a better idea of what is appropriate with scientific data.

Of the two pages comprising the final report, nearly one full page is devoted to "Problems Encountered." This section deals predominantly with a peripheral issue: "publicity and harassment by a religious group called the Watchmen" (Turner, 1996). This lengthy inclusion of gossip within an ostensibly scientific report is baffling. Proponents of TT must be aware of religious opposition to their activities on various grounds. Why a substantial fraction of their research discussions should be devoted to an attempt to discredit religious interference demonstrates the political and sociological controversy surrounding TT, not the scientific content of their activity.

When this project was announced, it was touted as a scientific effort to demonstrate the efficacy of TT. As we wrote in response to correspondents to our July/August 1996 article (Selby and Scheiber, 1996b), when we reviewed the research proposal, we became fairly certain that credible scientific results could not be anticipated from a research design that appeared to have been constructed merely to vindicate TT. Curiously, the report does not state any clear and meaningful conclusion, and yet the author writes: "Additional research is currently being conducted to assist us in *arriving at a maximal protocol for the administration of TT to subjects*" (emphasis added). Also, in the final paragraph she writes: "Therapeutic Touch is a nursing measure which is nonpharmacologic and produces no side effects. This therapy can be used to decrease subjects' perception of pain as either a one time or series of days intervention." None of this can be concluded from this study.

Also in our response, we expressed our concerns that the outcome would inevitably be presented as supportive of TT due to the open-ended, poorly defined experimental design. The final report does not say how many outcomes were evaluated and what criteria determined those that were included. If many potential outcomes were considered, random selection alone could have produced statistical significance. The report says that pain measured at day three was significantly reduced by TT ($p = 0.038$). What are we to conclude about any of the other five days? Nor does it provide any evidence that statistical adjustment for multiple comparisons was considered.

While the Visual Analogue Pain Estimation Scale (VAS) showed no statistical difference in subjective pain perception between the TT and sham groups, the results were significant when measured by the McGill scale, both measured on day one versus day six. It is possible that this inconsistency can be attributed to random positive results for the McGill scale due, once again, to multiple comparisons without proper statistical adjustment. Otherwise, it is unclear why two measures of the same effect produced different results.

The original design called for 150 burn patients, each randomly assigned to either the TT or sham group (Turner, 1994); only 131 were actually recruited. Additionally, "not all of these subjects actually remained in the study for the full six-day period." Who dropped out and why? What was the distribution between the TT and sham groups? Were the clinical characteristics of the dropouts from the two groups comparable? No charts or tables are included in the final report, thus precluding any independent evaluation of complete data. This information is as crucial as it is essential to know whether the experimental and control groups were balanced regarding relevant clinical variables. For example, did one group or the other not contain more seriously ill patients? The inadequacy of the report underscores a lack of understanding of experimental design required to demonstrate validity of a hypothesis.

In our article, we raised concerns about the use of "mimic TT as a control." Since the intention to heal is held out as a vital component of TT we raised the question, "What if the mimic TT practitioner feels compassion for the burn patient and accidentally performs actual TT?" Since the human "energy field" (presumably manipulated by TT) cannot be objectively quantified, there is no independent means to assess when manipulation is occurring. The final report states: "The greatest lesson learned from this process is that the inclusion of a true control group in addition to a sham and treatment group is required because a strong placebo effect occurs from the special attention given to patients in the "sham treatment." This observation is correct in its characterization of the placebo effect on patients participating in any such experiment. No practitioner or test of TT has shown that anything other than the placebo effect is taking place. The UAB study continues to support this assertion.

REFERENCES

Calvert, R. 1994. " Dolores Krieger, Ph.D., and Her Therapeutic Touch." *Massage* 47: 57–60.

Selby, C., and B. Scheiber. 1996a. "Science or Pseudoscience? Pentagon Grant Funds Alternative Health Study." *Skeptical Inquirer* 20 (4): 15–17.

———. 1996b. "Letters to the Editor." *Skeptical Inquirer* 20 (6): 62.

Turner, G. J. et al. 1994. "The Effect of Therapeutic Touch on Pain and Infection in Burn Patients (N94-020A1)." *Grant Agreement* (Grant No. MDA 905-94-Z-0080), Uniformed Services University of the Health Sciences, approved 9/20/94, accepted 11/9/94.

————. 1996. "Final Progress Report." *Tri-Service Nursing Research Grant Final Report* (May 20). Obtained through an FOIA from Uniform Services University of the Health Sciences.

Turner, G. J., J. A. Clark, K. D. Gauthier, and M. Williams. 1998. "The Effect of Therapeutic Touch on Pain and Anxiety in Burn Patients." *Journal of Advanced Nursing* 28 (1): 10–20.

21.

Therapeutic Touch: Evaluating the "Growing Body of Evidence" Claim

Béla Scheiber

A feature article in the January 23, 1997, issue of *Eugene Weekly* (Oregon) entitled "A Healing Touch" made the following claim:

> TT (therapeutic touch) is one of the most studied and documented complimentary modalities in use throughout the world. More than 200 studies have tested the technique's effectiveness on conditions including wound healing, chronic anxiety, tension headaches, and postchemotherapy nausea and vomiting.

Such claims can be found in newspapers and magazines throughout the country. In fact this claim was first encountered by the Rocky Mountain Skeptics (RMS) during our efforts at challenging the leaders of the nursing profession in the state of Colorado (Scheiber, 1993, 1994; Rosa, 1995). On January 30, 1992, the Colorado Board of Nursing (CBN) was asked by representatives of RMS the following question: "How can Board recognized, credentializing organizations be made responsible and accountable for the content of continuing education classes?" We listed several questionable nursing practices only one of which was Therapeutic Touch.

Originally published in *Scientific Review of Alternative Medicine* (fall/winter 1997). Copyright © 1997 Prometheus Books. Reprinted with updates with permission from author and publisher. Updated but based on an earlier author's version which appeared in the *Skeptical Inquirer* (1993) and an earlier version in the *Rocky Mountain Skeptic* (1993) (copyright by Rocky Mountain Skeptics). The author is greatly indebted to the many members of the Rocky Mountain Skeptics for their efforts and contributions to the RMS TT project. Much of the material referred to in this article is the result of their effort, including (but not limited to) Bill Ardorfer, Randy Bancroft, Linda Rosa, Larry Sarner, Béla Scheiber, Carla Selby, and Martin Tobias.

In a letter from CBN dated March 10, 1992, we were notified of the formation of a "subcommittee to address the question and present a recommendation back to the Board." The subcommittee's conclusions were presented to the full Board May 28 which then informed us in a letter dated June 8, 1992, that, "after review of the research literature and discussion, the subcommittee had made the recommendation that the Board should continue to award continuing education credit to such programs. After discussion, the Board voted to reaffirm its previous determination that therapeutic touch was an acceptable study area for continuing education credit."

While we were not invited to testify at the subcommittee's hearings, others were allowed to present a favorable case for TT in front of the full Board. Among the four witnesses was Janet Quinn, Ph.D., R.N., FAAN, who is an Associate Professor and Senior Scholar at the University of Colorado Health Sciences Center School of Nursing. Professor Quinn provided the Board a reading list (Quinn, 1992) of 200 entries among which were over two dozen authored by her including her master's thesis and doctoral dissertation (both done at New York University under Dorothy Krieger, the leading TT advocate).

In their recommendation to the CBN, the subcommittee wrote in part:

> Based on an increasing volume of research [see below for an analysis] and clinical literature supporting the effectiveness of Therapeutic Touch in the easing of human suffering and the stimulation of healing, the State Board of Nursing of Colorado, like other State Boards of Nursing all over the country, should continue to be an advocate for the public safety and for patient's rights to access the full range of caring and healing interventions by continuing to acknowledge continuing education units earned for the study of Therapeutic Touch. Therapeutic Touch, as a nursing intervention, is being taught to nurses through many colleges and universities, and by the National League for Nursing through its continuing education videotape series on Therapeutic Touch. It is completely within the mainstream of modern nursing practice. [See appendix 4.]

In a letter dated September 10, 1992, to the Board, RMS requested all documents that were presented by the subcommittee so that we could independently evaluate the evidence that they felt was so compelling. We wondered just what was the "increasing volume of research and clinical literature supporting the effectiveness of Therapeutic Touch"? We found that of the 200 entries found in Dr. Quinn's list, the works could be characterized and enumerated as follows (see also figure 1):

- Appearances in the popular press (13)
  (e.g., *Woman's Day, McCalls, People, American Baby, New Realities*)
- Unrelated publications, incidental mentions, and popular works (30)
  (e.g., *How to Meditate, The Tao of Physics, The Aquarian Conspiracy*)
- Articles in journals with scant or suspicious reputations (35)
  (e.g., *The American Theosophist, International Journal of Parapsychology, Re-Vision*)
- Non-peer-reviewed book (39)
  (e.g., *Spiritual Aspects of the Healing Arts, The Many Facets of Touch*)
- Unrefereed articles in newsletters and trade publications (31)
- Dissertations, master's theses, and research reports (19)
- Authentic-sounding research papers (33)

The last two categories constitute only 26 percent of the total, and we placed them in the "possible" category of valid research. In a further breakdown of these there were:

- Correspondence responding to attacks (2)
- Dissertations and theses which are oblique to the topic (6)
- Surveys with no original work in them (5)
- Probable surveys, with no original work (6)
- Repackagings of earlier works (3)
- Possible authentic research papers (16)
- Genuine research reports (14)

A closer look at the thirty constituting the last two categories showed:

- Research or responses not supportive of TT (15)
  (e.g., Quinn, 1989)
- Possibly authentic research papers (5)
- Supportive dissertations and theses (4)
  (Heidt, 1979; Quinn, 1982; Guerrero, 1986; Pomerhn, 1987)
- Supportive papers (6)
  (Heidt, 1981; Keller, 1983; Krieger, 1975; Quinn, 1984; Heidt, 1990; Kramer, 1990)

We were not able to locate the five in the "possibly authentic" subcategory so we were generous here. Note that of those constituting the

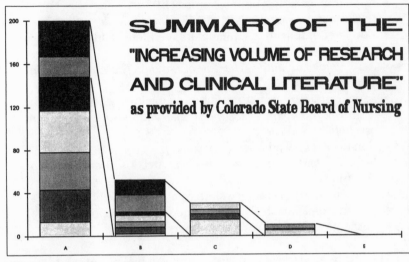

A Total references provided (200)

  A—>B Dissertations, masters theses, research reports (19)
  Authentic-sounding research papers (33)

    B—>C Possible authentic research papers (16)
    Genuine research reports (14)

      C—>D Supportive dissertations & theses (4)
      Supportive papers (6)

D—>E Validated or replicated research (0)

above list, half of them dispute the TT hypothesis such as Quinn (1989). Of the ten that have been identified as supportive research, many have received some scrutiny prior to the CBN's subcommittee meeting:

- Experimental designs in dispute (5)
- Could not be replicated (1)
- Unevaluated research (4)
- Validated or replicated research (0)

A capsule summary of many of these:

- Heidt (1979) (sample size = 90; attempted replication by Hale [1986] failed to confirm)
- Quinn (1982) (sample size = 60; claims to investigate only difference between contact and noncontact techniques)
- Guerrero (1986) (small sample size = 30)
- Pomerhn (1987) (small sample size = 40)
- Heidt (1981) (criticized by Clark [1984]: no objective data and no control for placebo effect)

- Keller (1983) (criticized by Bullough and Bullough [1993]: poor design)
- Krieger (1975) (criticized by Clark [1984]: poor design and subject selection)
- Quinn (1984) (criticized by Clark [1984]: no objective measures used, failed to be replicated in a better designed experiment by Quinn [1989])
- Kramer (1990) (Small sample; "observer participant")

Working independently of us, Peter Kramer, Ph.D. (biochemistry), investigated a similar claim by Krieger that there is a large body of evidence which addresses the above concerns. On April 22, 1993, he queried MEDLINE for references to "THERAPEUTIC TOUCH" and found: 294,425 hits on "THERAPEUTIC"; 2,600 hits on "TOUCH," 52 hits on "THERAPEUTIC TOUCH" (Kramer, 1993). He then classified the 52 into three categories:

- Basic research (5)
- Descriptive accounts, reviews, letters, research other than basic research (43)
- Nonapplicable topics, or undetermined (4)

His findings:

Of the vast body of retrieved verbiage concerning TT, only five articles actually reported results of basic research (or at least attempts at performing basic research) investigating TT. One of these failed to show any effect of TT but it did not involve human subjects. One paper dismissed negative results as the consequence of medications administered to patients. The remaining three articles claimed positive results but did not adequately design experimental controls to prevent effects of suggestion.

Finally, a $355,225 government grant was awarded several years ago to the University of Alabama at Birmingham to study the effect of TT on burn patients (Selby and Scheiber, 1996). Joan Turner was the UAB nurse who was the principal investigator. She was quoted in the *Birmingham News* as saying: "If we can successfully complete this study, this will be the *first real* scientific evidence there is for therapeutic touch" (Butgereit, 1994, emphasis added). [See also appendix 1 and 2, as well as chapters 13, 18, 19 and 20 in this volume].

REFERENCES

Bullough, V. L., and B. Bullough. 1993. "Therapeutic Touch: Why Do Nurses Believe?" *Skeptical Inquirer* 17: 169–74.

Butgereit, B. 1994. "Therapeutic Touch: UAB to Study Controversial Treatment for Pentagon." *Birmingham News*, November 17, pp. 1A, 10A.

Clark, M. J. 1984. "Therapeutic Touch: Is There a Scientific Basis for Practice? Reply." *Nursing Research* 33 (5): 296–97.

Clark, P. E., and M. J. Clark. 1984. "Therapeutic Touch: Is There a Scientific Basis for the Practice?" *Nursing Research* 33 (1): 3741.

Guerrero, M. A. 1986. "The Effects of Therapeutic Touch on State-Trait Anxiety Level of Oncology Patients." *Masters Abstracts International.* University Microfilms No. 1326756. 24 (3).

Hale, E. H. 1986. "A Study of the Relationship Between Therapeutic Touch and the Anxiety Levels of Hospitalized Adults." *Dissertation Abstracts International.* University Microfilms No. 8618897, 47:1928B.

Heidt, P. 1979. "An Investigation of the Effects of Therapeutic Touch on Anxiety of Hospitalized Patients." *Dissertation Abstracts International.* University Microfilms No. 8010289, 40:52063-5207B.

———. 1981. "Effect of Therapeutic Touch on the Anxiety Level of Hospitalized Patients." *Nursing Research* 30 (1): 32–37.

———. 1990. "Openness: A Qualitative Analysis of Nurses' and Patients' Experiences of Therapeutic Touch." *Image: Journal of Nursing Scholarship* 22 (3): 180–86.

Keller, E. 1983. "The Effects of Therapeutic Touch on Tension Headache Pain." *Masters Abstracts International.* University Microfilms No. 1322168, 22 (4): 372-373.

Kramer, N. A. 1990. "Comparison of Therapeutic Touch and Casual Touch in Stress Reduction of Hospitalized Children." *Pediatric Nursing* 16 (5): 483–85.

Kramer, P. 1993. Letter to the Bristol Press and Rocky Mountain Skeptics (April 24).

Krieger, D. 1975. "Therapeutic Touch: The Imprimatur of Nursing." *American Journal of Nursing* 75 (5): 784–87.

Pomerhn, A. 1987. "The Effect of Therapeutic Touch on Nursing Students' Perceptions of Stress During Clinical Experiences." *Masters Abstracts International.* University Microfilms No. 1330821, 25 (4):362.

Quinn, J. F. 1982. "An Investigation of the Effects of Therapeutic Touch Done without Physical Contact on State Anxiety of Hospitalized Cardiovascular Patients." *Dissertation Abstracts International.* University Microfilms No. DA 82-26-788, 43:1797-B.

———. 1984. "Therapeutic Touch as Energy Exchange: Testing the Theory." *Advances in Nursing Science* 6 (2): 42–49.

———. 1989. "Therapeutic Touch as Energy Exchange: Replication and Extension." *Nursing Science Quarterly* 2 (2): 79–87.

———. 1992. "Therapeutic Touch and Related Findings." Document submitted to the Colorado Nursing Board.

Rocky Mountain Skeptics. 1993. "Evidence Used to Defend Therapeutic Touch." *Rocky Mountain Skeptic* 10 (6): 7–8.

Rosa, L. 1995. "Therapeutic Touch: Skeptics in Hand to Hand Combat over the Latest New Age Health Fad." *Skeptic* 3 (1): 40–49.

Scheiber, B. 1993. "Colorado Board of Nursing Supports Therapeutic Touch, Skeptics Continue Challenge." *Skeptical Inquirer* 17 (3): 327–30.

———. 1994. "University of Colorado Report Critical of Therapeutic Touch." *Skeptical Inquirer* 18 (3): 232–34.

Selby, C., and B. Scheiber. 1996. "Science or Pseudoscience?: Pentagon Grant Funds Alternative Health Study." *Skeptical Inquirer* 20 (3): 15–17.

Turner, J. G., A. J. Clark, D. K. Gauthier et al. 1998. "The Effect of Therapeutic Touch on Pain and Anxiety in Burn Patients." *Journal of Advanced Nursing* 18 (1): 10–20.

22.

Complementary Healing Intervention and Dermal Wound Reepithelialization: An Overview

Daniel P. Wirth

A comparative analysis was conducted on a series of five experiments which examined the effect of complimentary healing to the reepithelialization rate of full thickness human dermal wounds. The treatment intervention focused primarily on Noncontact Therapeutic Touch, which was administered within randomized, double-blind, placebo-controlled experimental protocols. An important methodological component of the studies was that in general the complementary healing practitioners were separated or isolated from the participants and subjects. This design element, coupled with the fact that in four of the five experimental subjects were blinded to the nature of the active treatment modality, resulted in the preclusion of suggestion, expectation, and the placebo effect; the factors which have confounded most prior complementary healing research. The results of the experiments indicated significance for the treatment group in the initial two studies in the series, and nonsignificant and reverse significant results for the control group in the remaining three experiments. Several factors were postulated as important considerations in the differential results obtaining including: (1) cancellation and inhibitory elements, (2) carryover and learning effects, and (3) potential experimenter and placebo effect factors. Although the five studies represent a seminal research effort within the field of complementary healing, the overall results of the series are inconclusive in establishing the efficacy of the treatment interventions examined.

Originally published in *International Journal of Psychosomatics* 42, nos. 1–4 (1995): 48–53. Copyright © 1995 by International Psychosomatics Institute.

INTRODUCTION

The complex biological processes involved in wound regeneration and repair have fascinated and confounded medical researchers since antiquity. The management and treatment of cutaneous wounds was first documented by the ancient Egyptians and recorded in the Smith Surgical Papyrus, one of the oldest known medical treatises, dated at 3000–2500 B.C.E. [1-3] Ancient Sanskrit and Greek writings also made reference to fundamental tenets of wound care, such as the importance of cleanliness, the use of aseptic procedures, and the application of dressings which drained and protected the wound from potential pathogens.[4-6] Although early physicians such as Hippocrates, Herophilus, Celsus, Galen, and others utilized many of the basic principles essential to good wound care, much of our understanding of the biological processes involved in wound healing has been determined within only the last 100 years.[7-11] Studies conducted jointly by health scientists and clinical researchers have established the biochemical, neovascular, and neurological processes necessary for the reconstruction of connective tissue.[5,9,12,13] While the research indicates that the basic mechanisms for tissue regeneration are found in the cells of even the most primitive animals, the repair of human tissue has traditionally been limited to the epithelium, endothelium, skin, bones, and various organs.[12]

Although research in the area has indicated that complex physiological, immunological, and homeostatic factors can influence the human wound healing process,[5,13,14] few studies exist which have examined the potential psychophysiological components of wound regeneration or repair. While the anecdotal complementary healing literature has recognized the potential of alternative or psychophysiological techniques for accelerating the rate of wound healing.[15,16] this premise has only recently been examined experimentally.[17] Among the first controlled laboratory studies to analyze the effect of complementary healing intervention on wound repair was a series of experiments conducted in the early 1960s by Grad and associates[18,19] in which a laying on of hands approach was utilized to increase the rate of reepithelialization of skin biopsy wounds in a murine model. For the next twenty-five years, however, no other studies were conducted in this area until replication efforts initiated in the late 1980s examined the effect of complementary healing intervention on human dermal wounds. This research consisted of a series of five experiments which analyzed the rate of reepithelialization of full thickness human dermal wounds treated primarily with a derivative of the laying on of hands method known as Noncontact Therapeutic Touch.[20-24] The rest of this article is a review of these five studies and indicates that although statistically significant effects were obtained in two of the five studies, the majority demonstrated either statistical nonsignificance or a reverse effect wherein the control condition was significantly more effective than the treatment condition.

TREATMENT INTERVENTION

The primary complementary healing method examined in this series was the medically recognized nursing intervention known as Therapeutic Touch. The TT technique was evaluated either in isolation (S1, S2, S3, S5) or in combination with other complementary healing methods (S4) (table 1). TT was originally derived from the ancient healing practice of the laying on of hands and was first formally conceptualized by Dr. Dolores Krieger and Dora Kunz.[25,26] The method is performed utilizing either direct physical contact (TT) or a noncontact approach (NCTT).[22] The theoretical foundation of TT is based on the Rogerian conceptual model wherein the practitioner and patient are viewed as inseparable components of a complementary multidimensional energy field.[27] Although support for the TT method is based largely on anecdotal evidence and individual case studies, present experimental research has suggested that TT can accelerate the regeneration rate of salamander forelimbs,[28] elevate serum hemoglobin in humans,[26] induce a state of deep relaxation as demonstrated by EEG, EKG, and GSR,[29] decrease "A-state anxiety" and subjective measures of tension headache pain,[30-32] as well as decrease overall muscle tension as indicated by multi-sites EMG analysis.[33,34]

METHODOLOGICAL OVERVIEW

The central hypothesis examined in these studies was that complementary healing intervention can accelerate the rate of reepithelialization of full thickness human dermal wounds. The treatment intervention was administered without physical contact utilizing subjects who were randomly divided into treatment and control groups and assigned to biopsy of the right or left lateral deltoid. An innovative methodological element particular to this series of studies was that in general the complementary healing practitioners were separated or isolated from the experimental participants and subjects with the use of a specially modified door, video monitor apparatus, or a one-way mirror. These design

Table I-The Five Studies

Study 1 (S1)
Subjects: n = 44; age range 21–32 yrs. (avg. = 26).
Wounds/Dressings: 8 mm biopsy wound/occlusive dressing.
Dependent Variable: rate of reepithelialization.
Experimental Design: healer administered treatment from behind door equipped with 10" opening for subject's arm.
Treatment Intervention: NCTT; one healer.
Results: significant for the treatment group.

Study 2 (S2)
Subjects: n = 24; age range 35–63 yrs. (avg. = 47).
Wounds/Dressings: 4 mm biopsy wound/occlusive dressing.
Dependent Variable: rate of *reepithelialization*.
Experimental Design: exact replication of S1 except healer administered treatment from behind door equipped with one-way mirror.
Treatment Intervention: NCTT; one healer.
Results: significant for the treatment group.

Study 3 (S3)
Subjects: n = 25; age range 18–35 yrs. (avg. = 28).
Wounds/Dressings: 4 mm biopsy wound/non-occlusive dressing.
Dependent Variable: rate of reepithelialization.
Experimental Design: within subject crossover design with two sections and four conditions. Healer administered treatment: (1) through one-way mirror; (2) through one-way mirror with plastic sheet covering; (3) via video monitor image with subject in adjacent room on the same floor as the healers; and (4) via video monitor image with subject in separate room below the healers. Subjects also participated in a 1 1/2 hr biofeedback/visualization/relaxation component.
Treatment Intervention: 2 NCTT healers working simultaneously.
Results: nonsignificant.

Study 4 (S4)
Subjects: n = 15; age range 37–61 yrs. (avg. = 43).
Wounds/Dressings: 4 mm biopsy wound/non-occlusive dressing.
Dependent Variable: rate of reepithelialization.
Experimental Design: within subject crossover design with two sections and four conditions including: (1) NCTT treatment in-person while subjects used guided imagery with specific intent to heal wounds, distant LeShan and Intercessory Prayer healers utilized, NCTT healers received Reiki treatment; (2) same as condition 1 except with guided imagery with specific intent to relax; (3) same as condition 2 except mimic practitioners utilized and no distant or Reiki treatment; and (4) same as condition 3 except with guided imagery with specific intent to heal wounds. Ten min biofeedback element included for all four conditions.
Treatment Intervention: Two NCTT healers, LeShan healing group, Intercessory Prayer healing group, Reiki healer.
Results: significant for the control group.

Study 5 (S5)
Subjects: n = 32; age range 23–41 yrs. (avg. = 31).
Wounds/Dressings: 4 mm biopsy wound/occlusive dressing.
Dependent Variable: rate of reepithelialization.
Experimental Design: identical design as S2; healer administered treatment from behind door equipped with one-way mirror.
Treatment Intervention: NCTT; one healer.
Results: significant for the control group.

elements, coupled with the fact that in four of the five studies (S1, S3, S5) subjects were blinded to the nature of the active treatment modality, resulted in the preclusion of suggestion, expectation, and the placebo effect. Although many of the methodological design features were similar between experiments, the results demonstrated by the individual studies varied widely. Differences in experimental protocol and related methodological factors, as demonstrated in the table, were postulated to be important consideration for the differential results obtained.

DISCUSSION

In analyzing the above table, it is apparent that while the five experiments noted introduce a number of innovative methodological design features to the field of complementary healing research, the combined results are less than conclusive in establishing the efficacy of the treatment intervention for the reepithelialization of full thickness dermal wounds. The statistically significant effects demonstrated in the initial two studies, for example, are contrasted and negated by the nonsignificant and reverse significant effects of the remaining three experiments.

A collective analysis of the five studies indicates that similar design features and, in select cases, the same healer and subject population were utilized in order to increase the potential for a statistically significant treatment effect. The outcome of this approach, however, resulted in either nonsignificant or reverse significant effects. The last study in the series (S5), for example, utilized an identical methodological protocol and the same healer as the second study (S2). Yet, the results indicated reverse significance for the control condition. The fourth experiment in the series (S4) incorporated the same subject population as S2. Yet, it also demonstrated reverse significant effects. It was postulated that an integral component of the significance of S2 could have been the fact that the subjects were experienced meditators and practitioners of self-regulatory techniques. In view of this observation, S3 and S4 were designed to incorporate a self-regulatory, biofeedback, visualization element with either a specific intent to relax or a specific intent to heal the wounds.[22,23] The nonsignificance demonstrated in S3 and the reverse significance indicated by S4, however, failed to establish the efficacy of these methods for accelerating the rate of reepithelialization of full thickness dermal wounds.

The potential factors which could have contributed to the reverse and nonsignificant results obtained in S3-S5 include inhibitory, cancellation, carryover, learning, experimenter, and placebo effect confounds.[22-24] An analysis of the data obtained in S5, for example, indicated that the reverse significance demonstrated by the control group could have been due to the ill health of the healer which might have inhibited the wound healing process for the treatment group. Prior anecdotal research has indicated that if the healer is emotionally upset or physically ill, a transference of the state from practitioner to the patient might occur, thereby resulting in not only a nonsignificant treatment effect but, in extreme cases, a disturbance or inhibition of the patient's normal rate of healing.[35-37] This theoretical premise appears to be supported by the fact that the treatment group subjects reported experiencing the same physiological symptoms during the study as the NCTT healer and also concomitantly demonstrated no fully healed wounds. In contrast, the control group subjects exhibited four fully healed wounds with no accompanying ill effects.

In addition, an assessment of the methodological protocol and data obtained in S3 and S4 indicated that the use of multiple healers working simultaneously might have served to reduce or cancel the effectiveness of the treatment intervention. Previous research and anecdotal case reports have in fact suggested that a cancellation or reduction effect might occur when incompatible healers are combined.[22,28] Although the healers utilized in the two studies appeared to be compatible, there was a degree of ego investment involved as to which healing system was superior.

Prior research has established that many forms of complementary healing, including NCTT, Reiki, LeShan, and Intercessory Prayer, can produce physiological effects which might not appear until several days after the patient has received a treatment.[38-42] It was therefore speculated that the significant results demonstrated by the control group subjects during the second section of S4 could have been indicative of a potential carryover treatment effect from the first section. This assertion seems to be supported by the fact that the treatment group demonstrated nonsignificance during the first section of the study, yet indicated significant results when they were in the subsequent control condition a few days later.

Another possible explanation for the reverse significant results of S4 could be that the control group subjects in the second section demonstrated increased proficiency in the use of the self-regulatory healing techniques introduced during the initial treatment condition. Since the techniques were designed to increase the rate of wound healing, the continued utilization of the methods by the subjects during the following control condition could have resulted in the significance demonstrated. Such a learning effect postulate has been established by previous research which indicates that the longer individuals practice self-regulation methods, the more proficient they become at influencing their physiology or, in this case, increasing the rate of reepithe-lialization.[43-46]

Experimenter and/or placebo effect confounds were also intro-duced to explain the reverse significant results of S4. The experimenter effect is essentially a research construct wherein an experimenter has the potential to influence the outcome of a study due to knowledge of the methodological design and their conscious or unconscious inten-tions with other experimental participants and subjects.[47,48] The placebo effect, in comparison, is an integral component of medical research and is commonly defined as a physiological response within the subjects which is mediated by suggestion of improvement and their expectation or belief that the treatment administered will produce a positive therapeutic effect.[49-51] Since this was the only experiment in the series where the subjects and experimenters had complete knowledge of the nature and purpose of the study, as well as the experimental design, it was suggested that these factors could have influenced the results obtained. It should be noted, however, that the double-blind design and the randomized allocation of treatment and control groups should have equally distributed the influence of any potential experi-menter and placebo effect factors between groups. Nevertheless, the mere introduction of these elements into the methodological protocol raises the possibility that they might have influenced the efficacy of the treatment intervention.

The inhibitory, cancellation, carryover, learning, experimenter, and placebo effect explanations introduced above are, at best, theoretical postulates for the reverse significant and nonsignificant effects demon-strated in S3 through S5. An equally valid explanation, however, is that the healing interventions utilized might have been ineffective with the results simply indicating the range of possible outcomes inherent within the research design. Although the final three studies failed to replicate the significance demonstrated in the initial two experiments, the series as a whole nonetheless contained some rather pioneering methodological approaches to the study of complementary healing. The separation or isolation of the practitioner from the subject in four of five studies, for example, coupled with the fact that the subjects were unaware of both group assignment and the nature of the active treatment modality, resulted in the preclusion of suggestion, expecta-tion, and the placebo effect—the factors which have confounded most prior complementary healing research studies.

While the five experiments examined represent a seminal research effort within the field of complementary healing, the overall results remain inconclusive in establishing the efficacy of the treatment inter-ventions examined. Further research is needed in order to either confirm or repudiate the central hypothesis that complementary healing intervention is effective in accelerating the rate of reepithelialization of full thickness human dermal wounds.

REFERENCES

1. Majno, G. *The Healing Hand: Man and Wound in the Ancient World.* Cambridge, Mass.: Harvard University Press, 1975.

2. Breasted, J. H. *The Edwin Smith Surgical Papyrus.* Chicago: University of Chicago Press, 1930.

3. Steinbock, R. T. *Paleopathological Diagnosis and Interpretation: Bone Diseases in Ancient Human Populations.* Springfield, Ill.: Charles C. Thomas, 1976.

4. Bhishagratna, K. K., trans. *Sushrata Samhita. Vols 1–3.* Varanasi, India: Chowkhambra Sanskrit Office, 1963.

5. Brown, H. "Wound Healing Research Through the Ages." In *Wound Healing: Biochemical and Clinical Aspects.* Edited by I. K. Cohen, R. F. Diegelmann, and W. J. Lindlad. London: W. B. Saunders Co., 1992.

6. Garrison, F.J. *An Introduction to the History of Medicine.* Philadelphia: W. B. Saunders Co., 1929.

7. Richards, D.W. "Hippocrates of Ostia." *JAMA* 204 (1968): 1049–56.

8. Adams, F., trans. *The Genuine Works of Hippocrates.* London, 1849.

9. Cohen, I. K., R. F. Diegelmann, and W. J. Lindlad. *Wound Healing: Biochemical and Clinical Aspects.* London: W. B. Saunders Co., 1992.

10. Meinecke, B. "Aulus Cornelius Celsus: Plagiarist or Artifix Medicinae." *Bulletin of the History of Medicine* 10 (1941): 288–298.

11. Siegel, R. E. *Galen's System of Physiology and Medicine.* Basil: Karger, 1960.

12. Hunt, T. K., and J. E. Dunphy. *Fundamentals of Wound Management.* New York: Appleton-Century-Crofts, 1979.

13. Cajal, R. Y. May, R. M. trans., ed. *Degeneration and Regeneration of the Nervous System.* New York: Shafner, 1959.

14. Bell, C. *The Nervous System of the Human Body.* London: Longman, 1830.

15. Krieger, D. *Accepting Your Power to Heal: The Personal Practice of Therapeutic Touch.* Santa Fe, N.Mex.: Bear and Co., 1993.

16. Cousins, N. *The Healing Heart.* New York: W. W. Norton and Co., 1983.

17. Holend-Lund, C. "Effects of Relaxation with Guided Imagery on Surgical Stress and Wound Healing. *Research in Nursing and Health* 11 (1988): 235–44.

18. Grad, B., R. J. Cadoret, and G. J. Paul. "An Unorthodox Method of Treatment of Wound Healing in Mice." *International Journal of Parapsychology* 2 (1961): 5–19.

19. Grad, B. "Some Biological Effects of the Laying on of Hands: A Review of Experiments in Animals and Plants. *Journal of the American Society for Psychical Research* 59 (1965): 95–127.

20. Wirth, D. P. "The Effect of Noncontact Therapeutic Touch on the Healing Rate of Full Thickness Dermal Wounds. *Subtle Energies* 1 (1990): 1–20.

21. Wirth, D. P., J. T. Richardson, W. S. Eidelman, and A. C. O'Malley. "Full Thickness Dermal Wounds Treated with Noncontact Therapeutic Touch: A Replication and Extension. *Complementary Therapies in Medicine* 1 (1993): 127–32.

22. Wirth, D. P., M. J. Barrett, and W. S. Eidelman. "Noncontact Therapeutic Touch and Wound Reepithelialization. *Comp. Therap. Med.* 2 (1994): 187–92.

23. Wirth, D. P., and M. J. Barrett. "Complementary Healing Therapies." *International Journal of Psychosomatics* 41 (1994): 61–67.

24. Wirth, D. P., J. T. Ricardson, R. D. Martinez, W. S. Eidelman, and M. E. Lopez. "Noncontact Therapeutic Touch Intervention and Full Thickness Cutaneous Wounds: A Replication. *Complementary Therapies in Medicine*, in press.

25. Wirth, D. P., R. J. Chang, W. S. Eidelman, and J. B. Paxton. Hematologic Indicators of Complementary Healing Intervention. *Complementary Therapies in Medicine,* in press.

26. Krieger, D. The Imprimatur of Nursing. *American Journal of Nursing* 5 (1975): 784–87.

27. Malinski, V. M., ed. *Explorations on Martha Rogers' Science of Unitary Human Beings.* New York: Appleton-Century-Crofts, 1986.

28. Wirth, D. P., C. A. Johnson, J. S. Horvath, and J. D. MacGregor. "The Effect of Alternative Healing Therapy on the Regeneration Rate of Salamander Forelimbs." *Journal of Scientific Exploration* 6 (1992): 375–91.

29. Krieger, D., E. Peper, and S. Ancoli. "Therapeutic Touch: Searching for Evidence of Physiological Change." *American Journal of Nursing* 4 (1979): 660–62.

30. Heidt, P. R. "Effect of Therapeutic Touch on the Anxiety Level of Hospitalized Patients. *Nursing Research* 30 (1981): 32–37.

31. Quinn, J. F. "Therapeutic Touch as Energy Exchange: Testing the Theory." *Advances in Nursing Science* 6 (1984): 42–49.

32. Keller, E. and V. M. Bzdek. "Effect of Therapeutic Touch on Tension Headache Pain." *Nursing Research* 35 (1986): 101–105.

33. Wirth, D. P., and J. R. Cram. "Multi-site Surface Electromyographic Analysis of Noncontact Therapeutic Touch." *International Journal of Psychosomatics* 40 (1993): 47–55.

34. Wirth, D. P., and J. R. Cram. "The Psychophysiology of Nontraditional Prayer." *International Journal of Psychosomatics* 41 (1994): 68–75.

35. Wirth, D. P. "Healing Expectations: A Study of the Significance of Expectation Within the Healing Encounter." Unpublished master's thesis. John F. Kennedy University, 1987.

36. Frank, J. D. *Persuasion and Healing.* Baltimore: John Hopkins Press, 1973.

37. Meek, G. W. *Healers and the Healing Process.* Wheaton, Ill.: Theosophical Publishing House, 1977.

38. Krieger, D. *Therapeutic Touch: How to Use Your Hands to Help or to Heal.* Englewood Cliffs, N. J.: Prentice-Hall, 1979.

39. Haberly, H. *Reiki: The Hawayo Takatas Story.* California: Archedign Publishers, 1990.

40. Baginski, B. *Reiki: Universal Life Energy.* Life Rhythms, 1988.

41. LeShan, L. *The Medium, the Mystic, and the Physicist.* New York: Viking Press, 1974.

42. Dossey, L. *Healing Words.* New York: Harper Collins, 1993.

43. Achterberg, J., G. F. Lawlis. *Bridges of the Bodymind.* Champaigne, Ill.: I.P.A.T., 1980.

44. Achterberg, J. and Lawlis, G.F. *Imagery and Disease.* Champaigne, Ill.: I.P.A.T., 1984.

45. Basmajian, J. V., ed. *Biofeedback: Principles and Practice for Clinicians.* Baltimore: Williams and Wilkins, 1983.

46. Fotopoulos, S. S., and W. P. Sunderland. "Biofeedback in the Treatment of Psychophysiological Disorders." *Biofeed. Self-Regulation* 3 (1978): 331–61.

47. Rosenthal, R. "Interpersonal Expectance: The Effects of the Experimenter Hypothesis. In *Artifact in Behavioral Research.* Edited by R. Rosenthal and R. Rosnow. New York: Academic Press, 1969.

48. Rosenthal, R., and D. B. Rubin. "Interpersonal Expectancy Effects: The First 345 Studies." *Behavioral and Brain Sciences* 3 (1978): 377–415.

49. White, L., B. Tursky, and G. E. Schwartz, eds. *Placebo, Theory, Research, and Mechanisms.* New York: The Guilford Press, 1985.

50. Wirth, D. P. "The significance of Belief and Expectancy within the Spiritual Healing Encounter." *Social Science and Medicine* 41 (1995): 249–60.

51. Wirth, D. P. "Implementing Spiritual Healing in Modern Medical Practice." *Advances* 9 (1993): 69–81.

23.

The Pseudophysics of Therapeutic Touch*

Victor J. Stenger

Much of alternative medicine, including Therapeutic Touch, is grounded on vitalism, the notion that living organisms possess some unique quality, an *élan vital*, that gives them that special quality we call life. Belief in the existence of a living force is ancient and remains widespread to this day. Called *prana* by the Hindus, *qi* or *chi* by the Chinese, *ki* by the Japanese, and ninety-five other names in ninety-five other cultures (Brennen, 1988), this substance is said to constitute the source of life that is so often associated with soul, spirit, and mind. Wheeler (1939) reviewed the history of vitalism in the West and defined it as "all the various doctrines which, from the time of Aristotle, have described things as actuated by some power or principle additional to mechanics and chemistry." Modern theories of vitalism include those of Driesch (1914) and Bergson (1919).

In ancient times, the vital force was widely identified with breath, which the Hebrews called *ruach*, the Greeks *psyche* or *pneuma* (the breath of the gods), and the Romans *spiritus*. As breath was gradually acknowledged to be a material substance, words like "psychic" and "spirit" evolved to refer to the assumed nonmaterial and perhaps supernatural medium by which organisms gain the qualities of life and consciousness. The idea that matter alone can do the job has never proved popular.

Chi or qi remains the primary concept in traditional Chinese medicine, still widely practiced in China and experiencing an upsurge of interest in the West. Chi is a living force that is said to flow rhythmically

*This chapter is based on an earlier work by the author which appeared as "The Physics of 'Alternative Medicine': Bioenergetic Fields," in *Scientific Review of Alternative Medicine* 3, no. 1 (spring/summer 1999). Copyright © 1999 Prometheus Books. The author is grateful for very helpful comments from Benedict Adamson, Dr. Stephen Barrett, Paul Bernhardt, Keith Douglas, Robert G. Grimes, Jim Humphreys, Peter Huston, and Dr. David Ramey.

through so-called "meridians" in the body. Acupuncture and acupressure are used to stimulate the flow at special acu-points along these meridians although their location has never been consistently specified. The chi force is not limited to the body but is believed to flow throughout the environment (Huston, 1995). When building a house, many believers rely on a master to decide on an orientation that is well-aligned with this flow.

As modern science developed in the West and the nature of matter was gradually uncovered, a few scientists sought scientific evidence for the nature of the living force. After Newton had published his laws of mechanics, optics, and gravity, he spent many years looking for the source of life in alchemic experiments. His search was not irrational, given the knowledge of the day. Newtonian physics provided no basis for the complexity that is necessary for any purely material theory of life or mind. This requires quantum physics. Since Newtonian gravity had an occult quality about it with its invisible action at a distance, perhaps the forces of life and thought had similar immaterial properties. Still, Newton and others who followed the same trail never managed to uncover a signal for a special substance of spirit or life.

In the late nineteenth century, prominent scientists, including William Crookes and Oliver Lodge, sought scientific evidence for what they called the "psychic force" that they believed was responsible for the mysterious powers of the mind being exhibited by the mediums and spiritualist hucksters of the day. They thought it might be connected with the electromagnetic "aether waves" that had just been discovered and were being put to amazing use. If wireless telegraphy was possible, why not wireless telepathy? This was a reasonable question at the time. However, while wireless telegraphy thrived, wireless telepathy made no progress in the full century of uncorroborated experiments in "parapsychology" that followed (Stenger, 1990).

Conventional medicine follows conventional biology, conventional chemistry, and conventional physics in treating the material body—a complex, nonlinear system assembled from the same atoms and molecules that constitute (presumably) nonliving objects such as computers and automobiles. Medical doctors are in some sense glorified mechanics who repair broken parts in the human machine. Indeed, any stay in the hospital reinforces this image since you are hooked to devices that measure blood pressure, temperature, oxygen saturation, and many other physical parameters. You are almost always treated with drugs that are designed to alter your body's chemistry. You usually get better, every time but once, but, unless you are a physicist, you tend to view the whole experience rather negatively.

No surprise, then, that alternative practitioners such as touch therapists find many eager listeners when they announce that they go beyond materialism and mechanism and treat the really important part of the human system—the vital substance of life itself. People's religious sensibilities and images of self-worth are greatly mollified when they are told that they are far more than an assemblage of atoms—that they possess a living field that is linked to both God and cosmos. Furthermore, the desperately ill will quite naturally seek out hope wherever they can find it. So a ready market exists for therapists who claim that they can succeed where medical science fails.

UNIFIED BIOFIELD THEORY

The hypothetical vital force is often referred to these days as the bioenergetic field. Touch therapists along with acupuncturists, chiropractors, and many other alternative practitioners tell us that they can affect cures for many ills by "manipulating" this field thereby bringing the body's "life energies" into balance.

The use of "bioenergetic" in this context is somewhat ambiguous. This term is applied in conventional biochemistry to refer to the readily measurable exchanges of energy within organisms, and between them and their environment, which occur by normal physical and chemical processes. This is not, however, what the new vitalists have in mind. They imagine the bioenergetic field as a holistic living force that goes beyond reductionist physics and chemistry.

By "holistic" here, I am not referring to trivial homilies such as the need to treat the patient as a whole and recognize that many factors, such as the psychological, emotional, and social, contribute to well-being along with the physical body. While this is often the example used by those who claim to practice holistic medicine, they imply that something much more is at work in their treatments. Treating the whole person does not contradict any reductionist principles. Neither does the fact that the parts of a physical system interact with one another. Reductionism is not about a universe of isolated objects. The holism that goes beyond reductionism implies a universe of objects that interact simultaneously and so strongly that none can ever be treated separately. This concept enters into the discussion of bioenergetic fields where that field is imagined as some cosmic aether that pervades the universe and acts instantaneously, faster than the speed of light, over all of space.

Therapeutic Touch and other forms of "holistic healing" are now widely practiced within the nursing community (Rosa, 1994, 1998; Scheiber, 1997; Ulett, 1997; Pryjmachuk, 1998). It seems to be based on a theoretical system called "The Science of Unitary Human Beings" proposed by Martha Rogers (1970, 1986, 1989, 1990). According to Rogers, "energy fields are postulated to constitute the fundamental unit of the living and nonliving." The field is "a unifying concept and energy signifies the dynamic nature of the field. Energy fields are infinite and pandimensional; they are in continuous motion" (Rogers, 1990, p. 30). However, as Stranwick notes [see chapter 5 in this volume], the energy field that Rogers talks about is apparently not the same one that touch therapists imagine.

The exact nature of the bioenergetic field is not unambiguously specified, even as a speculative hypothesis, in Rogers or the other literature on holistic healing. On the one hand, the biofield seems to be identified with the classical electromagnetic field; on the other it is confused with quantum fields or wave functions. For example, Stefanatos (1997, p. 227) writes: "The principles of energy medicine originate in quantum physics. Bioenergetic medicine is the study of human and animal bodies as dynamic electromagnetic fields existing in an electromagnetic environment" (1997, p. 227).

AURAS AND DISCHARGES

Perhaps the most specific model for the bioenergetic field is as some special form of electromagnetism. Advocates claim that measurable electromagnetic waves are emitted by humans.

In the *Journal of Advanced Nursing*, Patterson relates "spiritual healing" to the belief that "we are all part of the natural harmonious energy of the universe." Within this universal energy field is a human energy field "that is intimately involved with human life, often called the 'aura' " (Patterson 1998, p. 291).

Some self-described psychics claim that they can "see" a human aura. The claim has not been substantiated (Loftin, 1990). Indeed, humans do have auras that can be photographed with infrared-sensitive film. However, this can be trivially identified as "black body" electromagnetic radiation. Everyday objects that reflect very little light will appear black. These bodies emit invisible infrared light that is the statistical result of the random thermal movements of all the charged particles in the body. The wavelength spectrum has a characteristic smooth shape completely specified by the body's absolute temperature. As that temperature rises, the spectrum moves into the visible. The sun, for example, radiates largely as a "black body" of temperature 6,000 K, with a broad peak at the center of the visible spectrum in the yellow. At their much lower body temperatures, humans radiate mostly in the infrared region of the spectrum that is invisible to the naked eye but easily seen with infrared detection equipment.

The inability of the wave theory of light to explain the black body spectrum led in 1900 to Planck's conjecture that light comes in bundles of energy called "quanta," thus triggering the quantum revolution. These quanta are now recognized as material photons. It is somewhat ironic that holists find such comfort in quantum mechanics which replaced etherial waves with material particles. Surely black body radiation is not a candidate for the bioenergetic field, for then even the cosmic microwave background, 2.7K radiation left over from the big bang, would be "alive." Black body radiation lacks any of the complexity we associate with life. It is as featureless as it can be and still be consistent with the laws of physics. Any fanciful shapes seen in photographed auras emanating from humans can be attributed to optical and photographic effects uncorrelated with any property of the body that one might identify as "live" rather than "dead," and the tendency for people to see patterns where none exist.

Stefanatos tells us that the "electromagnetic fields (EMF) emanating from bacteria, viruses, and toxic substances affect the cells of the body and weaken its constitution" (1997, p. 228). So the vital force is identified quite explicitly with electromagnetic fields and said to be the cause of disease. But somehow the life energies of the body are balanced by bioenergetic therapies. "No antibiotic or drug, no matter how powerful, will save an animal if the vital force of healing is suppressed or lacking" (Stefanatos, 1997, p. 229). So health or sickness is determined by who wins the battle between good and bad electromagnetic waves in the body.

Now it would seem that all these effects of electromagnetic fields in living things would be easily detectable, given the great precision with which electromagnetic phenomena can be measured in the laboratory. Physicists have measured the magnetic dipole moment of the electron (a measure of the strength of the electron's magnetic field) to one part in ten billion and calculated it with the same accuracy. They surely should be able to detect any electromagnetic effects in the body powerful enough to move atoms around or do whatever happens in causing or curing disease. But neither physics nor any other science has seen anything that demands we go beyond well established physical theories. No elementary particle or field has been found that is uniquely biological. None is even hinted at in the data from our most powerful detectors.

Besides the infrared black body radiation already mentioned, electromagnetic waves at other frequencies are detected from the brain and other organs. As mentioned, these are often claimed as "evidence" for the bioenergetic field. In conventional medicine, they provide powerful diagnostic information. But these electromagnetic waves show no special characteristics that differentiate them from the electromagnetic waves produced by moving charges in any electronic system. Indeed, they can be simulated with a computer. No marker has been found that uniquely labels the waves from organisms "live" rather than "dead."

Kirlian Photography is often cited as evidence for the existence of fields unique to living things. For example, Patterson (1998) claims that the "seven or more layers within an aura, each with its own color," have been recorded using Kirlian photography.

Semyon Davidovich Kirlian was an Armenian electrician who discovered in 1937 that photographs of live objects placed in a pulsed high electromagnetic field will show a remarkable surrounding "aura." In the typical Kirlian experiment, an object such as a freshly cut leaf is placed on a piece of photographic film that is electrically isolated from a flat aluminum electrode with a piece of dielectric material. A pulsed high voltage is applied between another electrode placed in contact with the object and the aluminum electrode. The film is then developed.

The resulting photographs indicate dynamic, changing patterns with multicolored sparks, twinkles, and flares (Ostrander, 1970; Moss, 1974). Dead objects do not have such lively patterns! In the case of a leaf, the pattern is seen to gradually go away as the leaf dies, emitting cries of agony during its death throes. Ostrander and Schroeder described what Kirlian and his wife observed: "As they watched, the leaf seemed to be dying before their very eyes, and the death was reflected in the picture of the energy impulses." The Kirlians reported that "we appeared to be seeing the very life activity of the leaf itself" (Ostrander, 1970, p. 200).

As has been amply demonstrated, the Kirlian aura is nothing but corona discharge, reported as far back as 1777 and completely understood in terms of well-known physics. Controlled experiments have demonstrated that claimed effects, such as the cries of agony of a dying leaf, are sensitively dependent on the amount of moisture present. As the leaf dies, it dries out, lowering its electrical conductivity. The same effect can been seen with a long dead but initially wet piece of wood (Pehek, 1976; Singer, 1981; Watkins, 1988, 1989).

Once again, like the infrared aura, we have a well-known electromagnetic phenomenon being paraded in front of innocent lay people who may be unfamiliar with basic physics, as "evidence" for a living force. It is nothing of the sort. Proponents of alternative medicine would have far fewer critics among conventional scientists if they did not resort to this kind of dishonesty and foolishness. (For more discussion of Kirlian photography, see Stenger, 1990, pp. 237–41).

QUANTUM HEALING

"Quantum" is the magic incantation that appears in virtually everything written on alternative medicine. It seems to be uttered in order to make all the inconsistencies, incoherencies, and incompatibilities of the proposed scheme disappear in a puff of smoke. Since quantum mechanics is weird, anything weird must be quantum mechanics.

Quantum mechanics is claimed as support for mind-over-matter solutions to health problems. The way the observer is entangled with the object being observed in quantum mechanics is taken to infer that human consciousness actually controls reality. As a consequence, we can all think ourselves into health and, indeed, immortality—if we only buy this book (Chopra, 1989, 1993). "Quantum healing" is based on a particularly misleading interpretation of quantum mechanics (Stenger, 1997). Other interpretations exist that do not require any mystical ingredients (see also Stenger, 1995).

"Einstein" is a name found frequently in the literature on energy therapy. Stephantos says: "Based on Einstein's theories of quantum physics, these energetic concepts are being integrated into medicine for a comprehensive approach to disease diagnosis, prevention, and treatment" (1997, p. 228).

Einstein's theories of quantum physics? What theories are these? While Einstein contributed mightily to the development of quantum mechanics, especially with his photon theory, modern quantum mechanics is the progeny of a large group of early twentieth century physicists. Planck, Bohr, de Broglie, Heisenberg, Schrödinger, Pauli, Born, Jordan, and Dirac each made contributions to quantum mechanics at least as important as Einstein's. Einstein's immortality rests securely enough on his two theories of relativity.

Referring to well-known promoters of quantum mysticism Fritjof Capra and Ken Wilber, Stefanatos tells how "Einstein's quantum model replaced the Newtonian mechanistic model of humankind and the universe" (1997, p. 227). Thus holistic healing is associated with the rejection of classical Newtonian physics. Yet, holistic healing retains many ideas about the aether and action at a distance from eighteenth and nineteenth century physics. Its proponents appear blissfully unaware that these ideas have been rejected by modern physics.

Never mind that Einstein was not the inventor of quantum mechanics and objected strongly to its anti-Newtonian character, saying famously, "God does not play dice." Never mind that electromagnetic fields were around well before quantum physics and it was Einstein himself who proposed that they are composed of reductionist particles. And never mind that Einstein did away with the aether, the medium that nineteenth-century physicists thought was doing the waving in an electromagnetic wave, and a few others thought might also be doing the waving for "psychic waves." The bioenergetic field described in holistic literature seems to be confused with the aether. Or, perhaps no confusion is implied. They each share at least one common feature—nonexistence.

As the nineteenth century drew to a close, experiments by Michelson and Morley had failed to find evidence for the aether. This laid the foundation for Einstein's theory of relativity and his photon theory of light, both published in 1905. Electromagnetic radiation is now understood to be a fully material phenomenon. Photons have both inertial and gravitational mass (even though they have zero rest mass) and exhibit all the characteristics of material bodies. Electromagnetism is as material as breath and an equally incredible candidate for the vital field.

Much as we might wish otherwise, the fact remains that no unique living force has ever been conclusively demonstrated to exist in scientific experiments. Of course, evidence for a life force might someday be found but this is not what is claimed in the literature that promotes Therapeutic Touch and the myriads of other forms of alternative medicine. There you will see the strong assertion that current scientific evidence exists for some entity beyond conventional matter and that this claim is supported by modern physical theory—especially quantum mechanics. Furthermore, the evidence is not to be found in the data from our most powerful telescopes or particle accelerators, probing beyond existing frontiers. Rather, it resides in vague, imprecise, anecdotal claims of the alleged curative powers of traditional folk remedies and other nostrums. These claims simply do not follow from any reasonable application of scientific criteria.

The bioenergetic field plays no role in the theory or practice of biology or scientific medicine. Vitalism and bioenergetic fields remain hypotheses not required by the data, to be rejected by Occam's razor until the data demand otherwise.

REFERENCES

Ball, T. S., and D. A. Dean. 1998. "Catching up with Eighteenth-Century Science in the Evaluation of Therapeutic Touch." *Skeptical Inquirer* 22 (4): 31–34.

Bergson, H. 1911. *Creative Evolution*. New York: Macmillan.

Brennen, B. A. 1988. *Hands of Light: A Guide to Healing Through the Human Energy Field*. New York: Bantam New Age Books.

Driesch, H. 1914. *History and Theory of Vitalism*. New York: Macmillan.

Huston, P. 1995. "China, Chi, Chicanery: Examining Traditional Chinese Medicine and Chi Theory." *Skeptical Inquirer* 19 (5): 38–42, 58.

Loftin, R. W. 1990. "Auras: Searching for the Light." *Skeptical Inquirer* 14 (4): 403–409.

Meehan, T. C. 1985. "The Effect of Therapeutic Touch on the Experiences of Acute Pain in Postoperative Patients." Unpublished doctoral dissertation, New York University.

Moss, T. 1974. *The Probability of the Impossible*. Los Angeles, Calif.: Tarcher.

Ostrander, S., and L. Schroeder. 1970. *Psychic Discoveries Beyond the Iron Curtain*. Englewood Cliffs, N.J.: Prentice-Hall.

Patterson, E. 1998. "The Philosophy and Physics of Holistic Health Care: Spiritual Healing as a Workable Interpretation." *Journal of Advanced Nursing* 27: 287–93.

Pehek, J. O., H. J. Kyler, and D. L. Faust. 1976. "Image Modulation in Corona Discharge Photography." *Science* 194: 263–70.

Pryjmachuk, S., D. P. O'Mathúna, W. Spencer, M. Stanwick, and S. Matthiesen. 1998. "Therapeutic Touch: Misusing Science to Justify Non Science." Submitted to *Research in Nursing and Health*.

Rogers, M. 1970. *The Theoretical Basis for Nursing*. Philadelphia, Pa.: F.A. Davies.

———. 1986. "Science of Unitary Human Beings." In *Explorations of Martha Rogers' Science of Unitary Human Being*. Edited by V. M. Malinski. Norwark: Appleton-Century-Crofts.

———. 1989. "Nursing: A Science of Unitary Human Beings." In *Conceptual Models for Nursing Practice*. 3d ed. Edited by J. P. Riehl-Sisca. Norwark: Appleton & Lange.

———. 1990. "Nursing: Science of Unitary, Irreducible, Human Beings." In *Visions of Rogers' Science-Based Nursing*. Edited by E. A. M. Barrett. New York: National League for Nursing.

———. 1992. "Nursing Science and the Space Age." *Nursing Science Quarterly* 5 (1): 27–34.

Rosa, L. A. 1994. "Therapeutic Touch." *Skeptic* 3 (1): 40–49.

Rosa, L., E. Rosa, L. Sarner, and S. Barrett. 1998. "A Close Look at Therapeutic Touch." *JAMA* 279: 1005–10.

Scheiber, B. 1997. "Therapeutic Touch: Evaluating the 'Growing Body of Evidence' Claim." *Scientific Review of Alternative Medicine* 1 (1): 13–15.

Singer, B. 1981. "Kirlian Photography." In *Science and the Paranormal*. Edited by O. Abell, B. Singer. New York: Scribners.

Stefanatos, J. 1997. "Introduction to Bioenergetic Medicine." In *Complementary and Alternative Veterinary Medicine: Principles and Practice*. Edited by A. Schoen, S. Wynn. Mosby-Year Book.

Stenger, V. J. 1990. *Physics and Psychics: The Search for a World Beyond the Senses*. Amherst, N.Y.: Prometheus Books.

———. 1995. *The Unconscious Quantum: Metaphysics in Modern Physics and Cosmology*. Amherst, N.Y.: Prometheus Books.

———. 1997a. "Quantum Quackery." *Skeptical Inquirer* 21 (1): 37–40.

———. 1997b. "Quantum Mysticism." *Scientific Review of Alternative Medicine* 1 (1): 26–30.

Ulett G. 1997. "Therapeutic Touch: Tracing Back to Mesmer." *Scientific Review of Alternative Medicine* 1 (1): 16–18.

Watkins, A., and W. Bickel. 1986. "A Study of the Kirlian Effect." *Skeptical Inquirer* 10 (3): 244–57.

———. 1989. The Kirlian Technique: Controlling the Wild Cards." *Skeptical Inquirer* 13 (2): 172–84.

Wheeler, L. R. 1930. *Vitalism: Its History and Validity*. London: Witherby.

Section 3.
Appendices

Appendix I.

Memorandum from Uniformed Services University of the Health Sciences

Memorandum

To: LTC. William L. Daniels
           Director, Research Administration
           Uniformed Services University of the Health Sciences

From: Dr. Joan Turner (LTC, USAR, NC)
           Professor, University of Alabama School of Nursing

Date: July 28, 1994

Subject: N94-020 "The Effect of Therapeutic Touch on Pain and Infection in Burn Patients"

In response to your agency's invitation dated June 30, 1994, we are submitting a revision of proposal N94-020 "The Effect of Therapeutic Touch on Pain and Infection in Burn Patients." Enclosed you will find the original and twelve copies. In this revision is reflected our thoughtful consideration of the Scientific Review Panel's critique. Changes and/or elaborations as a result of the panel's review are highlighted in boldface type in the proposal and are outlined in this memorandum as follows.

1. *Criticism*—"The precision and accuracy of the biological parameters are not addressed. . . ."

Response—It was a fairly simple matter to obtain the accuracy of the proposed biologic parameters (i.e., sensitivity and specificity). Having done that, we reconsidered the whole notion of obtaining selected biologic parameters on only 20 percent of the subject population. Although test results may have been useful to investigators as a means of supporting or refuting the conceptual framework and as pilot data for subsequent study, we opted to discard the notion of physiological measures that would ultimately not meet power requirements. The only other options would be to draw venous blood samples on all 150 subjects. This option was discarded because: 1) it would require venipuncture (a painful procedure) on 80 percent or $N = 120$ subjects, and 2) it would have required another $30,000 to be added to the budget.

2a. *Criticism*—"There is mention of medication for pain but how this will be controlled needs to be addressed in sufficient detail."

Response—In this study, Therapeutic Touch (TT) is conceptualized as an *adjunct*, rather than a replacement, to administration of physician-ordered analgesia. We feel this approach is particularly appropriate in light of the fact that pain is not consistently relieved [*sic*] by analgesia alone for many burn patients. Patient receipt of pain medication per twenty-four hour period will be recorded (see Patient Data Sheet, Page 6, Appendix A [in original]). Totals of pain medication received by subjects (expressed as morphine equilivants [*sic*]) will be treated statistically as both a covariate and an outcome variable. It is hypothesized that subjects who receive TT will receive significantly less pain medication.

2b. *Criticism*—". . . the proposal needs to address the degree or depth and percent of burns in relationship to potential problems, e.g., infection, more pain, etc."

Response—As discussed in the BACKGROUND section (page 37), the relationship between pain *perceived* by the burn victim and the depth and percentage of the burned area is complex. For example, Choiniere and colleagues (1989) reported the following: (1) the onset of pain varied among burn patients, (2) burn patients who were more anxious or depressed tended to report more pain at rest, (3) variables such as age, socioeconomic status and educational level were not good predictors of perceived pain, (4) the most severe pain tended to be reported during procedures such as dressing changes, and (5) there was no correlation between pain scores and burn sizes or the extent of injury.

The relationship between infection and depth and percentage of burn injury appears to be somewhat more straightforward. In essence, the greater the body surface involved and the greater the depth of the burn wound, the greater the chance of nosocomial infection (NI). Patient characteristics such as age, type, and severity of underlying illness and external factors such as the skill of the surgical team during debridement and skin grafting affect the risk of NI. Because underlying illness, extreme age, and factors such as being ventilator-dependent have the potential for greatly increasing risk for NI, subject selection criteria (p. 46) dictate disqualifying subjects who are over the age of sixty-five, have a preexisting health problem such as diabetes or one that compromises immunologic or neurologic function, or are ventilator-dependent. Finally, the percent of total body surface burned and burn depth, like demographic variables and total pain medication, will be treated as covariates during data analysis (see page 51).

3. *Criticism*—"The proposal is not clear as to exactly what intervention the control group is receiving. . . ."

Response—A placebo intervention consisting of a mimic TT treatment has been designed and is described in the DESIGN AND METHODS section (p 49). All control subjects will receive mimic treatment.

4. *Criticism*—"The number of subjects needed to participate . . . (in) 8 months may be difficult to achieve."

Response—One way to increase the subject population would be to include burn patients from another facility. However, after careful deliberation, this option was discarded because utilization of another site would introduce a host of confounding variables such as differing medical treatment, nursing management, and other environmental factors. Thus, to keep our study population as homogeneous as possible, we will not use another data collection site. However, the PI and coinvestigators have the resources and skills necessary to initiate data collection upon notification of funding while simultaneously recruiting other project staff. Thus, we have modified the projected timeline so that data can be collected over the entire twelve months of funding. As a failsafe, this same group could continue to collect data should we be short of the required number of subjects at the end of the funding period.

5. *Criticism*—"There may not be enough power . . . to make conclusions based on the biologic measurements. . . . The measurements of endorphins and suppressor T-lymphocytes and their *connectedness* with the intervention are crucial."

Response—As stated in the response to Criticism 1, we have discarded the plan for collecting blood for biologic measures. Collection of biologic measures will be pursued in future proposals.

6. *Criticism*—"The effect of TT will be difficult to substantiate if a mimic group is not added. . . ."

Response—A mimic group has been added and is described in the DESIGN AND METHODS section, page 49.

7. *Criticism*—"The review of the literature states that the results of Meehan's 1993 study demonstrated that TT relieves pain." It is the impression of the panel members that this study did not support this finding.

Response—In the 1993 Meehan study, "Therapeutic Touch and Postoperative Pain: A Rogerian Research Study," it is reported that a reduction (in pain) occurred in the TT group, whereas there was no reduction in the MTT (mimic TT) scores (Meehan, p. 73). The author also reported that SI (standard intervention, i.e., narcotic analgesia) "is much more effective than TT" (Meehan, p. 74). Meehan further reported that subjects in the TT group waited a significantly longer time before requesting further pm analgesia medication compared with subjects in the MTT group (Meehan, pp. 74–75). In the discussion section of the article, she suggested that "it is possible that TT may reduce the need for narcotic analgesia, or if TT is administered with narcotic analgesia, it may potentiate the effect" (Meehan, p. 75).

Using the results of this study as one of the background studies for this project, we reasoned that the TT project intervention used by Meehan was perhaps not strong enough (the strength of the TT intervention that relieved a tension headache might not be strong enough to impact the more severe postoperative pain). For this project, we have therefore designed a stronger TT intervention.

Secondly, Meehan's suggestion that TT may reduce the need for narcotic analgesia or potentiate its effect was used as the basis for designing the TT intervention as an adjunct to narcotic analgesia. In the pain induced by burn injury narcotic analgesia alone has not consistently produced pain relief Thus an effective adjunct to narcotic analgesia is needed for these patients.

Although it was not identified as a criticism and does not affect the total sample size required, we wanted to mention the reason we have changed the effect size for the power analysis. More extensive review of studies utilizing TT for pain relief revealed a 66 percent decrease in perceived headache pain reported by researchers. Since we are dealing with a different type of pain, but a stronger intervention, we estimate that the percentage decrease in pain in our study will be approximately 30 percent. Utilizing this to calculate an effect size of 0.33, we can increase power to 0.82 (see discussion under Power Analysis, p. 46).

In summary, we are grateful to the Review Panel and your agency for allowing us the rare opportunity to revise and resubmit for funding consideration. We found the critique valuable and have made every effort to revise accordingly. We look forward to your feedback.

Appendix 2.

Tri-Service Nursing Research Grant Final Report

Date: May 20,1996

Principal investigator: Joan G. Turner, D.S.N., R.N., C.I.C. (LTC, USAR, NC)

Grant number: MDA 905-94-Z-0080

Title: The Effect of Therapeutic Touch on Pain and Infection in Burn Patients

Date project initiated: 1 October 94

Period covered by this report: From 21 October 94 T0 30 March 96

FINAL PROGRESS REPORT

I. SYNOPSIS

A. Purpose with Specific Aims

1. Recruit 150 subjects aged 15 to 65 years of age, and randomly assign them to either the treatment or control group.
2. Compare the effects of therapeutic touch (TT) on the outcomes of pain perception and nosocomial infection (NI).
3. Develop and test a TT protocol for use as an adjunct to narcotic analgesia in lowering pain levels and the incidence of infection in burn patients.

B. Methods—This study was a randomized clinical trial utilizing Roger's conceptual model

C. Results with regard to Specific Aims

1. A total of 131 patients were recruited during the eighteen months of the study. Not all of these subjects actually remained in the study for the full six-day period.

2. Statistical analysis revealed the following findings.

   A. In the group completing the study, three NIs occurred among subjects during or after TT and one NI occurred in the sham group. This total infection rate is far below national averages for bum patients.

   B. When subjects' perception of pain was compared on days one versus six, and adjusting for numerous covariables such as pain medication, the treatment group had a more favorable score than did the sham subjects utilizing the McGill pain rating scale ($p = 0.018$).

      When pain was measured by the Visual Analogue Scale (VAS), no statistically significant difference was found between groups.

      When pain was measured immediately before and after TT or sham on day three, subjects in the TT group again showed a statistically significant better outcome ($p = 0.038$). Anxiety, as measured by a VAS between days one and six, was lower among treatment than sham subjects ($p = 0.06$).

      Physiologic indicators: A very small percentage of subjects had complete data sets, i.e., blood samples for days one and six. The only statistically significant finding in T-cell counts was the fact that the control group had a greater rise in T-8s from day one to six than did the experimental group ($p = 0.036$). The interpretation of this finding is that it is possible that TT acts to suppress cytotoxic cell production.

      Many of the subjects who were willing and available to have both day one and six blood draws showed very small numbers of endorphins (as measured by the laboratory scale). A nonparametric test showed that there was no statistically significant difference between controls and experiment subjects.

D. Additional research is currently being conducted to assist us in arriving at a maximal protocol for the administration of TT to subjects.

II. PROBLEMS ENCOUNTERED

One of the biggest barriers to collection of physiologic measures related to the fact that many patients did not have either central or venous lines by the time day six of the study occurred. Frequently, they requested not to be "stuck again."

The greatest lesson learned from this process is that the inclusion of a true control group in addition to a sham and treatment group is required because a strong placebo effect occurs from the special attention given to patients in the "sham" treatment.

Another problem related to the fact that admissions to the burn unit for the study period were decreased over previous years. With fewer admissions and stringent subject selection criteria, we were unable to enroll a total of 150 subjects (N = 131).

Another problem encountered was publicity and harassment by a religious group called the Watchmen. Because of the controversial nature of Therapeutic Touch, newspaper, radio, and TV publicity followed awarding of the original grant (see enclosed examples). As a result of the publicity, a religious group called the Watchmen was alerted, and subsequently took measures to stop the research and/or discredit it. Among the actions taken by this group were:

1. Complaining that Federal money was used to fund the project to Senator Shelby, (AL) who subsequently staged a congressional inquiry and made several calls to the UAB Center for Nursing Research regarding same.
2. Contacting University officials suggesting scientific misconduct *in* the project. (No details on this have ever been given).
3. Held a televised press conference charging that Therapeutic Touch is not effective and therefore no further research needed to be done.
4. Formed a National Therapeutic Touch Study group and placed misleading advertisements in local papers (see enclosed advertisement) to contact our research subjects.
5. Have made repeated requests to the Provost at UAB to meet with investigators on the project and University officials before findings from the research are released.

III. SIGNIFICANCE TO MILITARY NURSING

Therapeutic Touch is a nursing measure which is non pharmacologic and produces no side effects. This therapy can be used to decrease subjects' perception of pain as either a one time or series of days intervention.

IV. PUBLICATIONS, ABSTRACTS, AND PRESENTATIONS RESULTING FROM THIS PROJECT

1. "Therapeutic Touch Research at UAB" by Ann J. Clark Ph.D., R.N., at Invited Advanced Healers' Conference, Pumpkin Hollow Farm, Garyville, NY, July, 1995.
2. Research in Progress. "The Effect of Therapeutic Touch on Pain and Infection in Burn Patients" by Ann J. Clark, Ph.D. R.N. Networking session at the annual conference, Nurse Healers, Professional Associates, Kona-Kailua, HI, October 19, 1995.
3. "Therapeutic Touch Research" to be presented by Ann J. Clark, Ph.D., R.N., at the Troy State Nurses' Alumni Association, Montgomery AL, May 25,1996.
4. "Therapeutic Touch for Burned Patients" to be presented by Ann J. Clark, Ph.D., R.N., at the annual conference Nurse Healers' Professional Associates, Waterville, Valley, NH, October 20, 1996.

Appendix 3.

Report of the Chancellor's Committee on Therapeutic Touch (Claman Report)

Date: July 6, 1994

To: Vincent Fulginiti, M.D., Chancellor, UCHSC

From: Henry N. Claman, Chair, Committee on Therapeutic Touch

Re: Report of the Chancellor's Committee on Therapeutic Touch (CCTT)

On the advice of the Academic Relevance Committee, Chancellor Fulginiti appointed a committee on Therapeutic Touch (referred to as TT). This committee is composed of:

- Robert Freedman, M.D., Professor of Psychiatry, UCHSC, Denver, CO
- David Quissell, Ph.D., Professor and Chair, Dept. of Basic Sciences and Oral Research, School of Dentistry, UCHSC, Denver, CO
- Joan Fowler-Shaver, Ph.D., R.N., Professor and Chairperson, Dept. of Physiological Nursing, University of Washington, Seattle, WA
- Ora Lea Strickland, Ph.D., Independence Foundation Research Chair and Professor, Nell Hodgson Woodruff School of Nursing, Emory University, Atalanta [sic], GA
- Henry N. Claman, M.D., Distinguished Professor of Medicine and Immunology, UCHSC, Denver, *Chair*

Dr. Fulginiti asked the TT Committee to consider the role of TT in the curriculum of the Center for Human Caring (CHC), School of Nursing (SN), UCHSC and the rationale for the practice and theory of TT.

The TT Committee, in whole or in part, met with:

- Chancellor Vincent Fulginiti, M.D.
- Janet Quinn, Ph.D., R.N., FAAN, Associate Professor of Nursing, CHC, UCHSC
- Jean Watson, Ph.D., R.N., FAAN, Distinguished Professor of Nursing, CHC, UCHSC
- Clair E. Martin, Ph.D., Dean, School of Nursing, UCHSC
- Representatives of the Rocky Mountain Skeptics and other skeptical members of the public.

The TT Committee reviewed the set of three videotapes featuring Dr. Janet Quinn and produced under the auspices of the National League of Nursing.

The TT Committee held an open meeting in April, 1994; forty-two people attended and fourteen people spoke about TT.

TT Committee members received letters, telephone calls, reprints, books and brochures from the TT practitioners (SN) as well as from other sources across the United States.

The meetings of the TT Committee occurred between January and June, 1994. This report was produced during May and June, 1994.

INTRODUCTION

TT is a method that perports to use the hands to help or to heal. It is a derivative of the laying on of hands. In the variety of TT used and taught at the CHC, SON, UCHSC, the practitioner's hands do not touch the patient or client. This has been called Non-Contact TT and it is the only form of TT that is considered in this report. TT is practiced by faculty members at the SON, as well as by nurses, physicians and others in the community at large, in Colorado and elsewhere. TT is taught in elective courses at the SON, and students there have written Ph.D. theses which primarily use or investigate TT. Some investigative work on TT has been done at the SON.

It is fair to say that both the theory and the practice of TT are controversial. TT is not a generally accepted healing modality. There is disagreement about its efficacy both within and outside the nursing profession. There are firm believers in the efficacy of TT as it is practiced as well as firm skeptics who question the validity of both the theory and the practice of TT. There is a significant but not extensive amount of literature—scientific, lay press, news media, etc.—which describes in detail both support of and nonbelief in TT.

In considering as many aspects as time permitted, the TT Committee made the following comments.

A. ACADEMIC FREEDOM

The teaching of Therapeutic Touch is an academic activity of the School of Nursing that is protected and regulated by Article X of the Laws of the Regents, as outlined in the 1988 Faculty Handbook of the University of Colorado. The Handbook makes clear that the educational aims of the University "can only be achieved in that atmosphere of free inquiry and discussion which has become a tradition of universities and is called academic freedom. For this purpose, academic freedom is defined as the freedom to inquire, discover, publish, and teach truth as the faculty member sees it. . . ." The Regents' Law thus puts the primary determination of what should be taught onto the individual faculty member. In this case, the decision of several faculty members of the School of Nursing to teach TT is clearly within the academic freedom given by the Regents to University members.

As the choice of what to teach is defined as a freedom, the limitations on this freedom must be narrowly interpreted. In the case of academic freedom, the Regents state that it is "subject to no control or authority, save the control or authority of the rational methods by which truth is established." This committee found that the scientific rationale for TT is not established and indeed can be questioned in several areas. However, the committee also found that the faculty members currently teaching TT have participated in empirical research on TT. Therefore, we conclude that the requirement of control or authority of rational methods has been met by these faculty.

The Faculty Handbook further states that: "The fullest exposure to conflicting opinions is the best insurance against error." The creation of the intellectual setting in which teaching occurs is not the prerogative of an individual faculty member, but it is a responsibility which has been clearly delegated in the Faculty Handbook to departmental chairs (Regent Action 12/20/84, Faculty Handbook, pp. 1–22, 1–23). The responsibility of the leadership of the School of Nursing to set the teaching of TT within the appropriate scholarly framework, in which the conflict of evidence and opinion is clearly delineated, is described in a subsequent section. A second related duty of the SON faculty stems from the use of TT in the clinical care mission of the School. The SON faculty's duty is to ensure that TT is good clinical care and to fully inform patients of the nature of TT, so that each can make an informed consent to the procedure, is also described in a subsequent section.

A final duty, which the Regents have relegated to the members of the University as a whole, is the duty to protect the scholarly efforts of faculty members from "direct or indirect pressures or interference from within the University, and the University will resist to the utmost such pressures or interference when exerted from without." The committee recognizes that the University of Colorado is a public institution and, as such, that scholarly and teaching activities of faculty members should be fully disclosed to members of the public, including their Regential and legislative representatives. Furthermore, it is appropriate that Regents, legislators, and members of the general public should freely comment on scholarly and teaching activities of faculty members. However, the protection of academic freedom by the University, as specified by the Regents, requires that the process of public debate not become one of interference or pressure on the scholarly activities of faculty members, to the extent that these activities are protected by academic freedom. Therefore, the creation of special committees to respond to public criticism of activities such as the teaching of TT should not be used as the instrument of interference or pressure. This committee thus wishes to make explicit that the teaching of TT is protected by the academic freedom set forth by the Regents. Furthermore, the regularly constituted bodies within the School of Nursing that review curriculum content and clinical practice are fully adequate to perform these functions, without interference or pressure from within or without the University.

B. CURRICULUM EVALUATION

Within the academic milieu it is expected that educational programs be evaluated in a consistent ongoing manner. It is the responsibility of the faculty and program administrators to develop and implement an evaluation plan that informs them and other program audiences about program inputs, processes and outcomes to aid in decision-making regarding the overall effectiveness of the program and its curriculum, the program's policies and procedures, and resource needs and utilization.

The TT Committee has determined that the Chancellor of the UCHSC at Denver has appropriately implemented University-level review of the Center for Human Caring and the members of the TT component of the curriculum. The School of Nursing has implemented appropriate evaluation of the TT component of the nursing curriculum by receiving ongoing evaluations of courses and faculty review of course syllabi. The School of Nursing programs also have been thoroughly reviewed externally by the National League for Nursing and received national accreditation. There is currently no evidence available to indicate that the TT component of the program should be discontinued based on evaluation data. However, when programs are under development or are of a nontraditional nature, it is the responsibility of the faculty and school administrators to implement more intensive evaluation strategies which involve the review of external experts in the field (see recommendations).

C. PUBLIC REPRESENTATION OF THERAPEUTIC TOUCH

Issue

The representation of TT within the scientific community is fledgling with few sustained programs of research. The majority of support for TT as a nursing therapeutic emanates from clinical efficacy observations by practitioners. Since the scientific basis for this therapy has yet to be substantially developed, it is important that it is being represented appropriately and accurately and that false claims or misleading statements are not made in the marketing and representation of courses of study at the University of Colorado.

Evaluation

The Committee evaluated the brochure, "Therapeutic Touch at the Center for Human Caring." In general, the claims made in the brochure are fair and adequate. Key claims noted include the following:

1. TT is a derivative of the laying on of hands but differs in that a religious context is not part of the representation and it is a skill that can be learned and taught.
2. TT is taught in an estimated eighty colleges and schools of nursing.
3. TT "may" decrease pain, decrease the amount of pain medicine people need, induce profound relaxation, and accelerate would healing.
4. Our understanding of how and why TT works is incomplete and the underlying theory of a human energy field remains to be demonstrated using traditional Western science.
5. Attempting to cure disease is not part of the view.
6. Natural processes for healing are stimulated.
7. There is no way to know what specific effects TT will have for an individual.
8. TT complements rather than replaces regular medical and nursing care.

9. There is no preconceived dose (number of treatments) over time and each treatment takes about ten to fifteen minutes.
10. TT is embedded in clarifying goals for health, exploring meanings of health problems and learning self-care.
11. The process for the therapist is to become calm, enter her/himself with the *intention* to assist healing and perform movements believed to allow interaction with an energy field.

No clearly misleading statements are made in the brochure. However, because of the thin scientific basis for claiming efficacy or mechanism, a rewording for claim 3 (above) is suggested; e.g., "Although not completely proven, over twenty years of clinical experience and research suggests that in certain contexts, TT might reduce pain and the amount of needed pain medication, perhaps improve wound healing and very often induce profound relaxation."

Under brochure section "Can TT cure my disease?," and in relation to claim #\6, since the "natural processes" are unspecified, it is recommended that wording of sentence 2 in this paragraph be something like: "The focus for TT is on healing, defined as stimulating wholeness of body, mind, and spirit."

Under the brochure section "What happens in a TT session?," and its relation to claim 11, since the mechanism is uncertain, omit from second last sentence of this section "which we believe allow her to interact with energy field" or substitute with "which promotes healing" or a less specific statement.

A question regarding claim 2 is how or where this is documented; i.e., eighty colleges and schools of nursing. The recommendation is to omit or refer to the proper source.

In sum, this brochure with suggested changes will convey the historical grounding for TT, the tentative research outcomes, and the lack of theoretical substantiation. It will also disavow replacement of conventional therapy, make no promises regarding individual response and generally explain the process. Thereby, the brochure can represent the reality of what is known about the phenomenon and is not deemed to constitute misrepresentation.

D. THE EFFICACY OF THERAPEUTIC TOUCH

There is disagreement about whether TT is effective. To date, there is not a sufficient body of data, both in quality and quantity, to establish TT as a unique and efficacious healing modality. There are major gaps in the literature regarding the actual efficacy of the practice of noncontact TT as a unique healing modality. This lack of data and consequently the perceived uncertainties of TT's possible unique beneficial attributes in the practice of the healing arts greatly compromise the general acceptance of TT and brings the potential to have a negative effect on the stature and reputation of the School of Nursing. Qualitative judgments and evaluation are not sufficient to document and establish TT as an efficacious therapeutic or healing modality. The development of verifiable data is essential if TT is to be accepted in the health sciences community. If an effect is observable, it can be measured. It is not adequate to state that TT involves mechanisms which exist beyond the five senses and which therefore cannot be proven by ordinary methods. Such comments are a disservice to science and the practice of healing and demonstrate a commitment to metaphysics and the mystical view of life rather than to a scientific or rational view of life. Therefore, it is not surprising that TT is looked upon by many individuals within and outside the community with concern and disbelief. It is inappropriate in the context of a health science center to teach and practice TT for another twenty years in the absence of validation of TT as an efficacious healing modality. As private practitioners are unlikely to undertake controlled studies, it is the academic practitioners of TT who have the obligation and responsibility to the community to critically assess TT. Studies of TT as an empirical phenomenon, if they are to be performed adequately, may require a critical mass of skilled individuals with academic expertise in different areas of both the social, nursing, and medical sciences.

From our study and analysis, it has become quite clear that the University of Colorado School of Nursing has a unique opportunity and responsibility to provide to the health sciences community a greater understanding of the actual nature and efficacy of TT. The School of Nursing has established itself as one of the major nursing schools in the country where TT is being practiced and taught as an effective alternative healing modality. TT has become an important academic component of the Center for Human Caring. Nonetheless, the critical evaluation of TT and the establishment of its efficacy as an unique healing modality has not been emphasized to the same extent as its practice and the training of new TT practitioners.

E. THE SCIENTIFIC BASIS FOR THERAPEUTIC TOUCH

The primary scientific explanation for the possible efficacy of TT is based on the concept of personal energy fields. TT proponents believe that each person is and/or has an energy field which extends beyond the edges of the physical body. This concept can be found in Oriental lore but TT proponents trace it mainly to Dr. Martha Rogers of NYU. Her metaphor that a person is an energy field has been made concrete by TT practitioners who believe (a) that this energy field can be perceived by trained TT practitioners, (b) that it is perturbed (or "imbalanced" or "congested") in people who need healing, (c) that practitioners of TT can modify this energy field by passing their hands over the body repeatedly, and (d) that such changing of the' energy field will promote relaxation, healing, and well-being.

Although TT practitioners state that the existence and nature of the energy field is an hypothesis which has not been confirmed in over twenty years, in practice they behave as if the energy field were a perceptible reality.

There is virtually no acceptable scientific evidence concerning the existence or nature of these energy fields. There is no ongoing research on this concept at the Center for Human Caring, nor are there any plans for such research, nor even any ideas about how such research might be conducted. In view of these facts, the Committee believes that assertions about the existence and modification of energy fields as the possible scientific basis of the teaching and practice of TT are premature.

F. SUMMARY

In terms of UCHSC School of nursing faculty teaching, research, and practice scholarship incorporating TT, the committee determined that in the main, this involves two faculty who have TT as their major scholarship domain and two elective courses within the curriculum of the School. The faculty involved have engaged in some empirically based research in this domain which, as with virtually all intervention research, can be criticized for its incompleteness and methodological flaws. It was deemed by the Committee that the domain of TT and the teaching and research done by members of the faculty is protected by Article X of the Laws of the Regents of the U of C, guaranteeing faculty the academic freedom to pursue worthy scholarship (see Section A). Further, the faculty within the School of Nursing have subjected this domain of scholarship to the same evaluation process as the remaining domains of the curriculum which was deemed by the Committee in accordance with usual curricular quality control (see Section B). A public document through which potential therapists and recipients are informed of the practice of TT was analyzed and it was determined that no misrepresentations of the phenomenon existed in the document (see Section C).

G. RECOMMENDATIONS

1. *The need for external input.*

As the TT program appears to be operating in settings which are somewhat isolated from other biomedical disciplines, the Committee believes that there is a need for cross-disciplinary input relative to approaches to teaching and research. Many academic programs have standing external review or advisory boards or committees, and this should be considered for TT. In the case of TT, representatives from the social as well as the health sciences should be useful.

2. *Research approaches for TT.*

In the field of TT as a whole, there is an urgent need for:

    a.   Information concerning the scientific basis of TT in terms of the existence, nature and modulation of a personal energy field.

    b.   Information concerning the efficacy of TT as an adjunct to healing, in comparison to other options such as no treatment or placebo TT or another form of relaxation or biofeedback, etc.

Faculty in the School of Nursing should decide if research in TT is to be part of its widely promulgated program of TT. This Committee believes that research into the scientific basis and the practical efficacy of TT is highly desirable and that the UCHSC SON is a logical place for this research effort. Proponents of TT need to reach beyond their own practices to develop true interdisciplinary approaches to understanding TT. In such endeavors, it is highly desirable to use, as much as possible, quantitative methods rather than relying heavily on descriptive phenomenology.

In terms of the *underlying scientific basis of TT*, i.e., energy fields, TT proponents need to collaborate with engineers and biophysicians, perhaps with experts in biofeedback, autonomic physiology, and electrophysiology to seek empirical validation.

In terms of establishing the *efficacy of TT* as a healing modality according to accepted methods used in other fields, the following items come to mind.

    • Approaches to assessment of outcome could be developed in collaboration with the UCHSC Center for Health Services

Research. This center is an acknowledged leader in the field of outcomes research. Such collaboration could aid in the design of studies, in decisions as to which clinical situations should be explored and which control groups might be used (e.g., TT vs. no treatment, vs. placebo, vs. another relaxation modality, etc.), and which methods of assessment are best.

- If TT is as dramatically helpful in reducing posttraumatic pain and inflammation as is claimed in anecdotal reports, interdisciplinary studies could be carried out in collaboration with:
    1. UCHSC pain clinics which study chronic pain.
    2. The Dept. of Obstetrics & Gynecology, which operates a clinic for women with chronic pelvic pain.
    3. The Dept. of Emergency Medicine and/or the Dept. of Orthopedics for the study of the reduction of posttraumatic pain or inflammation.
- If TT is effective in helping to relieve stress and fatigue, there is an internationally recognized program in Chronic Fatigue Syndrome studies at the National Jewish Center here in Denver, where patients are eager to find relief for their problems.

It is not difficult to think of other collaborative situations in which SON faculty which practice TT could fruitfully interact with other health science disciplines.

3. Teaching and practice of TT.

TT is potentially a source of considerable income. Training in TT is not complex and arduous and the practice of TT does not require a large investment in equipment or personnel.

The Chancellor should recommend to the Dean of the School of Nursing that the Faculty of the School of Nursing ensure:

- that the proper type of informed consent be obtained from patients prior to TT, i.e. consent for standard treatment vs. consent for research.
- that TT practice represents good nursing practice. A special concern is that the TT program avoid as much as possible being perceived as a New Age cult procedure.
- that proper academic standards be maintained for courses and degree requirements in the teaching of TT.
- that public representation of TT and their promotion of TT practice in brochures, videotapes, etc., be accurate.
- that adequate formal records of treatment and reimbursements be kept.

With these considerations in mind, the Committee believes that the School of Nursing could establish Therapeutic Touch as a beneficial adjunct treatment to work along with regular medical and nursing care.

Appendix 4.

Recommendations from a [Colorado] State Board of Nursing Subcommittee to Investigate the Awarding of Continuing Education Units to Nurses for the Study of Therapeutic Touch and Other Nontraditional and Complementary Healing Modalities

Because Nursing is both a science and an art, nurses require access to and familiarity with many belief systems and knowledge bases, including, but not limited to, the traditional sciences. Nurses conduct scientific research on nursing interventions and phenomenon of concern to nurses, such as pain, suffering, and healing. Nurses also use the insights and experiences gained from studying peoples of other cultures and learning other perspectives to alleviate suffering and promote health and healing, which may lack modern scientific investigation. Always at the heart of nursing practice is the well-being of the patient, using approaches which help without causing harm. An openness to all possible approaches to the relief of human suffering and the compassionate, caring use of touch have been the cornerstones of excellent nursing practice since the time of Florence Nightingale.

Based on an increasing volume of research and clinical literature supporting the effectiveness of Therapeutic Touch in the easing of human suffering and the stimulation of healing, the State Board of Nursing of Colorado, like other State Boards of Nursing all over the country, should continue to be an advocate for the public safety and for **patient's rights to access the full range of caring and healing interventions by** continuing to acknowledge continuing education units earned for the study of Therapeutic Touch. Therapeutic Touch, as a nursing intervention, is being taught to nurses through many colleges and universities, and by the National League for Nursing through its continuing education videotape series on Therapeutic Touch. It is completely within the mainstream of modern nursing practice. Moreover, we encourage the Board to continue to acknowledge continuing education efforts undertaken by nurses in related complementary healing modalities, even when scientific investigation of such modalities is incomplete, for two reasons. First, the lay public is becoming increasingly sophisticated in these complementary modalities and nurses should be familiar enough with them to be able to provide adequate information at the request of patients. Second, these modalities can be used as meaningful adjuncts to, and not replacements for, standard medical and nursing care.

We wish to remind all concerned that individual patients always have the right to refuse *any* intervention, medical or nursing, which is not consistent with their values or beliefs. The State Board of Nursing will undoubtedly continue to serve as an advocate and protector of that right.

Appendix 5.

Chronology of Therapeutic Touch

Jack Stahlman

1836-1866:   Period of the Transcendental movement.

1875:   Foundation of the Theosophical Society.

1888:   Publication of Blavatsky's *The Secret Doctrine*.

1909:   Publication of the Theosophical work *The Science of Psychic Healing*.

1916:   Kunz begins her studies under the tutelage of Theosophical seer C. W. Leadbeater.

1925:   Publication of the Theosophical work *The Etheric Double: The Health Aura of Man*.

1927:   Publication of C. W. Leadbeater's highly influential work *The Chakras*.

Early 1930s: Dora Kunz works with Otelia Bengtsson, M.D., honing her skills as a seer and a reader of auras.

1961-1963:   Bernard Grad conducts experiments with the healer Oskar Estabany.

For a thorough discussion of the history of Therapeutic Touch, see Mr. Stahlman's article in chapter 1 of this volume.

Late 1960s: Kunz and Krieger assist Oskar Estabany in healing clinics.

1970:   Publication of *Nursing's Conceptual Model* (Rogers).

1971:   Krieger completes first pilot study into healing via the laying-on of hands.

1972:   Krieger completes first full-scale study into healing via the laying-on of hands.

1973:   Krieger presents results of her early research to the American Nurses Association's Ninth Council of Nurse Researchers.

1973:   First published critique of Krieger's early research (Schlotfeldt).

1974:   Transition from the "laying-on of hands" to TT's contemporary form.

1975:   Krieger publishes "Therapeutic Touch: The Imprimatur of Nursing" in the *American Journal of Nursing*, introducing TT to the nursing profession at large.

1975 (fall):   First university course teaching TT begun at New York University.

1975:   First published critical response to the practice of TT in a widely circulated nursing journal by Walike.

1980:   Publication of *Nursing: A Science of Unitary Man* (Rogers).

1984:   Publication of Clark and Clark's critical review of TT research.

1986:   Publication of *Science of Unitary Human Beings* (Rogers).

1988:   Initial involvement of the Rocky Mountain Skeptics in TT.

1988:   Formation of the Society of Rogerian Scholars.

1990:   Publication of *Nursing: Science of Unitary, Irreducible Human Beings: Update* (Rogers).

1990:   Incorporation of TT into the College of Nurses of Ontario Implementation Standards of Practice.

1992:   Rocky Mountain Skeptics present their concerns to the Colorado Board of Nursing regarding the awarding of continuing education credits towards fringe nursing practices including TT.

1992:   Publication of *Nursing Science and the Space Age* (Rogers).

1992:   U.S. Dept. of Health grants of $200,000 to treat patients and train students in TT at D'Youville Nursing Center.

1993:   Rocky Mountain Skeptics provide testimony to the Colorado Senate's HEWI Committee.

1994:   Addition of "energy field disturbance" to the list of *NANDA* diagnoses.

1994:   Department of Defense grant of $335,000 to study effects of TT on burn patients.

1994:   Rocky Mountain Skeptics provide testimony at a private hearing of the University of Colorado Health Science Center's Chancellor's Committee on TT.

1996:   The James Randi Educational Foundation posts $742,000 award for any TT practitioner who can demonstrate the ability to detect human energy fields.

1996:   Testing of a TT practitioner by Robert Glickman and James Randi in Philadelphia.

1998:   Publication of the critical study "A Close Look at Therapeutic Touch" in *JAMA*.

Appendix 6.

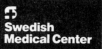
**Swedish
Medical Center**

SEPTEMBER 9, 16, 23 & 30, 1991

DESCRIPTION: Come take a closer look at Therapeutic Touch. Based on the age old technique of laying-on of hands, this four week seminar will explore the technique that helps to lessen pain and anxiety, promote health, accelerate the natural healing process and maintain a higher level of wellness. You will learn and experience enough to begin using therapeutic touch in your daily life and appropriate health practices.

TARGET AUDIENCE: Nurses, Physicians, and other health care professionals

OBJECTIVES:
1. Contrast the history of Therapeutic Touch and other healing modalities.
2. Participate in becoming aware of one's own energy field and the energy field of another.
3. Identify the feeling state of being centered and it's psychophysiologic effects.
4. Identify the five phases of Therapeutic Touch.
5. Identify the implications for using Therapeutic Touch in patient care.

CE CREDIT: 12 contact hours are available and approved by the Colorado Nurses' Association which is accredited as an approver of continuing education for nursing by the American Nurses' Association's Board on Accreditation.

DATES/TIME: Mondays, September 9, 16, 23 & 30, 1991 - 6:00 to 9:00 p.m.

LOCATION: 2nd Floor Conference Center, Swedish Medical Center, 501 E. Hampden Avenue, Englewood, Colorado

FACULTY: Colleen Whalen, RN, BSN, Critical Care Nurse Manager
Dona Leiper, RN, BSN, Private Practice Therapeutic Touch

PLANNING COMMITTEE: Colleen Whalen, RN, BSN and Nancy Savidge, RN, BA

FEE: $50.00 (Fee for SMC/Craig/Spalding/Vail Valley Medical Center employees is $25.00)

TO REGISTER: Complete the registration form and send a check made payable to: Swedish Medical Center, 501 E. Hampden Avenue, P.O. Box 2901, Dept. 8615, Englewood, CO 80150-0101, or you may register by phone when using your Mastercard, Visa or Discover card. CANCELLATION request must be received ten days prior to the offering for tuition refund. Swedish Medical Center reserves the right to cancel an offering; a full refund would be made.

That's Not All! **Beginning in October a "Department of Energy" branch will be launched through Employee Health and Fitness. This is a network created to help support those caregivers who are actively involved in holistic health touch and energy work. LOOK FOR UPCOMING DETAILS!**

- CLIP AND MAIL -
THERAPEUTIC TOUCH
September 9, 16, 23 & 30, 1991

NAME_____SOCIAL SECURITY_____
ADDRESS_____CITY_____STATE_____ZIP_____
PLACE OF EMPLOYMENT_____AREA OF PRACTICE_____
TELEPHONE (DAY)_____(EVE)_____AMT ENCLOSED_____
BILL MY VISA___MASTERCARD___DISCOVER___CARD#_____EXP DATE_____

339

Appendix 7.

Task Force to Colorado State Board of Nursing

Regarding Therapeutic Touch

UNIVERSITY OF COLORADO HEALTH SCIENCES CENTER SCHOOL OF NURSING

DATE: April 8, 1992
LOCATION: Room 2918, UCHSC, School of Nursing
TIME: 9-10:30 a.m.

Members:
Sally Phillips, Colorado State Board of Nursing
Coleen Whalens, Swedish Medical Center
Ginette Pepper, UCHSC and Swedish Medical Center
Fran Reeder, UCHSC
Mary Jo Cleveland, The Children's Hospital
Tom Cabral (unable to attend), Wheatridge Regional Center

1. Sally Phillips, Chair of the Colorado State Board of Nursing gave the charge to the committee from the Board of Nursing. The membership of this group was directed by the Board. Those individuals reported to give continuing education credit by Rocky Mountain Skeptics were to be convened. The purpose is to explore CE offerings at respective institutions, review research and writings on this healing modality, and prepare a summary report back to the Board. Janet Quinn and Fran Reeder represent the University of Colorado School of Nursing continuing education endeavors as well as the practice of Therapeutic Touch. C. Whalens and G. Pepper represent Swedish Medical Center, no one was able to be located to represent Presbyterian/St. Luke's, a representative from Children's Hospital attends as a practice site, Tom Cabral was to attend as a community member representative. Chair, Sally Phillips represents the State Board of Nursing.

   Sally Phillips reviewed facts from the March Board Meeting, The Skeptics comments, and board discussion as a framework. The goal of this meeting is to submit a summary on Therapeutic Touch as continuing education for nurses and compile research and writings on the modalities.

2. Each representative presented an overview of C.E. offerings and practice of Therapeutic Touch in their institutions. Specific issues addressed were ethical practice (informed consent), client outcomes (effectiveness), bibliographies used in courses, enrollment issues (number of nurses, types of nurses, etc.).

3. Based on these reports, the group moved to a discussion on how to report data to the Board. Fran Reeder talked of two of her clients who would be eager to address the Board, demonstrate how they used touch and its effectiveness. Jane Quinn was designated to pull together the reference list from everyone.

Appendix 8.

STATE OF COLORADO

BOARD OF NURSING
Karen D. Brumley
Program Administrator

1560 Broadway, Suite 670
Denver, CO 80202
Phone (303) 894-2430

Department of Regulatory Agencies
Steven V. Berson
Executive Director

Division of Registrations
Bruce M. Douglas, Director

Roy Romer
Governor

February 10, 1993

Bela Scheiber, President
Rocky Mountain Skeptics
Box 7277
Boulder, CO 80306

Dear Mr. Scheiber:

At its January 28-29, 1993 meeting, the Colorado Board of Nursing considered various issues raised by the Rocky Mountain Skeptics. Specifically, Skeptic members Carla Selby and William Alderfer presented to the Board and made four requests of the Board including a request that the Board withdraw accreditation for all courses advocating "not-traditional or complementary healing modalities." After extensive discussion, the Board voted to reaffirm the decision made at the May, 1992 Board meeting to approve therapeutic touch as acceptable content for continuing education. The vote was 8 members in favor, 1 opposed (Thomas Haga), and one abstaining.

The Board recognizes and appreciates the Skeptics viewpoint that the Board "must rely upon science and only upon science and the scientific method to provide you with the standards to judge proposed treatments and techniques." Unfortunately, new treatments, procedures, and methods do not arrive with pre-developed scientific justification and research. The treatment must be performed in order to measure its effect. For the treatment to be performed, persons must learn how to perform the treatment. Accordingly, the Board approved of therapeutic touch as acceptable content for continuing education. It also noted that the subject must be studied by the researcher before the research can begin.

The Board may discipline a nurse upon proof the nurse "has willfully or negligently acted in a manner inconsistent with the health or safety of persons under his care" (C.R.S. 12-38-117(1)(c) and "has negligently or willfully practiced nursing in a manner which fails to meet generally accepted standards for such nursing practice" (C.R.S. 12-38-117(1)(f). Thus a nurse who told a patient that therapeutic touch would cure a terminal disease could be disciplined.

The Board agrees with the Rocky Mountain Skeptics that it is a responsibility both of the Board and each of its practitioners to carefully examine new ideas, practices, etc. It applauds the growing body of nursing research which is resulting from such analysis and research. However, it disagrees with the Skeptic's conclusions with

respect to therapeutic touch as acceptable content for continuing education. The Board will continue to be mindful of its statutory responsibility to protect the public health, safety, and welfare of the people of the State of Colorado and believes that nurses learning and practicing therapeutic touch are consistent with that mandate.

FOR THE BOARD OF NURSING

Karen D. Brumley, RN
Program Administrator

Appendix 9.

SALLY HOPPER
State Senator
21649 Cabrini Blvd.
Golden, Colorado 80401
Capitol: 866-4873
Home: 526-0785

Senate Chamber
State of Colorado
Denver

COMMITTEES:
Chairman of:
    Health, Environment,
        Welfare and Institutions
Member of:
    Judiciary

May 7, 1993

Board of Nursing
1560 Broadway, Suite 670
Denver, CO 80202

Dear Members of the State Nursing Board:

The Senate Health, Environment, Welfare and Institutions (HEWI) Committee members are concerned that the continuing education courses on non-traditional healing practices being approved by the Colorado Board of Nursing are not receiving sufficient review.

Since continuing education is a condition for renewing licensure for the various nursing professions under the jurisdiction of the board, the review and approval of appropriate courses closely concerns the health and safety of the citizens of this state. As such, the Senate HEWI Committee expects board members to thoroughly review alternative healing practices, such as therapeutic touch, neurolinguistic programming, and crystal healing, prior to approving the study of these healing methods for continuing education.

Please send copies of future board meeting agendas listing hearings of the above courses, and any other courses based on non-traditional healing practices to the Senate HEWI committee members.

Very truly yours,

Sally Hopper
Chairman of Senate HEWI

Appendix 10.

STATE OF COLORADO

BOARD OF NURSING

Karen D. Brumley
Program Administrator

1560 Broadway, Suite 670
Denver, CO 80202
Phone (303) 894-2430

Department of Regulatory Agencies
Joseph A. Garcia
Executive Director

Division of Registrations
Bruce M. Douglas, Director

Roy Romer
Governor

February, 1994

TO WHOM IT MAY CONCERN:

The Colorado Board of Nursing has addressed a number of issues that relate to continuing education over the past few years. Each issue required reevaluation of the purpose and worth of continuing education as a mandatory requirement for license renewal. At the September 23-24, 1993 meeting, the Board continued the discussion and voted to hold a rule-making hearing to abolish the continuing education requirement. After hearing testimony at the January 26, 1994 hearing, the Board voted unanimously to repeal the requirement. This document will provide clarification of the rationale behind the decision.

In 1981, the Board voted to require 20 hours of continuing education for nurses to renew their licenses in an attempt to assure that individual nurses would remain competent in their own practice settings. After 12 years of the requirement, the Board is increasingly concerned with continuing competency, not compliance with a continuing education requirement. The number of complaints and corresponding action related to substandard nursing care is significantly rising and board and staff time is increasingly devoted to disciplinary matters and monitoring the nursing practice of licensees. There is no research available either in Colorado or anywhere in the nation that shows any correlation between linking continuing education with license renewal and the continued competence of any licensed group. The Board believes it must concentrate its emphasis and resources in areas that are demonstrably related to public protection.

This should not be interpreted as a lack of Board support for licensees continuing their education. The Board endorses each licensee continuing his education; the Board does not support continuing education being linked to license renewal. The Board believes that each licensee is accountable for having the necessary knowledge, skills, and abilities to engage in the licensee's unique area of practice. Each nurse is responsible for self assessment and for obtaining the continuing education required for safe, effective practice in the nurse's individual circumstances. Employers have a large role in this process by providing the time and means for each licensee to obtain and maintain the competency required, serving as partners with the licensee in strategies which promote professional proficiency and accountability.

The Board believes it should use its resources (1) to assure that nursing educational programs prepare competent nurses, (2) to license only persons who meet minimal competency standards, and (3) to identify and intervene with nurses who are incompetent, unsafe, or who do not appropriately self-limit their own practice. The Board believes that the responsibility and accountability for increasing licensee knowledge, skills, and abilities is properly that of the licensee and the Board will hold each licensee accountable for continuing competency.

Appendix 11.

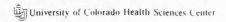

4200 East Ninth Avenue   University Hospitals   School of Nursing   School of Pharmacy
Denver, Colorado 80262   School of Medicine   School of Dentistry   Graduate School

November 17, 1993

TO: Vincent Fulginiti, M.D.
                   Chancellor, Health Sciences Center

FROM: Academic Relevance Committee

RE: The Center For Human Caring

The Center for Human Caring was organized in 1986 under the direction of Dr. Jean Watson, then Dean of the School of Nursing.   Campus and Presidential approval was obtained and it is stated by Dr. Watson that Regental approval was not needed at that time. The Center does not have a separate non-profit status and operates as an entity within the School of Nursing.

MISSION

The first Mission Statement in July 1986 listed the central purposes of the Center to be:

1. The study of human response to care-giving practices in a variety of settings.

2. The development of a theory of flexible health care relating to the importance of human responses with scientific and technological aspects of such care.

3. The incorporation of this theory into education.

4. Support of the development of human care-based practices.

5. The development of the Center as a local, regional and national resource for on-going study, research and dissemination of information.

In 1989 the Mission Statement was revised to delineate four essential purposes:

1. The work of nursing is the work of human caring.

2. The art and science of human caring is a framework for nursing, health care and health policy.

2

3. "To develop and disseminate educational, research and clinical strategies to re-establish the critical balance between techno-cure and human-care within the health care system".

4. "To restore the centrality of the arts and humanities in understanding the subjective human dimensions of nursing, health, illness and healing and in designing new strategies for caring and healing".

In July 1993, it was re-emphasized that the Center for Human Caring shares the missions of education, research, practice and service enunciated by the School of Nursing and the University of Colorado.

ORGANIZATION

The full-time Director, Dr. Watson, reports administratively to the Dean of the School of Nursing. A part-time Senior Scholar, a Scholar in Residence, 11 Project Directors and 12 Associates along with 2 full-time staff comprise the table of organization listed for 1991. Very few of these individuals draw salary or other support from state sources. In 1987, a combined local and national Visiting Board was set up for both the Center and the School of Nursing. Initially, there seems to have been no clear delineation between the functions of these two units, possibly because the positions of Director and Dean were held jointly by Dr. Watson. The Visiting Board minutes for 1988 and 1989 reflect the blending of the goals and interests of the School of Nursing and the Center for Human Caring without clear separation of missions or activities. After Dr. Watson relinquished the Deanship, the minutes of 1991 indicate that she outlined two directions for the Center - to formalize the international perspective on human caring, and to develop clinical demonstration models of caring. The most recent minutes available to our Committee, from April 23, 1993, note that Dr. Watson felt that the Center for Human Caring could serve as an organizational unit to develop new directions for nursing, such as the development of Centers offering "total care of patients".

FINANCES EXPEDITURES

	1991-92 Actual	1992-93 Actual	1993-94 Budget
Unrestricted Funds (State)	$26,901	$101,491[1]	$0
Restricted Funds (Grants, Contracts, Gifts)	89,856	105,900	164,616
Auxiliary Funds (Other Non-State Sources)	83,489	110,180	209,377
Totals	200,246	317,571	373,993

[1] Includes Dr. Watson's Salary

3

ACTIVITIES/PROGRAMS

1. Doctor of Nursing (ND) Degree- Although a degree from the SON, conceptual and instructional strategies intregal to the program were piloted through the Center.

2. Postgraduate Summer Institutes in Human Caring. These were begun in 1990 and have been given every year since. Tuition is charged and there have been 83 participants to date.

3. Continuing education courses.

4. Professional Development Certificate in Caring Praxis.

5. Advanced Postgraduate Study Program in Caring and Healing.

6. Visiting Fellows program.

7. Denver Nursing Project in Human Caring. This is a nurse managed clinic established in 1988 for persons who either have AIDS or who have a positive HIV test. Local support comes from the Veterans Affairs Medical Center, The Denver Department of Health and Hospitals and University Hospital as well as from a Health and Human Services Grant. Over 20,000 client visits have been recorded to date.

8. Nightingale Unit for Caring Excellence. A joint endeavor with Mercy Medical Center to develop a caring-healing nursing unit.

9. Baycrest Centre for Geriatric Care, Toronto, Canada. Funds from the Centre and the Ministry of Health of Canada have supported four pilot units based on caring theories.

10. State of Hawaii Department of Health on Kauai. A unit has been set up, with consultative assistance from Dr. Watson, to develop training programs for rural health professionals.

11. Visitors Program. Nearly 60 national and international visitors have arrived since January 1990.

12. Affiliations with national and international caring centers. These include centers in Scotland and Canada.

13. Fitness Center. An ongoing activity for students, staff and faculty on the Health Sciences Campus.

14. Therapeutic Touch. An activity that is taught and practied in a number of Center programs. Discussed below.

4

15. Massage Therapy. Initially begun through the Center, it is now part of University Hospital.

RESEARCH AND SCHOLARLY PRODUCTIVITY

Research proposals have been submitted in a variety of areas to foundations and federal granting agencies. To date, the Denver Nursing Project in Human Caring has been the most successful, being the recipient of a $450,000 grant for three years from the Division of Nursing of the Department of Health and Human Services.

Frequent publications have emanated from the Center members, many of which have appeared in peer reviewed journals. (See Attachment 1)

FUTURE OBJECTIVES

1. Establish full endowment.

2. Implement human caring-healing study programs.

3. Conduct faculty institutes in cooperation with the National League for Nursing and other academic and clinical sponsors.

4. Create new clinical demonstration models of caring and healing.

5. Establish and coordinate additional national and international affiliations.

ACCOMPLISHMENTS

The accomplishments of the Center for Human Caring, as listed by Dr. Watson this year, include:

1. A conceptual umbrella for nursing has been developed.

2. Reframing nursing theory and practice to encompass the whole person.

3. Worldwide acceptance of this theory based practice. ·

4. Faculty and nursing education and development.

CONCLUSIONS AND RECOMMENDATIONS

The Academic Relevance Committee has come to the following conclusions, and offers the following recommendations:

1. The Center for Human Caring has relevance to the academic programs and mission of the School of Nursing.

5

The major thrust of the Center, to emphasize and enhance the caring aspects of nursing, is praiseworthy, and it is clear that the Center concept has answered a need felt by many practicing nurses. Just as there has been a concern that medical practice which emphasizes only technology, tasks and skills might lead to dehumanizing what physicians do, nurses who have mastered technological skills unheard of even a few years ago are concerned that issues of patient control, participation and support may be overlooked. The philosophical underpinning of the Center approaches patient care with the recognition that mind and body both must be attended to, particularly in those diseases such as AIDS and terminal illnesses which do not have rapid or complete cures, and that a technological tour de force may not be sufficient for complete or even partial healing.

The target audience for this Center is the entire field of nursing education and nursing practice, whether this be undergraduate, graduate or postgraduate. The programs are not duplicative of others in the School of Nursing and it is clear that the Center is, or has the potential to be, one of the educational leaders in the field.

    2.   The Center is the sum of many parts and is not just a single program.

The totality of programs of the Center must be considered in the context of any evaluation. It has served as a focal point for nurses who wish to emphasize human caring in nursing, without excluding the technical and skills area of the profession. By acting to accumulate a critical mass of investigators and by offering graduate and postgraduate courses, the Center seeks to develop and disseminate knowledge in this field. The most signal success of the program has been the development by Dr. Ruth Neil of the Denver Nursing Project in Human Caring. This widely recognized and praised program is, in a sense, a demonstration of caring in action. Dr. Neil has emphasized that without the theoretical background promulgated by the Center for Human Caring, her program would not have been developed or matured. The Massage Therapy Program is another area that is being studied as a complement to traditional medical treatments. The Fitness Center, developed initially by the Center has proven itself to be a valuable campus resource.

Therapeutic Touch is the most controversial of the Center activities and will be discussed further below. It is important to realize, however, that the Therapeutic Touch activity is not a synonym for the Center for Human Caring. Therapeutic Touch is taught and practiced in a number of the Center programs, such as the Denver Nursing Program in Human Caring, The Summer Postgraduate courses and in graduate programs. In some of these, however, such as the Denver Nursing Program in Human Caring, it is a minor component of the much larger activity.

    3.   The governance structure of the Center needs to be improved.

The relationship of the Center and its Director to the Dean of the School of Nursing

6

needs to be clarified. The fact that the Center developed at a time when Dr. Watson was both Dean and Director may account for this vagueness. In our opinion, the Director of the Center must at all times be administratively and fiscally responsible to the Dean.   Annual budgets, mission statements, performance evaluations, curricula, program development and annual reports, among other items, should flow to the Dean for final approval. The Center should be a separate administrative entity within the School of Nursing but needs to be more responsible to the School.

There needs to be an annual or biennial outside review mechanism for the programs, functions and achievements of the Center. The review mechanism might consist of a group of outside individuals appointed by both the Director and the Dean charged with the creation of a thorough oversight report. In addition, there needs to be a Board of Directors for the Center approved by the Dean with a clearly defined set of missions. In the past, it appears that there was considerable confusion about the activities of the Board of Visitors whose function appeared to deal more with the School of Nursing than with the Center for Human Caring.

As programs develop, particularly those dealing with "caring in action" such as Dr. Neil's, the School of Nursing should consider the possibility of seed money for start up assistance, with the understanding that eventual self-funding should be obtained.

4.   The Center has been funded primarily by grants, contracts and gifts. Very little State money has been expended.   The further development of grant, gift and contract funding should be pursued vigorously.

5.   Consideration should be given to interaction with, rather than isolation from, other schools on the campus. Areas such as Bioethics, Geriatrics, the Cancer Center, Adolescent and Clinical Psychiatry programs come to mind as ones in which the concept of human caring can be broadened and not just be exclusive to nursing.

6.   The Center Directors should realize that they do themselves, their concepts and the School harm by the use of jargon that cannot clearly be understood, and by the espousal of theoretical constructs which appear devoid of proof.   Course titles such as Emerging Otologies, Developing Resources of the Inner Self-in-Context, and Existential Advocacy: An Ethic of Embodiment do not encourage widespread appeal or understanding.   The criticism of Therapeutic Touch has cast suspicion over the entire Center. If it is good therapy, it should be validated and encouraged. If not, it should be terminated. The sense of our Committee is that the scientific basis for Therapeutic Touch has not been validated and that efforts at this Center to do so have been inadequate.

7.   Our Committee believes that the following should be done with regard to Therapeutic Touch.   The Chancellor and the Dean of the School of Nursing should appoint a special committee of investigators to carefully read the very extensive literature on this subject, to view all the videos and relevant course material, and to witness actual demonstrations of this technique. It should solicit testimony from both critics and advocates. The members of the

7

committee should be investigators well-versed in the scientific method and should come from several disciplines on the Health Sciences Center campus with the exception of the School of Nursing. Nurses should be represented on the committee but it would be appropriate if they came from other nursing schools to avoid the appearance of conflict of interest. Our Committee cannot feasibly take on this time consuming and important task because of our charge to review approximately 35 other Centers on this campus, because two members of the Committee are faculty of the School of Nursing, and because not all members possess the background needed to fairly critique this program. Rather than superficially review this most contentious area, we feel that it should be done once and for all in depth, and in a thorough scientific manner. We believe that a focused committee with this single charge could come up with a useful report in a short time frame. If Therapeutic Touch is not recognized as a bonafide activity with academic relevance, then no further course work should be offered under the aegis of the University.

8. Finally, if and when the administrative relationships of the Center are clarified, the Center mission more focused, a frequent review mechanism established, the role of Therapeutic Touch investigated, and jargon and mysticism eliminated from course work, then seed money for a variety of programs, of which the Denver Nursing Project in Human Caring is the best example, might flow appropriately to the Center. Unless these issues are dealt with, the good ideas with which the Center started may be overlooked in a tide of mounting criticism of unorthodox and unproven or untestable viewpoints and hypotheses.

Appendix 12.

 University of Colorado Health Sciences Center

Office of the Dean

Campus Box C288	School of Nursing
4200 East Ninth Avenue	
Denver, Colorado 80262	
Telephone: (303) 270-7754	
Fax: (303) 270-8660	

M E M O R A N D U M

TO: Vincent Fulginiti, Chancellor

FROM: Clair Martin, Dean

SUBJECT: Report of the Chancellor's Committee on Therapeutic Touch

DATE: August 2, 1994

The School of Nursing accepts the "Report of the Chancellor's Committee on Therapeutic Touch" and has initiated the following activities in response to the recommendations of the report.

Therapeutic Touch is a topic that receives limited attention in the teaching, research, and practice programs of the School of Nursing. It is covered in an elective course available to students who wish to learn about it and it is made available to patients as a therapeutic modality complimentary to other therapeutic interventions. Initial research efforts have been designed to test the efficacy of Therapeutic Touch, including RO1 proposals to the National Institutes of Health (NIH). These research proposals have not been funded to date. Consultation with Dr. Joseph Jacobs, Director of the NIH Office of Alternative Medicine, was provided to the practitioners of Therapeutic Touch. It is within this context that the report recommendations are addressed.

Recommendation 1. The need for external impact.

The School of Nursing is preparing its Self-Study Report for a site visit and re-accreditation by the National League for Nursing. This process will critically explore the integrity and quality of all courses offered by the School in its baccalaureate, nursing doctorate and master's degree programs. The site visit is scheduled for 1995 and will provide external review and the critical reflection of School faculty. Therapeutic Touch courses are included in this review.

The School of Nursing has a strong, interdisciplinary advisory committee structure that provides external review of the School's activities vis-a-vis its goals in teaching, research and practice. This committee will review Therapeutic Touch.

The School of Nursing has one of the strongest research reputations of any national school. The record of NIH funding places the School among the top half dozen schools in the nation. There is a strong precedence for significant interdisciplinary participation in

351

2

planning, implementing and evaluating research projects. Dr. Marilyn Stember, Associate Dean for Research, has initiated planning for an interdisciplinary research team to investigate the efficacy of Therapeutic Touch. NIH funding will be sought for this program of research.

Recommendation 2. Research approaches for Therapeutic Touch.

The School of Nursing accepts responsibility to implement a research program designed to provide: (a) information concerning the scientific basis of Therapeutic Touch in terms of the existence, nature and modulation of a personal energy field, and (b) information concerning the efficacy of Therapeutic Touch as an adjunct to healing in comparison with other options such as no treatment, placebo Therapeutic Touch, or another form of relaxation or biofeedback. Teaching and practice of Therapeutic Touch will be limited to the extent that a program of research to explicate the underlying scientific basis of Therapeutic Touch and establish the efficacy of Therapeutic Touch is implemented. Exercising the academic freedom to teach and practice Therapeutic Touch will be balanced with responsibility to implement a program of research. This program of research will be subject to peer review as an integral part of the grant proposal process and as a consequence of written and verbal scholarly presentations to the professional community.

Recommendation 3. Teaching and Practice of Therapeutic Touch.

The School of Nursing provides assurance that informed consent for Therapeutic Touch will be secured from patients, that Therapeutic Touch practice represents good nursing practice, that proper academic standards will be maintained for the teaching of Therapeutic Touch, that public representation of and promotion of Therapeutic Touch is accurate and, furthermore, that adequate formal records of treatment and reimbursement are kept.

The above assurances are the responsibility of the Dean who will exercise oversight as appropriate within the context of academic freedom and responsibility of faculty and consistent with the traditions of the scholarly community.

/er

Appendix 13.

Rocky Mountain Skeptics, Inc.

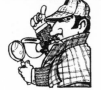

Box 7277
Boulder, Colorado 80306
(303) 444-5368
FAX (303) 447-8412

***

A Rational Alternative to Pseudoscience

Officers:
Béla Scheiber / president
    system analyst
Martin Tobias / vice president
    software engineer
Jeff Johnson / treasurer
    electrical engineer
Sherma Erholm / secretary
    educator

Board Members:
William Aldorfer
    technician
Erica Byrne
    chemical engineer
Douglas Dreher
    engineer
Meg Hedgecock
    librarian
George M. Lawrence
    physicist
Joan C. Ludeke
    cultural anthropologist
W N Reinhardt
    mathematician
Carla Selby
    anthropologist
Eric Steinberg
    consultant

Consultants:
Roger Culver
    astronomer
Michael Edwards
    magician
Mary Folsom
    writer
Ray Hyman
    experimental psychologist
Edward Karnes
    psychologist
James (The Amazing) Randi
    magician/MacArthur Fellow
Dr. John Renner, MD
    President CHIRI
    (Consumer Health Information
    Research Institute)
Eugenie C. Scott
    anthropologist
    Executive Director NCSE
Alan Shapley
    geophysicist

Vincent Fulginiti, M.D.
Chancellor, UCHSC
A095
University of Colorado HSC
Denver, Colorado

18 September 1994

Dear Dr. Fulginiti:

The Rocky Mountain Skeptics has carefully reviewed the report of Dr. Henry Claman's committee on Therapeutic Touch. The following are some of our major concerns with that document.

The University of Colorado HSC's, "Academic Relevance Committee report on the Center for Human Caring," of 17 November 1993 contained the recommendation that: "The Chancellor and the Dean of the School of Nursing should appoint a special committee of investigators to carefully read the very extensive literature on the subject (Therapeutic Touch)...[review all relevant materials]...witness actual demonstrations of this technique [and] solicit testimony from both critics and advocates. The members of the committee should be investigators well-versed in the scientific method...Rather than superficially review this most contentious area...it should be done once and for all in depth, and in a thorough scientific manner."

The report of the Committee on Therapeutic Touch (hereinafter referred to as "the report") does draw important conclusions about the non-scientific foundation of TT and the complete lack of any scientific evidence for the existence of the energy field upon which TT is based. Unfortunately, they are buried on the last pages, as if the authors hoped that these highly significant considerations would not be too evident. Specifically, Sections D and E, on the efficacy and scientific basis of TT focus on the principal issues with which the committee was charged but are the last items discussed. The rest of the report is either superficial or irrelevant.

The issue addressed in Section A, academic freedom, is pure apologia and a smoke screen. There is no reason to have entered into an elaborate and space-consuming defense of academic freedom since it was never under attack. Neither was the First Amendment. The issue has always been that TT must demonstrate scientific evidence for its claims of efficacy, "...once and for all in depth and in a thorough scientific manner..." before it or its advocates at the HSC promote it. The right to market for financial gain and to act on a belief as if it had a foundation in the physical world should have been addressed early and often in the report. Instead, the University is exhorted to continue its twenty-year policy of patience. We doubt that this would have been the case if, for example, a research biologist had attempted to market a video tape for many hundreds of dollars promoting a cure for AIDS based on only a few experiments which had yielded equivocal results.

The real meat of Section A is to be found at the section's end: "The responsibility of the leadership of the School of Nursing [is] to set the teaching of TT within the appropriate scholarly framework, in which the conflict of evidence and opinion is clearly delineated...to ensure that TT is good clinical care and to fully inform patients of the nature of TT, so that each can make an informed consent to the procedure." The RMS's insistent question here is, "Has the TT committee ensured that the SON has resolved the "...conflict of evidence and opinion...and ensured that TT is good clinical care?" We conclude that, although some of the most critical issues are briefly mentioned, the report so obscures them and addresses the suggested resolutions so ineptly that it--in fact--fails in its charge.

An almost incidental mention is made in Section A about the necessity for the academic world to be protected from outside pressure in the conduct of teaching and research. Yet the university in the Center for Human Caring was well and truly embarked on a path of potentially great embarrassment and even financial regression. May we immodestly point out that without the outside pressure exerted by RMS, neither the regents nor any other authority would have been aware of, much less been moved to investigate this potentially damaging situation?

One other major conclusion listed in Section A must be refuted. As the authors note, academic freedom is accompanied by an absolute requirement that it be "...subject to the authority of the rational methods by which truth is established." The report then concludes, quite incorrectly, that "...faculty members currently teaching TT have participated in empirical research...[and therefore] that the requirement of...authority of rational methods has been met..." The facts are quite different; those who teach, practice and promote TT have participated in what they *describe* as "empirical research." However, their description of such work as either "empirical" or "research" is without merit. They cite no experimental designs worthy of the name research and have submitted papers to no reputable peer-reviewed journals. Nor have these results been replicated by any scientists in other centers of the University or in other research facilities elsewhere. Apparently, these faculty are aware of the requirements of science research and know how to use the jargon. Unfortunately, this use is not supported by any actual research.

In Section C we have the frank admission that support for TT emanates from "...clinical efficacy observations by practitioners." These practitioners are not scientists conducting research but are, in fact, believers in what amounts to a religion. This religion gives as an article of faith, as initially formulated by Martha Rogers, that the human body "is an energy field" and that this energy can be manipulated by a properly trained person. Throughout Dr. Claman's report, the assumptions or beliefs noted immediately above are in full view.

Section C also contains a bizarre evaluation of a brochure produced by the CHC. We can find nowhere in the original charge to Dr. Claman's committee the request that his group act as marketing consultants to the CHC.

In Clair Martin's statement attached to the report he says, "...development of a scientifically based research program focused on the **efficacy** [our emphasis] of TT...funding will be sought from the NIH." This statement begs the real question. Before "efficacy" can be scientifically evaluated, research must determine whether such a thing as a human energy field exists at all and, if it does, whether or not it can be manipulated in any way by person or machine.

This would have been the ideal moment for Dr. Claman's paper to suggest an interdisciplinary, scientifically-based research program focused on answering the above delineated question. Efficacy can be evaluated only after something can be demonstrated to be measurable. Note that the NIH, through its Office of Alternative Healing, is offering funding for just such studies.

Finally and most important, there is a very serious conflict of interest delineated in the statement from Clair Martin. Dr. Jean Watson was the dean of the SON at the time that the Center for Human Caring was founded with her as the head. This center is the principal part of SON that is involved with TT at this time. Dr. Martin states that the entire SON and the CHC will be preparing for re accreditation by the National League for Nursing next year in partial fulfillment of the requirements of Dr. Claman's report. *Dr. Jean Watson is the president elect of the NLN.* She will assume the presidency proper sometime in 1995. Therefore **no** independent review of the CHC or SON will be taking place.

The Rocky Mountain Skeptics was encouraged by Dr. Fulginiti's presentation to the regents in November 1993. Conversely, we are more than a little dismayed by some serious failures of Dr. Claman's paper under discussion here. We will continue to closely monitor the Center for Human Caring and its promotion of a belief system masquerading as a legitimate nursing practice.

Sincerely,

Béla Scheiber
President

Carla Selby
Member of Nursing Practice Task Force

CC: Dr. Henry Claman
     Clair Martin, Dean
     University of Colorado Board of Regents
     Board Members of Rocky Mountain Skeptics
     CSICOP
     NCAHF

Appendix 14.

THE REGENTS OF THE UNIVERSITY OF COLORADO

Guy J. Kelley
Chair, Board of Regents
HEWLETT-PACKARD COMPANY
3404 EAST HARMONY ROAD, MS 79
FORT COLLINS, COLORADO 80525
TELEPHONE (303) 229-6970
FAX (303) 229-7247

April 24, 1995

President Bela Scheiber
Rocky Mountain Skeptics, Inc.
Box 7277
Boulder, Colorado 80306

Dear President Scheiber:

I received the copy of the letter you sent 18 September 1994 to Chancellor Fulginiti about the report on Therapeutic Touch (TT). I appreciate your watchful eye over activities like TT. The University of Colorado is an academic and research institution.

Activities at CU must be academically relevant and follow rational thought and investigation. CU is not a church. There is <u>academic</u> freedom not total freedom to engage in any activity with any process. Even if there is little hope of demonstrating the validity of a hypothesis, the validity of the process should not be in question.

Academicians need the freedom to explore, but the discipline to use processes of investigations which are reliable and valid. Academic freedom shouldn't lead to scientific anarchy.

I appreciate your concern and your efforts.

Best regards,

Guy J. Kelley
Chair, Board of Regents

GJK:vb

Contributors

Paul Bernhardt earned his Ph.D. in Educational Psychology from the University of Utah, his bachelors degree in Mechanical Engineering from Georgia Institute of Technology, and his masters degree in Social Psychology from the University of Utah. His research interests include testosterone correlates with behavior and experience and psychophysiological detection of deception. He is also a member of the Rocky Mountain Skeptics.

Dale Beyerstein teaches philosophy at Langara College, in Vancouver, B.C., Canada.

Bonnie Bullough, Ph.D., R.N., FAAN, was Dean of the School of Nursing and professor of nursing at State University of New York at Buffalo.

Vern L. Bullough, Ph.D., R.N., FAAN, is a visiting Professor of Nursing, University of Southern California, at Los Angeles.

Ann J. Clark, Ph.D., R.N., is Associate Professor and Director, Center for Nursing Research, University of Alabama School of Nursing.

Mary Jo Clark, P.N.P., who in 1984 was an assistant professor at the School of Nursing, Medical College of Georgia, Augusta, Georgia.

Philip E. Clark, 1st Lt. ANC, R.N., was a psychiatric staff nurse in 1984 at the Dwight David Eisenhower Army Medical Center, Fort Gordon, Georgia.

Stephen James Colgan, R.N., MRCNA, is a registered nurse. He received his Bachelor of Nursing from Deakin University, Warrnambool, Australia, in 1994 and is a Member of the Royal College of Nursing Australia (MRCNA).

Frank D'Amico, Ph.D.

William Evans, Ph.D., is Associate Professor in the Department of Communication at Georgia State University. His research interests include science and health communication, computer-supported content analysis, and news media. Information regarding Evans's projects and publications can be found on the web at http://www.gsu.edu/~jouwee/evans.html.

Dorothy K. Gauthier, Ph.D., R.N., is an Associate Professor at the University of Alabama School of Nursing, University of Alabama at Birmingham.

Robert Glickman, R.N., is a perioperative nurse at Frankford Hospital in Philadelphia. He was a founder and officer of PhACT, the Philadelphia Association for Critical Thinking. The author can be contacted via phact.org.

Andrea Gordon, M.D.

Ed J. Gracely, Ph.D., is Associate Professor of Community and Preventative Medicine at MCP Hahnemann University in Philadelphia and a member of PhACT. The author can be contacted via phact.org.

David Hudgens, M.A.

Ray Hyman is considered the leading constructive critic of academic parapsychology research and recently voted the fifth "Outstanding Skeptic of the Century." He is Professor Emeritus of Psychology at the University of Oregon and a founder of the Committee for the Scientific Investigation of Claims of the Paranormal and currently serves on its Executive Council.

Rebecca Long is a nuclear engineer and President of the Georgia Skeptics and the Georgia Council Against Health Fraud Inc. She is also a consultant to the Scientific Investigation of Claims of the Paranormal and member of the Rocky Mountain Skeptics.

Therese C. Meehan, R.G.N., R.N.T., Ph.D., is with the Department of Nursing Studies, University College Dublin, National University of Ireland, Earlsfort Terrace, Dublin 2, Ireland.

Joel H. Merenstein, M.D.

Dónal P. O'Mathúna, Ph.D., is Professor of Bioethics and Chemistry at Mount Carmel College of Nursing in Columbus, Ohio, and a Fellow of the Center for Bioethics and Human Dignity in Chicago. He is on the Board of Governors of the Ohio Council Against Health Fraud, and involved in various editorial capacities with the journals *Ethics and Medicine*, *Journal of Christian Nursing*, *FACT: Focus on Complementary and Alternative Medicine*, and *Scientific Review of Alternative Medicine*.

Steven Pryjmachuk, B.A., P.G.Dip.Ed, Msc, R.N., R.N.T., is a Nurse Teacher and Ph.D. student in the School of Nursing, Midwifery, and Health Visiting at the University of Manchester, UK.

James Randi is President of the James Randi Education Foundation, lecturer and author of numerous articles and books. In 1986 he was named a MacArthur Foundation Fellow and recently voted the number one "Outstanding Skeptic of the Century."

Béla Scheiber, B.S., M.B.S., received his degree in Mathematics from the University of Colorado. He is the founder and President of the Rocky Mountain Skeptics, member of the Executive Council of the Committee for the Scientific Investigation of Claims of the Paranormal, and a Charter member of the Council for Scientific Medicine. He is also involved in various editorial capacities with the journals *Skeptical Inquirer* and *Scientific Review of Alternative Medicine*. He can be contacted at http://bcn.boulder.co.us/community/rms.

Carla Selby is an Anthropologist by inclination and education. She is a consultant to the Committee for the Scientific Investigation of Claims of the Paranormal, a long-time member of the Board of the Rocky Mountain Skeptics and a Charter member of the Council for Scientific Medicine.

Jack Stahlman is a registered nurse who first encountered the practice of Therapeutic Touch while a nursing student in 1993. After graduating from the University of Washington with a master's degree in nursing in 1998, he moved to the mountains of western North Carolina, where he currently works as a psychiatric nurse practitioner.

Michael Stanwick, B.Sc.(Hons), is a retired school teacher now living in the UK.

Victor J. Stenger, Ph.D., is in the Department of Physics and Astronomy, University of Hawaii at Manoa. His other career has been as a writer and skeptic, and he has published three books: *Not By Design: The Origin of the Universe*, *Physics and Psychics: The Search for a World Beyond the Senses*, and *The Uncounscious Quantum: Metaphysics in Modern Physics and Cosmology.*

Joan G. Turner, D.S.N., R.N., C.I.C., is Professor at the University of Alabama School of Nursing.

Mahlon W. Wagner, Ph.D., is Professor Emeritus of Psychology at State University of New York at Oswego.

Monica Williams, B.A., M.A., is a medical student at the University of South Alabama, Mobile, Alabama.

Daniel P. Wirth, M.S., J.D., is associated with Healing Sciences Research International, Orinda, California.